Women's Health

TOTAL
FITNESS
GUIDE

2008

Women'sHealth
TOTAL FITNESS GUIDE
2008

SCULPT YOUR BEST BODY EVER!

From the Editors of Women'sHealth Magazine

RODALE

© 2008 by Rodale Inc.

All rights reserved. No part of this publication may be reproduced or transmitted in any form or by any means,electronic or mechanical, including photocopying, recording, or any other information storage and retrieval system, without the written permission of the publisher.

Women's Health is a registered trademark of Rodale Inc.

Printed in the United States of America
Rodale Inc. makes every effort to use acid-free ♾, recycled paper ♻.

ISBN-13 978–1–59486–877–1
ISBN-10 1–59486–877–8

2   4   6   8   10   9   7   5   3   1   hardcover

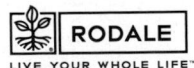

RODALE
LIVE YOUR WHOLE LIFE™

We inspire and enable people to improve their lives and the world around them
For more of our products visit **rodalestore.com** or call 800-848-4735

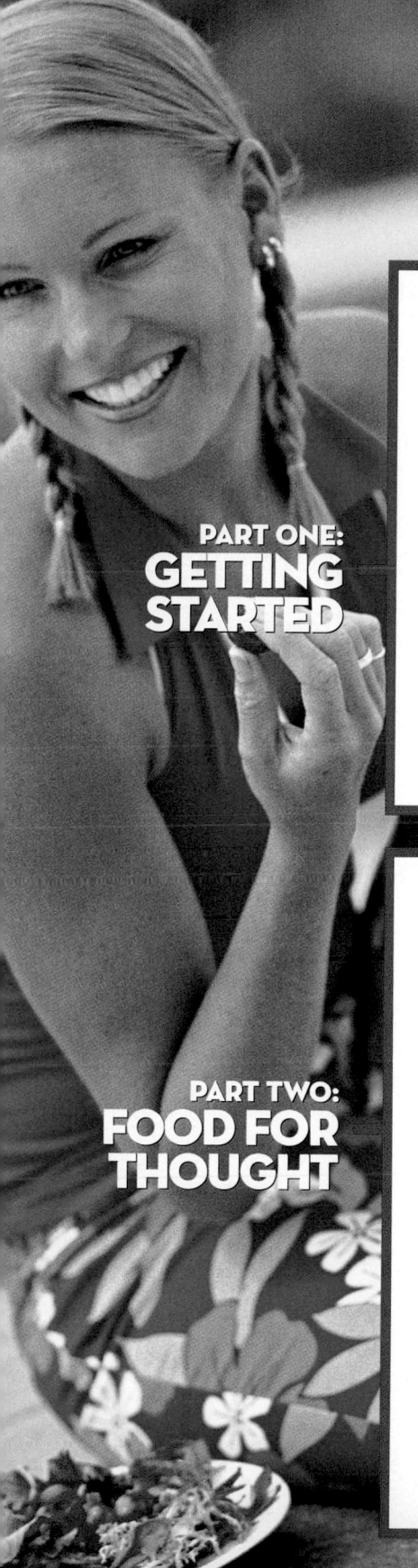

contents

contents

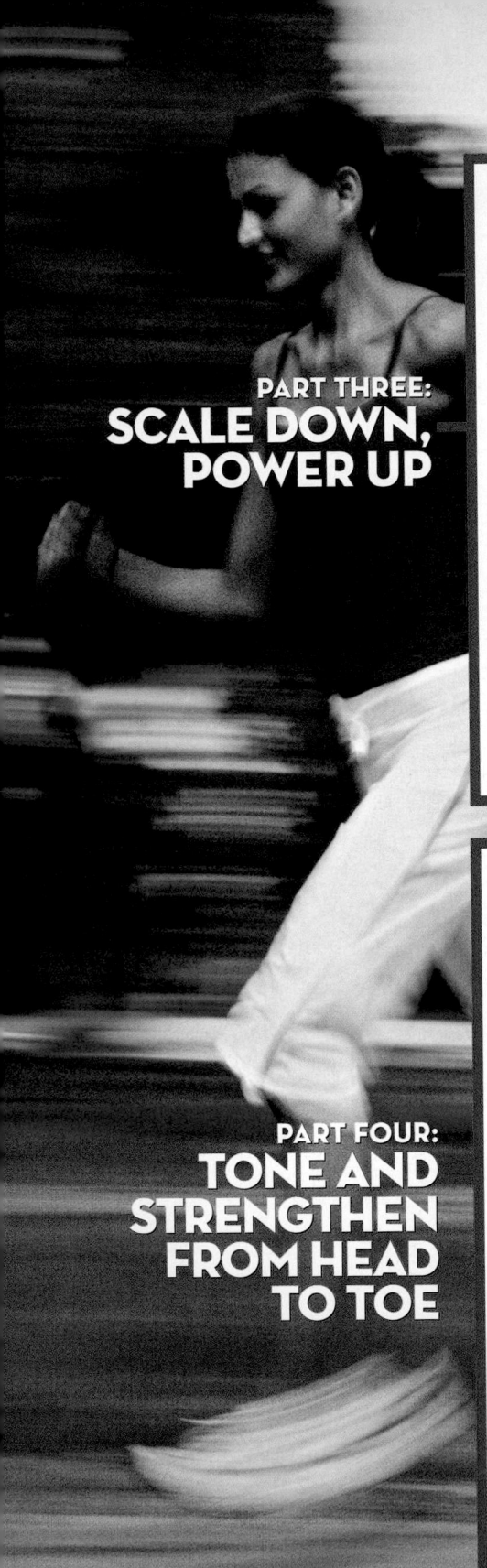

contents

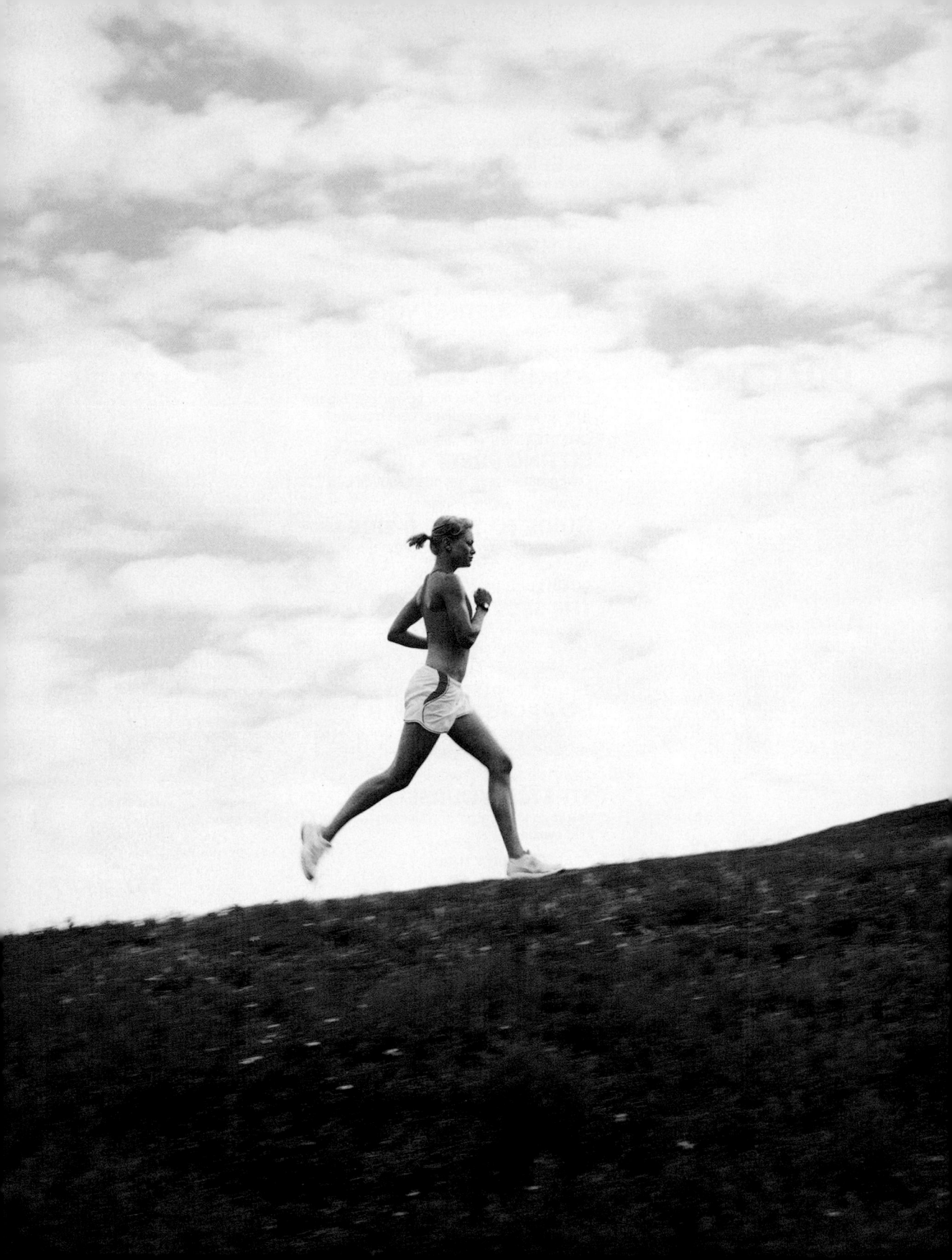

■ PART ONE

getting started

Whether you want to drop a few dress sizes, rack up more miles on the treadmill, or simply twist open those stubborn jar lids, we have the fitness plan for you. And lest you fall off the wagon, we also have the quickest and easiest way to scramble right back up there. So what are you waiting for?

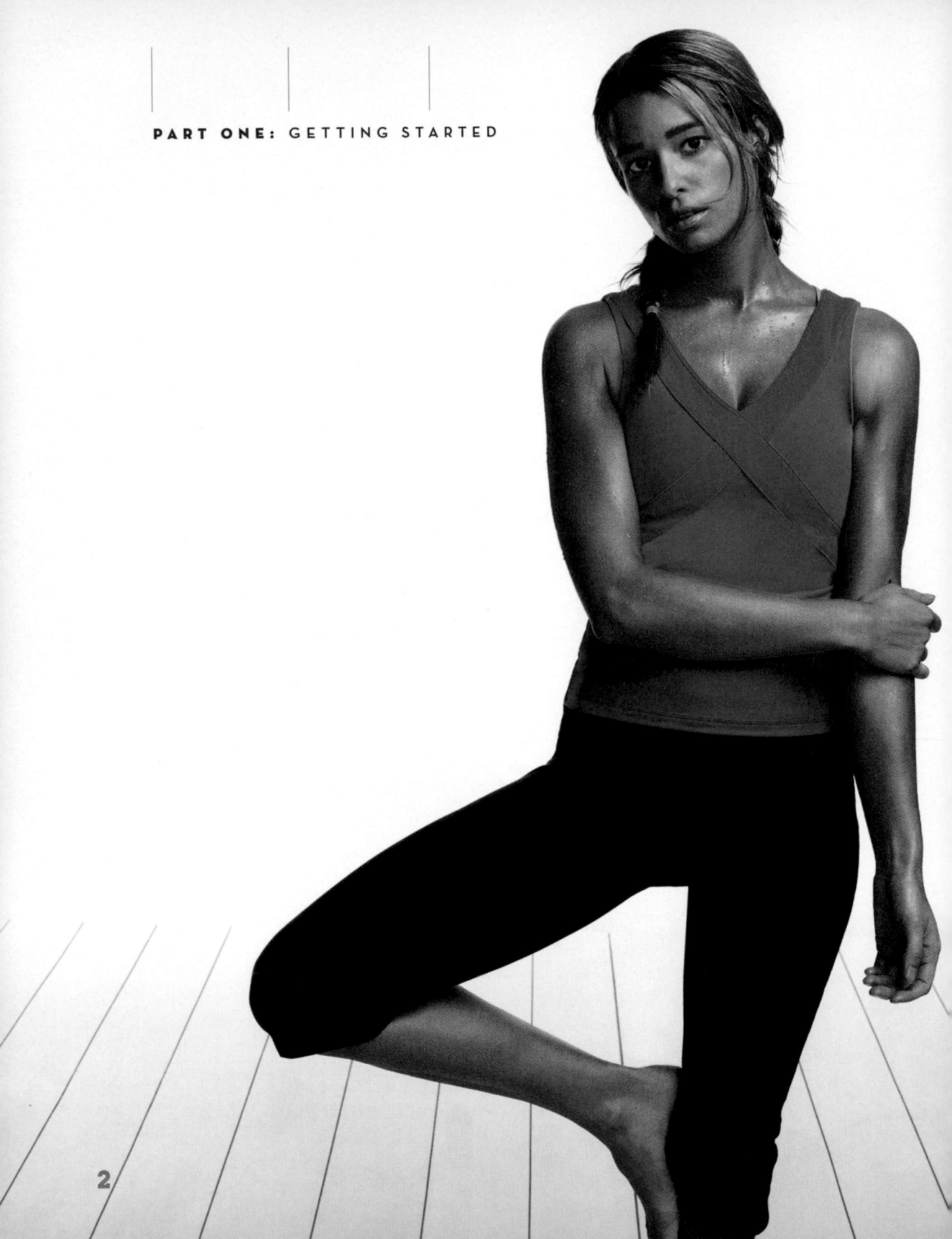

PART ONE: GETTING STARTED

CHAPTER ONE

GET FIT FOR GOOD

IN JUST 8 WEEKS, YOU CAN BE IN THE
BEST SHAPE OF YOUR LIFE WITH THIS ULTIMATE
FITNESS PLAN.

ARE YOU FINALLY READY to stick to that get-my-butt-in-shape-for-real promise you make at least twice a year? Well, we're here to help you keep your word. With the *Women's Health* Ultimate Fitness Plan, you can skip one of the most common get-fit missteps: setting a goal without a detailed plan for accomplishing it.

Why 8 weeks? Because during the first month of any new program, 80 percent of your strength gains are neuromuscular, which means your brain is mostly just getting used to moving those muscles, according to Wayne Westcott, Ph.D., C.S.C.S., fitness research director at the

South Shore YMCA in Quincy, Massachusetts. "So stopping there is like pulling the curtain right before the big show," he says. After 2 months, you'll realize your potential for fat loss and muscle tone.

Our Ultimate Fitness Plan is tailored to your personal fitness level in five areas: cardio, strength, flexibility, balance, and agility. You'll be working out 6 days a week, but none of the daily routines takes longer than an hour (some last less than 5 minutes)—so there's no excuse for not squeezing them in between bed and work or work and happy hour. To get started:

1. FIGURE OUT HOW FIT YOU ARE

On these pages you'll find five fitness challenges designed by a team of *WH* experts: Tim Church, M.D., Ph.D., M.P.H., an exercise science professor at Pennington Biomedical Research Center in Baton Rouge; Lori Incledon, C.S.C.S, author of *Strength Training for Women*; and Valerie Waters, a personal trainer in Brentwood, California, who works with the likes of Jennifer Garner. Take each test, then score yourself accordingly: Aspiring (you've got potential), Solid (pretty fit but could use a push), or Strong (woo-hoo!). All you need is a step (or stairs), a stability ball, a water bottle, a mat, and a roll of masking tape.

2. FOLLOW OUR 8-WEEK PLAN

The moves in this chapter fall into one of the five test categories and have three levels of difficulty. Do the level that corresponds with your test score for that category.

3. TEST YOUR PROGRESS

Repeat each test after 4 weeks to see whether you're ready for the next level. If you're already at the highest level—bravo, you've exceeded our expectations—monitor your progress (watching your scores soar is instant motivation). Also, keep challenging yourself by adding weight to strength moves or subtracting some rest time from cardio.

How fit is your heart?

3-MINUTE STEP

Stand in front of a 12-inch-high step with your feet hip-width apart. Step up with one foot and then the other. Step down the same way. Try to maintain a steady, unhurried pace: up, up, down, down. After 3 minutes, remain standing and check your heart rate by placing two fingertips an inch to the right of your windpipe. Count the beats for 1 minute.

CARDIO SCORING

AGE	ASPIRING	SOLID	STRONG
18 to 25	111 or higher	94 to 100	93 or lower
26 to 35	112 or higher	95 to 111	94 or lower
36 to 45	120 or higher	97 to 119	96 or lower
46 to 55	125 or higher	102 to 124	101 or lower

Got muscle?

UPPER BODY: STABILITY BALL PUSHUP

The goal is to perform 10 pushups with your arms shoulder-width apart and legs elevated on a 65-inch stability ball. The farther your torso is from the ball, the harder it'll be to complete the set. To start, try to do them with the fronts of your ankles on the ball. If that's impossible, try from your knees. Still too tough? Place the ball under your thighs.

Strength Scoring

ASPIRING: 10 or fewer with thighs on ball
SOLID: 10 or fewer with knees on ball
STRONG: 10 or fewer with ankles on ball

LOWER-BODY: 1-MINUTE SQUAT

Stand in front of a 12-inch step or box with your feet shoulder-width apart. Raise arms to shoulder height and hold them straight out in front of you. Drop your hips as though you're sitting in a chair until your butt grazes the step. Return to start and repeat as many times as you can in 1 minute, maintaining good form (head up, spine neutral, knees behind toes and pointed straight ahead).

Strength Scoring

ASPIRING: 20 or fewer
SOLID: 21 to 29
STRONG: 30 or more

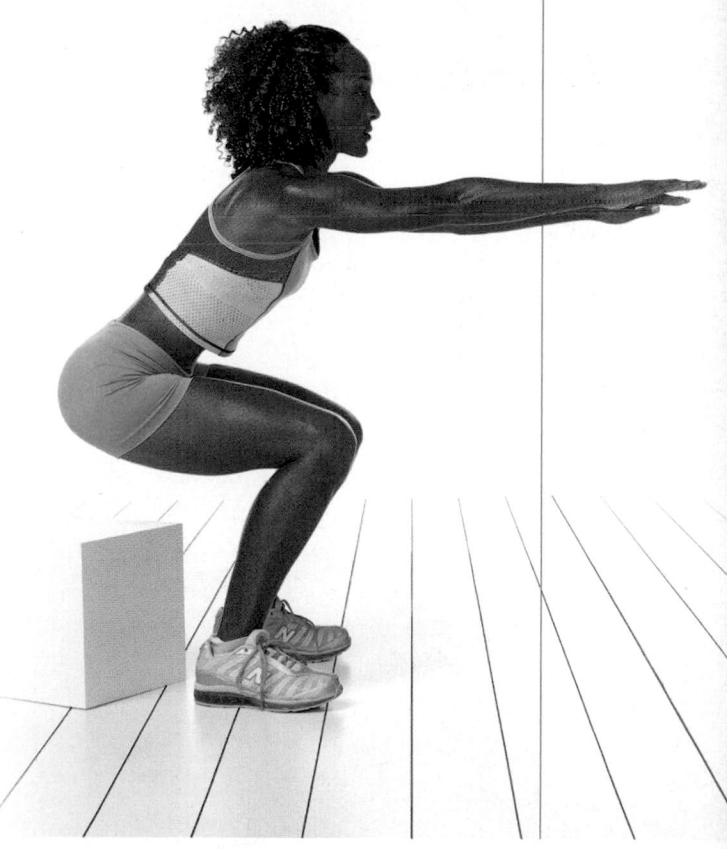

TEST #3

Can you bend it like Bikram?

DOWNWARD DOG

Begin on your hands and knees with palms shoulder-width apart and feet together. Push up through your toes, then lean into your palms and straighten your legs, lifting your tailbone toward the ceiling while pulling your navel toward your spine. Keeping your neck and spine aligned, focus on sinking your torso into the position so your ears are in line with your upper arms and your heels are as close to the floor as possible. With your elbows and knees locked, see how far down you can reach with your torso and heels.

Flexibility Scoring

ASPIRING: Heels up, ears above your arms

SOLID: Heels almost to floor, ears even with your arms

STRONG: Heels on floor, ears past your arms

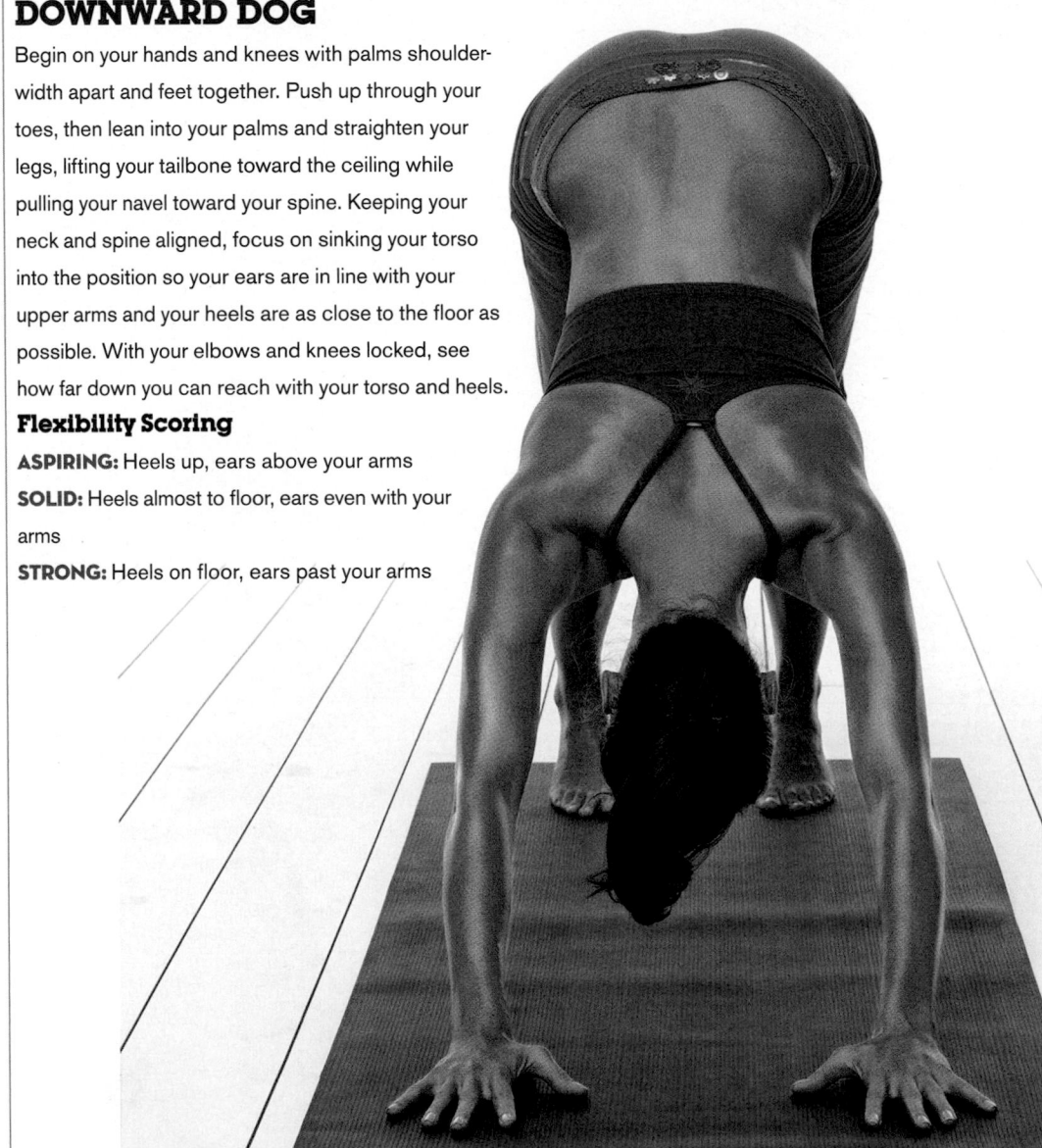

TEST #4

Are you well balanced?

FLAMINGO REACH

Place a water bottle 2½ feet in front of you. Stand with your feet together, arms at your sides. Draw your navel toward your spine and lift your left foot off the floor behind you and your arms straight overhead, in line with your shoulders. Bend forward at the waist, allowing your right knee to bend slightly as you reach your arms forward and down to touch the bottle. Return to standing and repeat as many times as possible up to 15, without letting your left leg touch the floor. If it does, the test is over. Repeat on your left leg. Take the average.

Balance Scoring

ASPIRING: 7 or less

SOLID: 8 to 11

STRONG: 12 or more

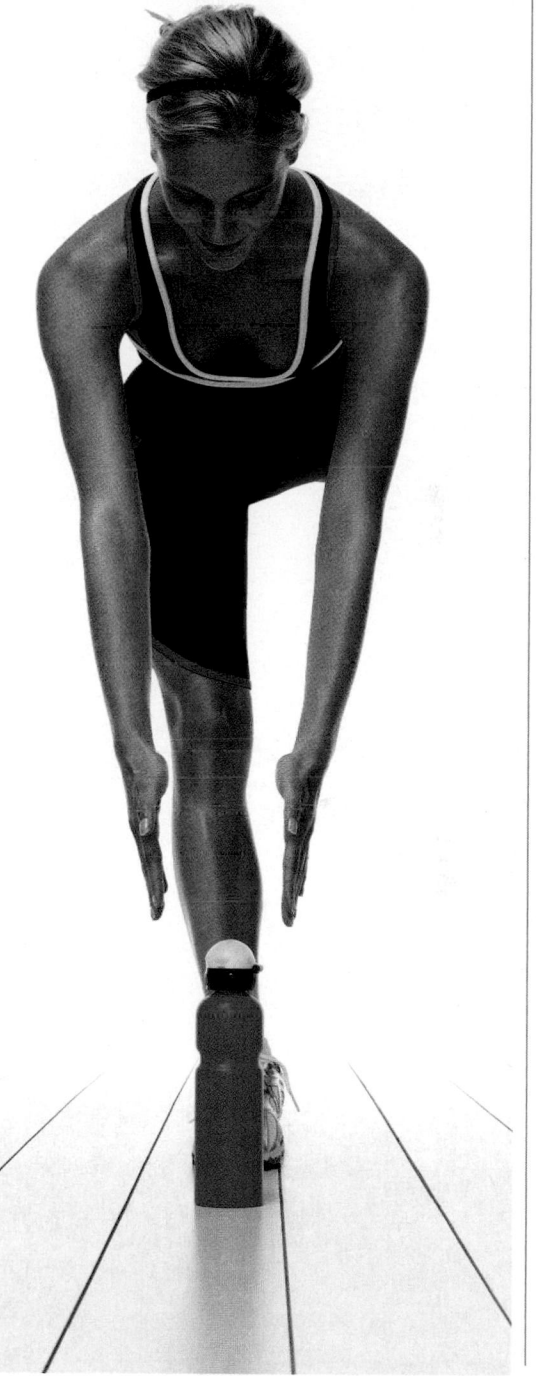

W|H

TEST #5
Do you have fast feet?

TWO LINE HOP

Place two pieces of tape on the floor parallel to each other, 12 inches apart. Stand with one foot on each line, arms at your sides. Lift your right foot. Hop from line to line (side to side) on your left foot as many times as you can in 15 seconds. Repeat on your right foot, and take the average.

Agility Scoring

ASPIRING: 21 or fewer

SOLID: 22 to 26

STRONG: 27 or more

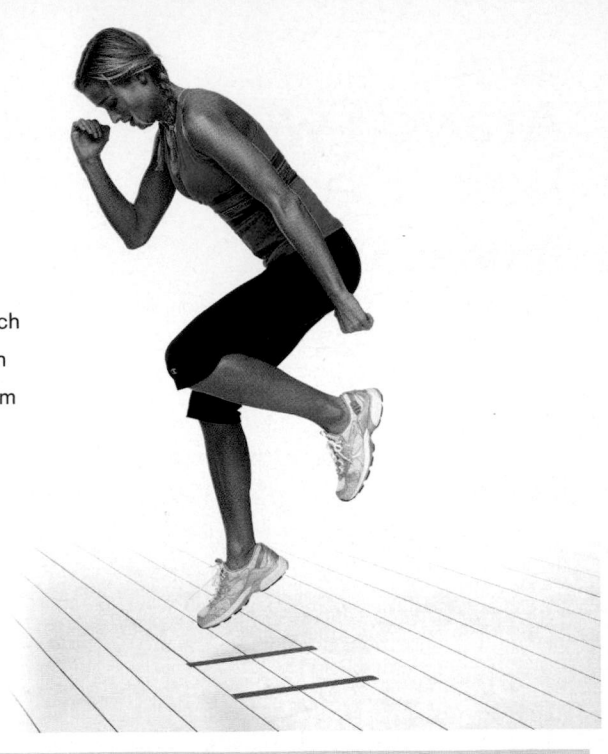

The Workout

Now that you know where you stand, it's time to start moving toward your goal—whether it's to lose inches from your thighs, shave minutes from your 5-K, or simply stop tripping over your own feet.

WH Ultimate Fitness Plan

Warm up with a 3-minute walk or easy jog. Then do today's recommended cardio (see Maximum Endurance Cardio Plan on the opposite page), followed by the moves on the Total Body Toning Plan chart on page 10.

CARDIO

These three workouts, designed by Leigh Crews, national spokesperson for the American Council on Exercise, will strengthen your heart and lungs, increase your fat-burning capacity, and raise what the pros call your lactate threshold (the point at which your cardiovascular system sputters and you have to slow down). Whether you're on a track, bike, or cardio machine, these workouts switch up the intensity to make you go farther, faster, and longer.

Maximum Endurance Cardio Plan

Weeks	Mon	Tues	Wed	Thurs	Fri	Sat	Sun
1 TO 2	Rest	**ASPIRING** Fat Burning **SOLID** Fat Burning **STRONG** Fat Burning	**ASPIRING** High Intensity (4x30s with 5:00 recovery) **SOLID** Roof Raising **STRONG** Roof Raising	**ASPIRING** Fat Burning **SOLID** Fat Burning **STRONG** Fat Burning	**ASPIRING** Roof Raising **SOLID** High Intensity (4x60s with 5:00 recovery) **STRONG** High Intensity (4x60s with 4:00 recovery)	**ASPIRING** Fat Burning **SOLID** Fat Burning **STRONG** Fat Burning	**ASPIRING** Fat Burning **SOLID** Fat Burning **STRONG** Roof Raising
3 TO 4	Rest	**ASPIRING** Fat Burning **SOLID** Fat Burning **STRONG** Fat Burning	**ASPIRING** Fat Burning **SOLID** High Intensity (4x60s with 4:00 recovery) **STRONG** High Intensity (4x90s with 4:00 recovery)	**ASPIRING** Roof Raising **SOLID** Fat Burning **STRONG** Fat Burning	**ASPIRING** Fat Burning **SOLID** Fat Burning **STRONG** Roof Raising	**ASPIRING** High Intensity (4x60s with 4:00 recovery) **SOLID** Roof Raising **STRONG** Roof Raising	**ASPIRING** Roof Raising **SOLID** Fat Burning **STRONG** Fat Burning
5 TO 6	Rest	**ASPIRING** Fat Burning **SOLID** Fat Burning **STRONG** Roof Raising	**ASPIRING** Roof Raising **SOLID** Roof Raising **STRONG** Fat Burning	**ASPIRING** Fat Burning **SOLID** Fat Burning **STRONG** High Intensity (4x90s with 4:30 recovery)	**ASPIRING** Fat Burning **SOLID** High Intensity (4x75s with 4:00 recovery) **STRONG** Fat Burning	**ASPIRING** High Intensity (4x75s with 4:15 recovery) **SOLID** Fat Burning **STRONG** Roof Raising	**ASPIRING** Fat Burning **SOLID** Roof Raising **STRONG** Fat Burning
7 TO 8	Rest	**ASPIRING** Fat Burning **SOLID** Fat Burning **STRONG** Roof Raising	**ASPIRING** Roof Raising **SOLID** High Intensity (6x90s with 3:30 recovery) **STRONG** High Intensity (7x90s with 3:00 recovery)	**ASPIRING** Fat Burning **SOLID** Roof Raising **STRONG** Fat Burning	**ASPIRING** High Intensity (4x90s with 4:00 recovery) **SOLID** Fat Burning **STRONG** Roof Raising	**ASPIRING** Fat Burning **SOLID** Roof Raising **STRONG** High Intensity (7x90s with 3:00 recovery)	**ASPIRING** Roof Raising **SOLID** Fat Burning **STRONG** Fat Burning

TOTAL FITNESS GUIDE 2008

W|H

1. FAT BURNING Hit a pace that's steady and moderate—fast enough that you're breathing harder than normal but can still carry on a conversation. On a scale of 1 to 10, with 10 being Marion Jones, aim for a 4 or 5. "This is the foundation of your training and where your body learns to burn maximum fat," Crews says.

ASPIRING: 25 to 30 minutes
SOLID: 35 to 40 minutes
STRONG: 45 to 50 minutes

2. ROOF RAISING Up the intensity to 6 to 8: You're able to speak, but only in spurts of three or four words. This type of hard, steady effort raises your aerobic ceiling, so eventually you'll be able to maintain a faster pace and burn more calories (even during your slower workouts).

ASPIRING: 25 to 30 minutes
SOLID: 35 to 40 minutes
STRONG: 45 to 50 minutes

3. HIGH INTENSITY Time to hit it hard. Move like there's a mad dog snapping at your heels—an effort of 9-plus. These intervals are 30 to 90 seconds long with 3 to 5 minutes of recovery at a moderate pace between efforts. See the cardio plan on page 9 for specific times based on your test level.

Total Body Toning Plan

EXERCISES SHOWN ON FOLLOWING PAGES >>

Weeks	Mon	Tues	Wed	Thurs	Fri	Sat	Sun
1 TO 2	Rest	**STRENGTH** (2 sets of 8 to 10 reps) **BALANCE FLEXIBILITY**	Rest	**STRENGTH** (2 sets of 8 to 10 reps) **BALANCE FLEXIBILITY**	Rest	**STRENGTH** (2 sets of 8 to 10 reps) **BALANCE FLEXIBILITY**	**AGILITY**
3 TO 4	Rest	**STRENGTH** (2 sets of 10 to 12 reps) **BALANCE FLEXIBILITY**	Rest	**STRENGTH** (2 sets of 10 to 12 reps) **BALANCE FLEXIBILITY**	Rest	**STRENGTH** (2 sets of 10 to 12 reps) **BALANCE FLEXIBILITY**	**AGILITY**
5 TO 6	Rest	**STRENGTH** (3 sets of 10 to 12 reps) **BALANCE FLEXIBILITY**	**AGILITY**	**STRENGTH** (3 sets of 10 to 12 reps) **BALANCE FLEXIBILITY**	Rest	**STRENGTH** (3 sets of 10 to 12 reps) **BALANCE FLEXIBILITY**	**AGILITY**
7 TO 8	Rest	**STRENGTH** (3 sets of 10 to 12 reps as quickly as you can keeping control) **BALANCE FLEXIBILITY**	**AGILITY**	**STRENGTH** (3 sets of 10 to 12 reps as quickly as you can keeping control) **BALANCE FLEXIBILITY**	Rest	**STRENGTH** (3 sets of 10 to 12 reps as quickly as you can keeping control) **BALANCE FLEXIBILITY**	**AGILITY**

Total Body Toning Plan

Strength

When you don't work muscles, they get weaker . . . and you get wider. But you can replace 5 to 10 years of lost muscle in just 8 weeks. Valerie Waters, a personal trainer in Brentwood, California, designed the following routine for netting lean, strong muscles fast. The exercises shown are the Solid variations. Follow your upper-body level for the upper-body moves and your lower-body level for the lower-body moves.

LOWER BODY
TOUCHDOWN LUNGE
WORKS GLUTES, HAMSTRINGS, AND QUADS

Stand with your feet hip-width apart, knees bent 45 degrees (**A**). Take a giant step back with your right leg, bending both knees until your back knee grazes the floor. Simultaneously, reach down and touch the floor on either side of your left ankle (**B**). Push back to start. Do one set, then switch sides.

ASPIRING: Don't return to start. Continue performing touchdowns in your lunge.

STRONG: Hold a 5- to 10-pound dumbbell in each hand.

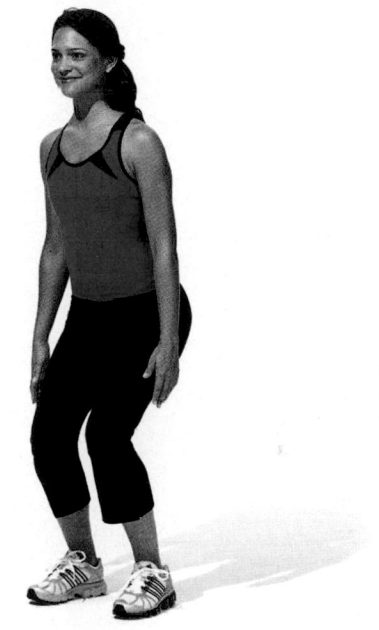

A

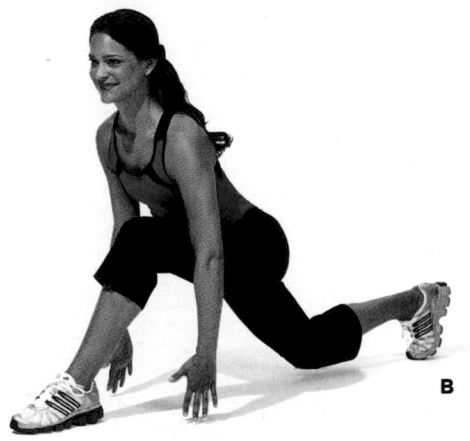

B

LOWER BODY
SIDE LIFTOFF
WORKS ABDUCTORS, ADDUCTORS, GLUTES, AND HAMSTRINGS

Stand with a staircase to your right, with your right foot parallel to the bottom step. Plant your right foot on the first or second stair with knee bent (**A**). Step up on your right foot, bringing your left foot up and tapping the step with your left toes (**B**). Lower back to start. Do one set, then switch sides.

ASPIRING: Start with both feet on the floor and step back to the floor with both feet on each repetition.

STRONG: In the "up" position, lift your outside leg to the side before lowering.

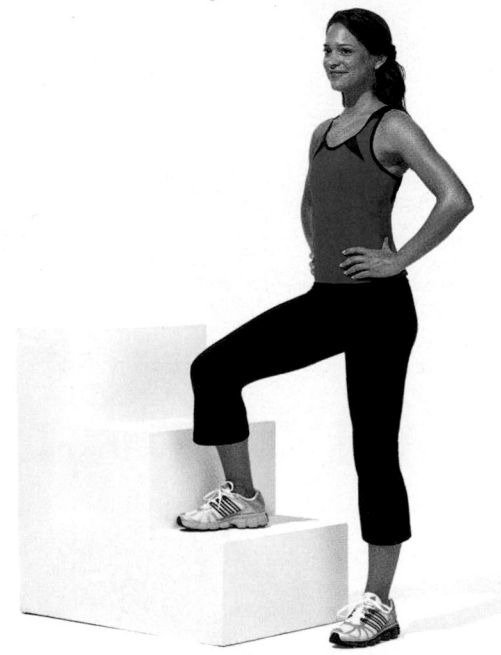

A

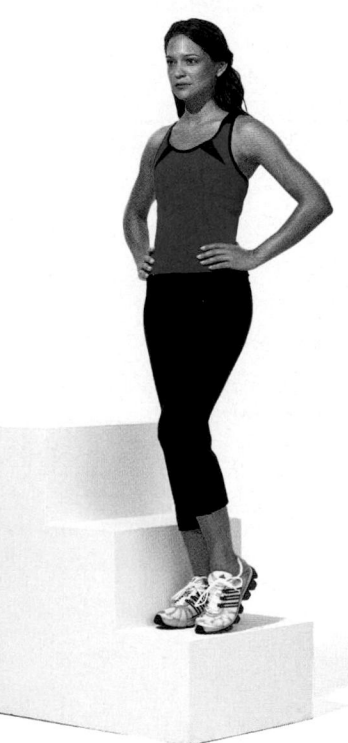

B

LOWER BODY

BALANCE SQUAT AND PULL
WORKS BACK, CORE, GLUTES, HAMSTRINGS,
AND QUADS

Tie an exercise band low on a sturdy table leg.
Face the table, holding the free end of the band in
your left hand. Pull the band taut. Lift your left leg
so you're balancing on your right (**A**). Lean forward
and reach toward where the band is tied (**B**). Stand
up and pull your left arm back (**C**). Row for one set,
then switch sides.

ASPIRING: Lower your foot between reps.

STRONG: Bend your standing leg so you're in a
90-degree squat.

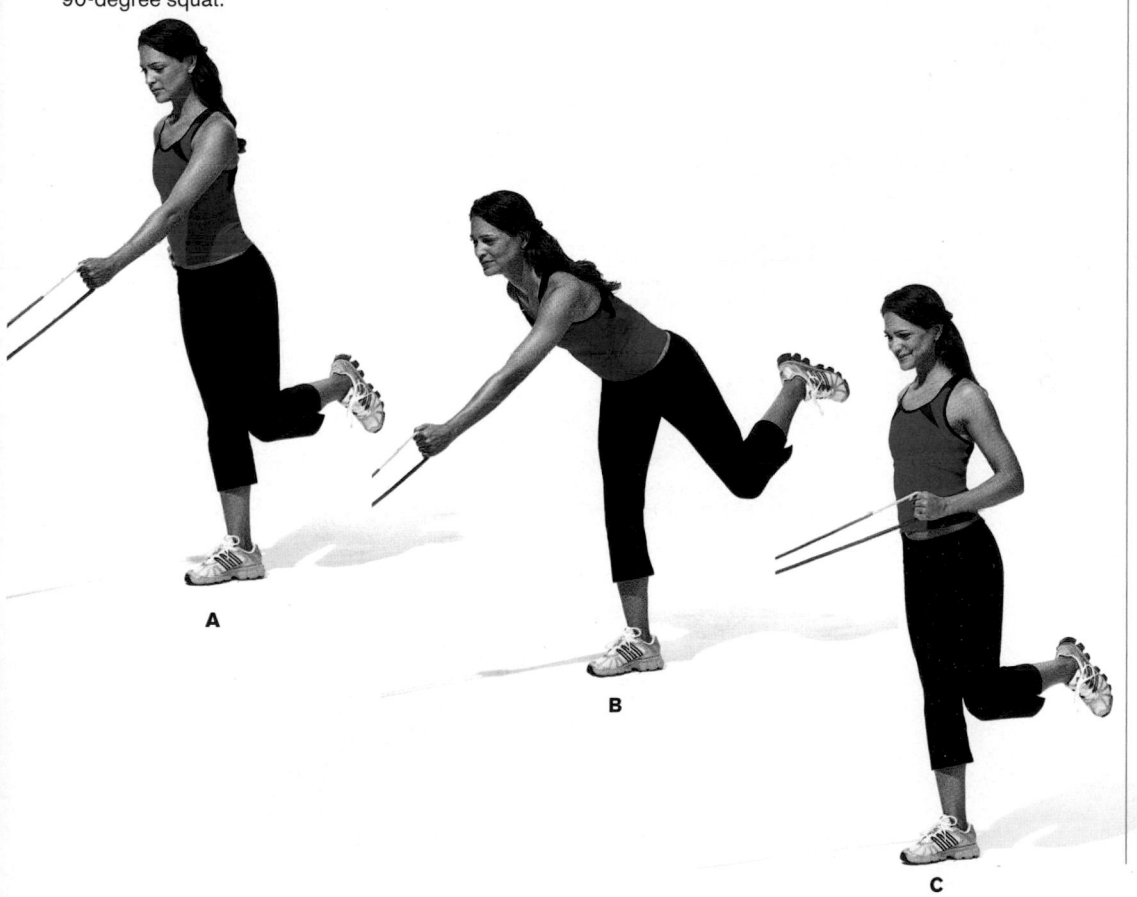

A

B

C

PUSH AND ROW

WORKS ARMS, CHEST, CORE, SHOULDERS, AND UPPER BACK

Grab 5-pound dumbbells and assume a modified pushup position: arms straight, knees on floor, ankles crossed (**A**). Bend your elbows and lower your chest until upper arms are parallel to the floor (**B**). Press back up, immediately pulling the left weight to your chest (**C**). Return to start and continue alternating arms for a full set.

ASPIRING: Do pushups minus the row.

STRONG: Do the move from your toes.

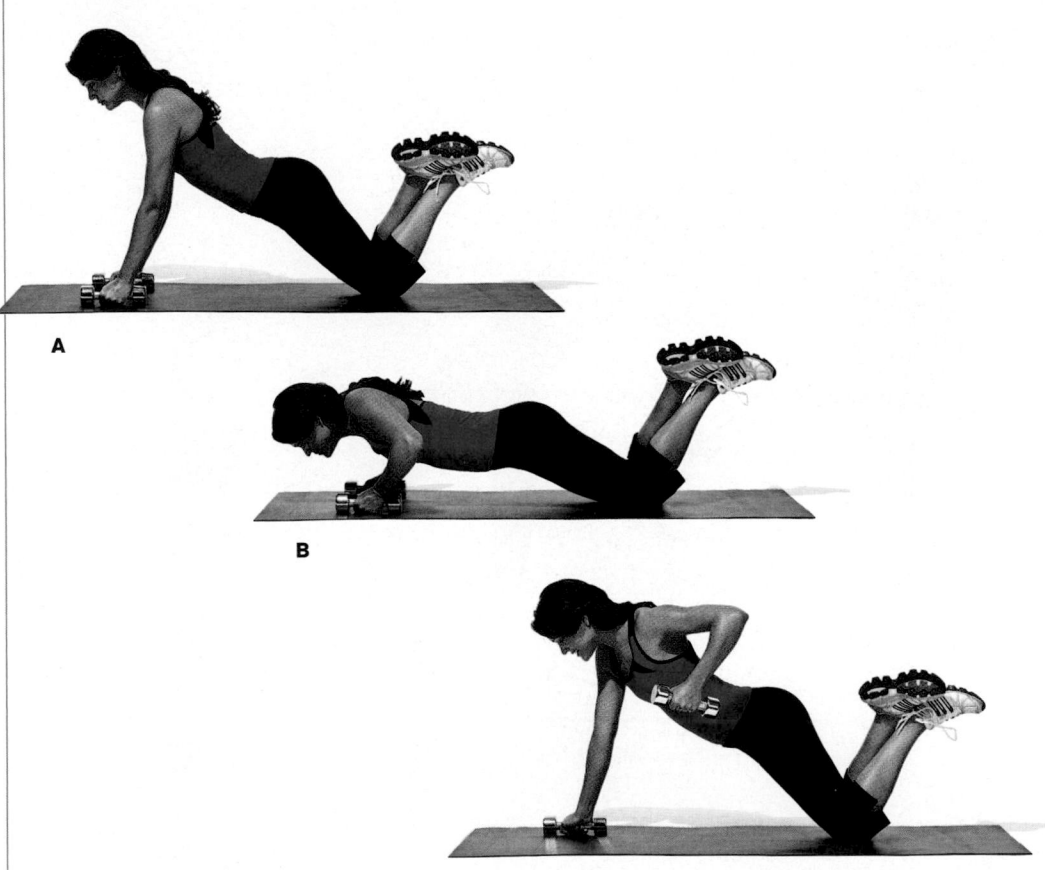

A

B

C

UPPER BODY
PEDALING PLANK
WORKS CORE

Get in a plank position: arms and legs straight, hands beneath shoulders (**A**). Pull your right knee toward your chest without lifting your butt (**B**). Extend your leg back out without letting your foot touch the floor. Do one set, then switch sides.

ASPIRING: Instead of bringing your knee to your chest, drop it to the floor.

STRONG: After extending your leg back to start, swing it out to the side. The full motion is: in, out, side, and back to start.

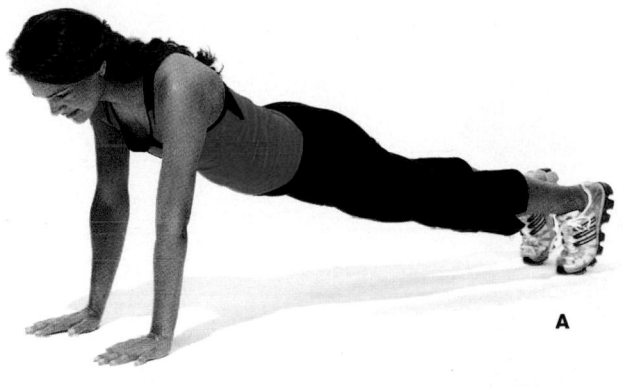

A

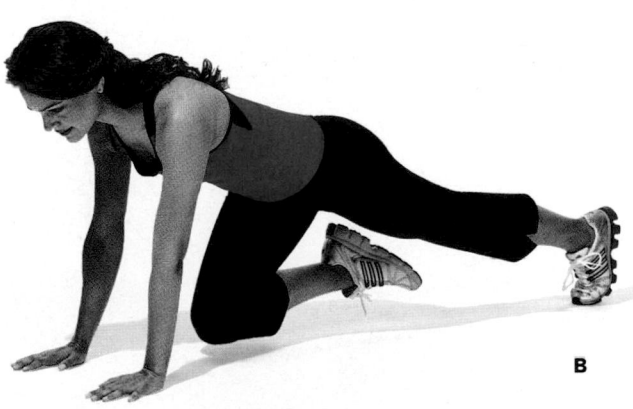

B

W|H

UPPER BODY

BRIDGE PRESS

WORKS CHEST, GLUTES, AND HAMSTRINGS

Grab a set of 8- to 10-pound dumbbells and lie
faceup on the floor with your knees bent, feet flat, and
arms at your sides. Hold weights down at chest level
with palms facing forward. Keeping your thigh still,
raise your left calf until it's in line with your right knee
(**A**). Lift your butt and hips off the floor as you press
the weights toward the ceiling (**B**). Return to start.
Do one set, then switch sides.

ASPIRING: Cross your ankle over your knee
instead of extending it.

STRONG: Lift your extended leg so the sole of
your foot faces the ceiling.

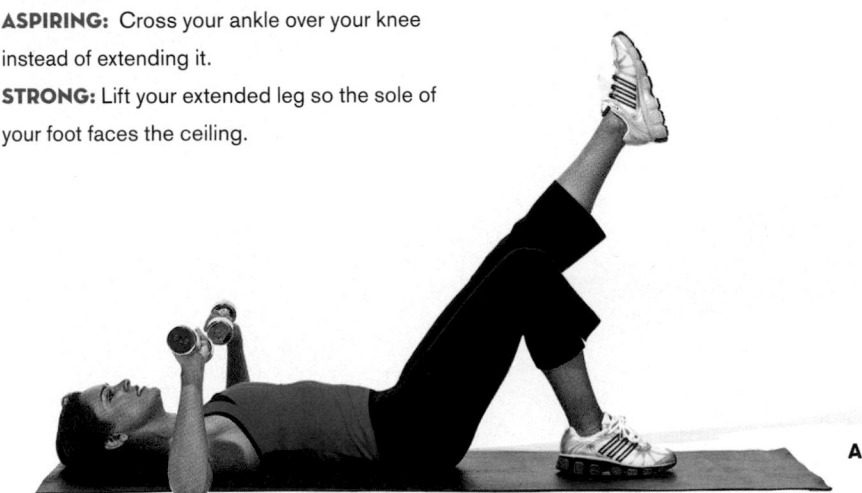

A

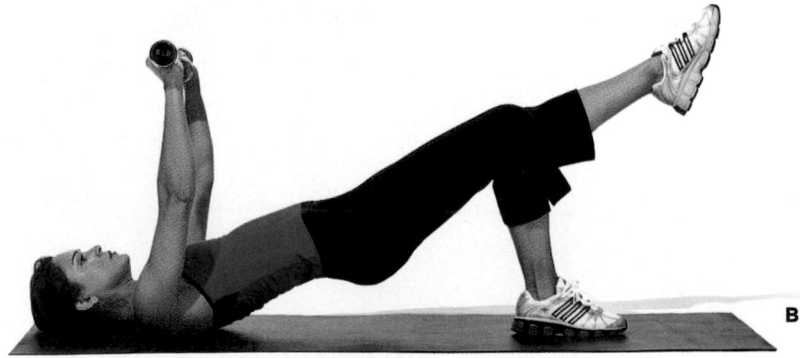

B

Balance

You can get rock steady with just a few moves that sharpen coordination. Do each move once, rest 1 minute, then repeat.

STABILITY BALL TWIST

Sit on a stability ball with your feet together and arms extended at shoulder height, palms down. Extend your left leg straight in front of you (**A**). Turn your torso to the left as far as possible, keeping your arms in line with your shoulders (**B**). Return to center and lower your leg. Then repeat on the right side.

ASPIRING: Keep both feet flat on the floor.

STRONG: Start with your feet wider than your shoulders.

TREE

From a standing position, place the sole of your right foot on the inside of your left thigh. Press your hands together in front of your chest or, if you can, raise them overhead, palms facing each other. Hold for 30 seconds to 1 minute. Switch legs.

ASPIRING: Place foot on calf instead of thigh.

STRONG: Close your eyes.

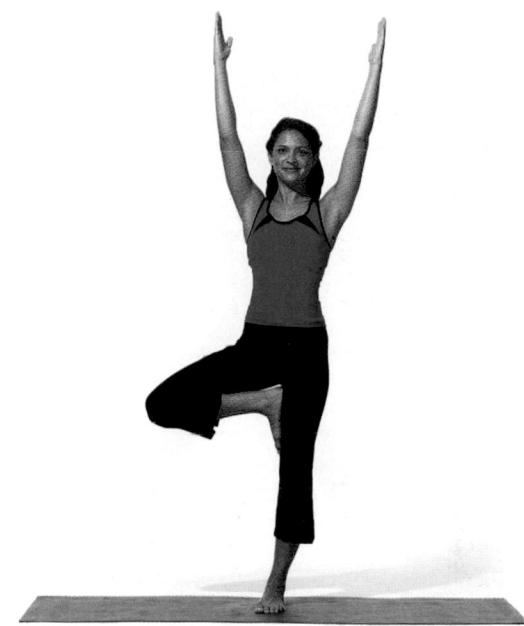

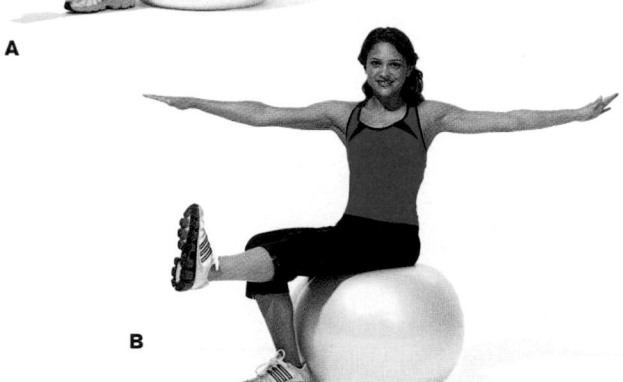

A

B

Flexibility

Taking your body through a full range of motion lubricates your joints and keeps you injury free. Do a Downward Dog (p. 6), holding for 30 seconds, followed by these moves. Rest 1 minute, then repeat.

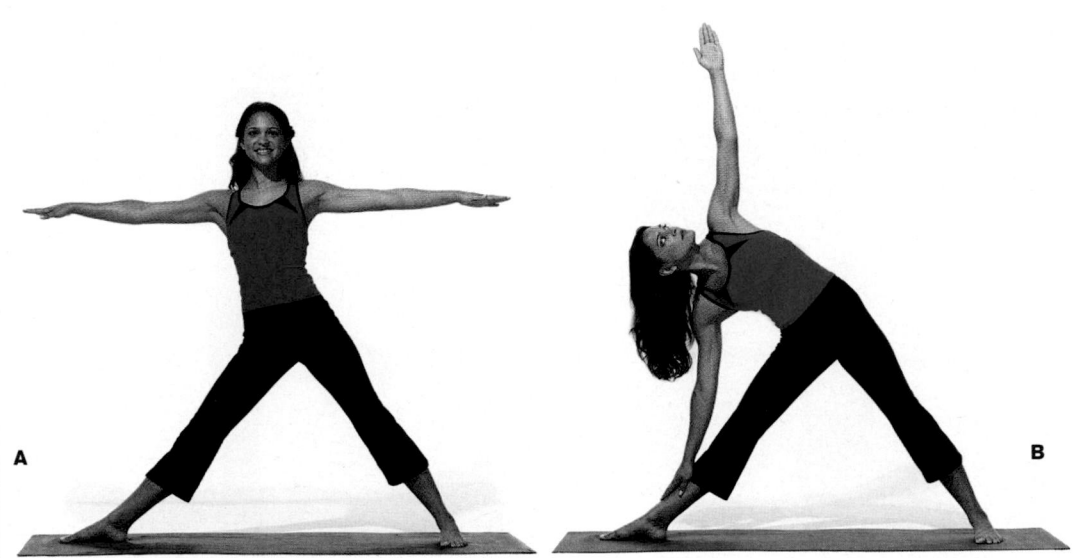

A

B

EXTENDED TRIANGLE

STRETCHES HAMSTRINGS AND HIP FLEXORS

With feet 4 feet apart, turn your right foot out 90 degrees and your left foot in slightly. Extend your arms at shoulder height, palms down (**A**). Bend to the right, keeping your arms in position. Grab your right ankle with your right hand. Stretch your left hand toward the ceiling, and look up (**B**). Hold, breathing deeply, for 30 seconds. Switch sides.

ASPIRING: Place hand below your knee.

STRONG: Stretch your top arm forward, palm facing down, over your top ear, so it's parallel to the floor.

WARRIOR I

STRETCHES BACK, GROIN, AND HAMSTRINGS

With feet 4 feet apart, turn your right foot out 90 degrees and your left foot in slightly. Extend your arms out at shoulder height, palms down. Turn your palms to face the ceiling and bring them toward each other until they're touching above your head, fingertips pointing up. Rotate your pelvis and chest to the right so they're facing in the same direction as your right toe. Bend your right knee 90 degrees. Hold, breathing deeply, for 30 seconds. Switch sides.

ASPIRING: Hold your arms overhead at shoulder width, with your palms facing each other but not touching. Bend your right leg only 45 degrees.

STRONG: Instead of lunging, keep your right leg straight and bend at the hips, lifting your left leg straight out behind you until your body forms a T. Hold for 30 seconds.

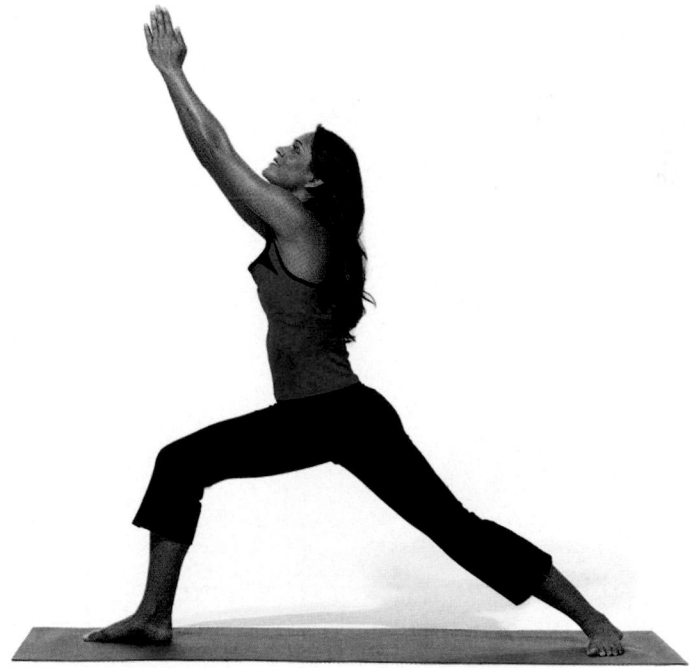

Agility

Life often requires grace—say, for navigating toy-strewn stairs while carrying a laundry basket. Some coordination can make everyday tasks easier and safer. Get nimble with two sets of 8 to 12 reps of these moves from Lori Incledon, C.S.C.S., author of *Strength Training for Women*.

SPLIT JUMP

From standing, take a big step back with your left foot. Bend your right knee and let your left knee sink (**A**). Jump up and switch legs (**B**). Immediately sink back down into the lunge. When your right knee touches the floor, jump again.

ASPIRING: Stand in a doorway, holding the doorframe for support.

STRONG: Extend arms out in front of you and clasp your hands.

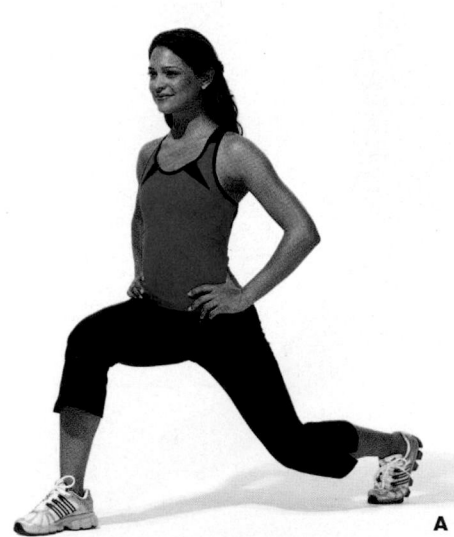

A

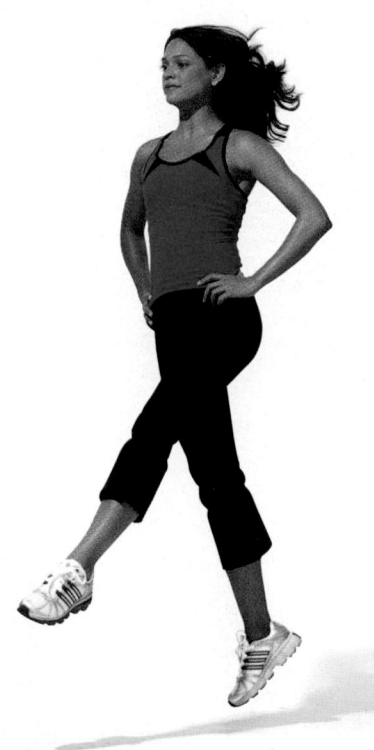

B

FROG HOP

Stand with a basketball between your feet (**A**). Jump up, gripping the ball with your feet, and bend your knees out to the sides. At the top of the jump, toss the ball with your feet and catch it with your hands (**B**). Return to start and repeat.

ASPIRING: Start with arms in front of your chest, ready to catch the ball.

STRONG: Ditch the ball. Stand with your legs a foot apart. Hold your arms straight out to the sides so your hands are at waist height, palms facing down. Keeping your hands in place, bend your knees 45 degrees and explode into the air, pulling your knees up to hit your palms.

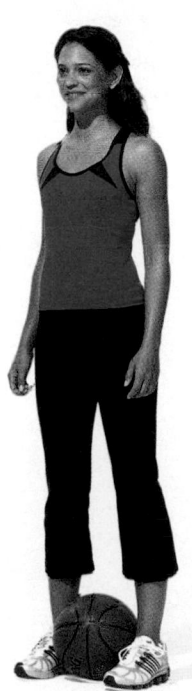

A

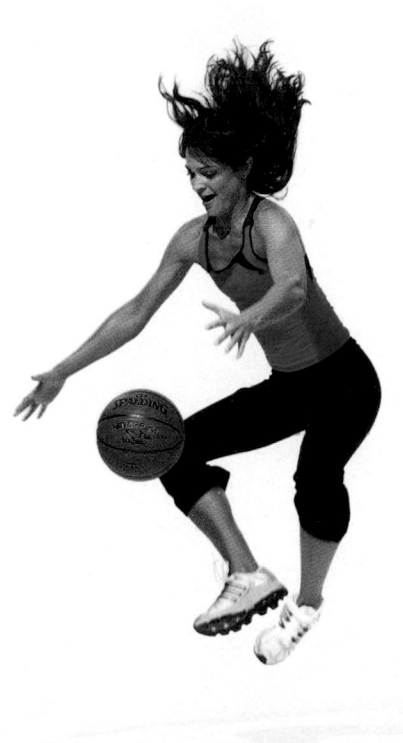

B

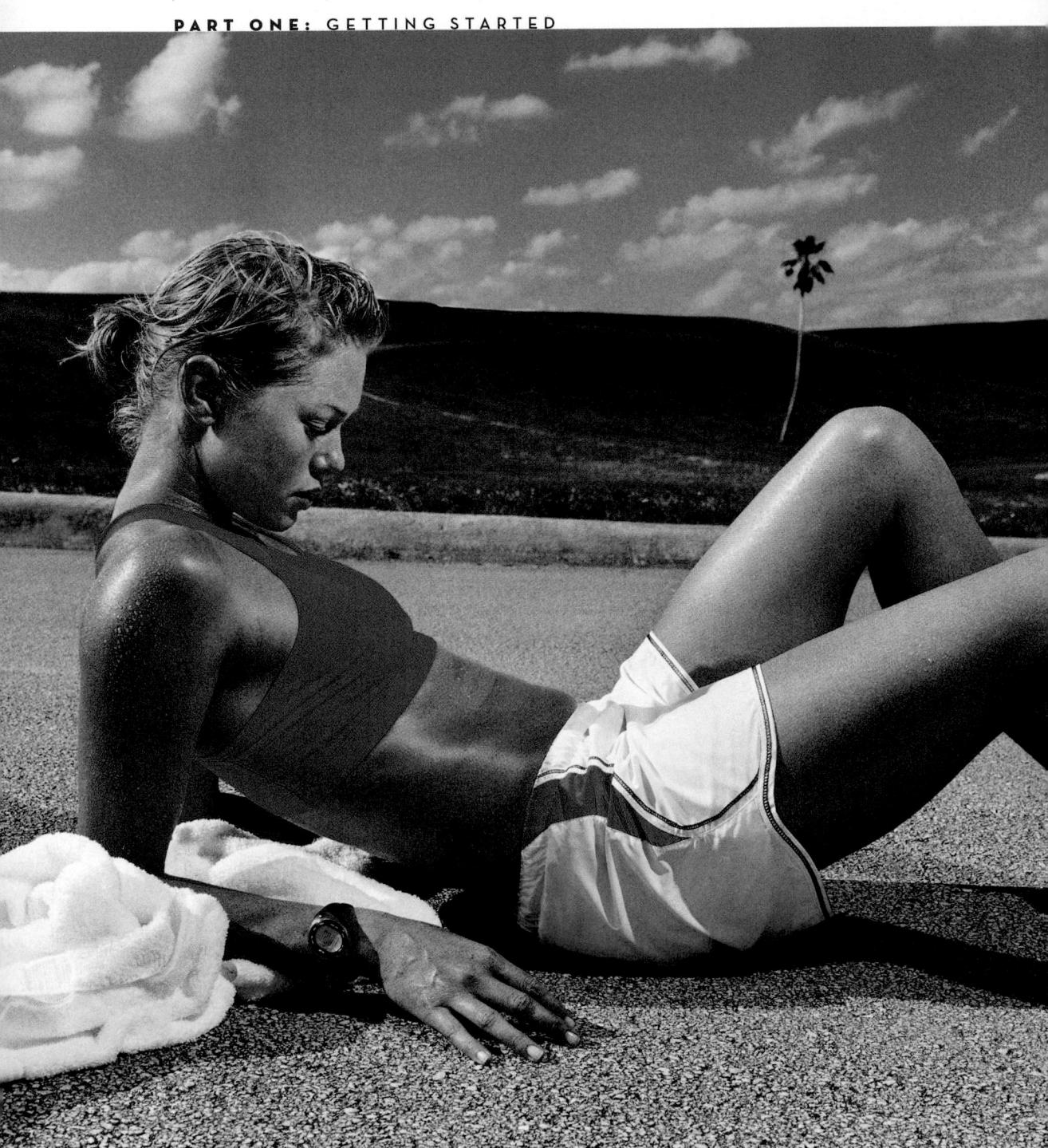

CHAPTER TWO

THE FITNESS BOUNCE-BACK PLAN

DON'T SWEAT IF YOU'VE TAKEN A BREAK FROM WORKING OUT. INSTEAD, FOCUS ON THE WAY TO BOUNCE YOUR BODY BACK INTO SHAPE– NO MATTER HOW LONG YOU'VE BEEN OUT OF IT

BY SARAH TUFF

SOME COMEBACKS–LIKE LEG WARMERS and TV dance contests—should stay packed up in the past. But your prime-time return to the gym is different. Slipping back into a fitness routine after a break can be daunting, especially when you consider that such breaks can cause you to lose up to 50 percent of your lean muscle mass and cardiovascular strength. "As soon as you stop participating in regular activity, your body starts detraining," says Lynn Millar, Ph.D., professor of physical therapy at Andrews University in Michigan. "But if you were fairly fit before the break, you'll bounce back quickly, because your muscular patterns were more deeply etched." Whether you've been planted on your butt for 2 weeks or 2 years, we have tips to help you ease your body up off the couch and back into your routine.

Your break: 2 weeks

Loss of muscle strength: Up to 12 percent
Loss of aerobic endurance: 7 percent
Comeback time: 1 week

What happened: Luckily, not too much. Your loss of muscular strength means that you can probably still do your standard sets of biceps curls, but you'll feel the burn earlier in your repetitions, says New York City athletic trainer Gene Schafer. Your ticker's a bit slower, too. "You've lost some of your endurance because your heart has not been stimulated to be efficient," says Mary Mundrane-Zweiacher, an athletic trainer in Dover, Delaware. "So if you were running 5 miles a day before the break, you might now get winded at the 4.5-mile mark instead of the end."

Get it back: You haven't lost much in terms of your fitness level, so you just need to step back and make a few small tweaks to your routine to get back on track. Here's how:

HIT PAUSE

Allow for 10 extra seconds to recover between sets. "This will allow your heart rate, which isn't quite at its normal level, to lower enough to give you a better next set, with better technique," Schafer says. "So you'll be able to complete your routine and see results faster."

FOCUS ON POWER MUSCLES

After a 2-week break, your glutes and quads are still strong enough to tackle tough exercise, Mundrane-Zweiacher says. "Squats, lunges, and stepups will set muscle fibers firing and rebuilding fast—without risking injury," she says. Working such a large muscle group will also get you back into a high calorie-burning mode. Run up a flight of steps (the longer the better) and at the top, stand with your feet shoulder-width apart and squat until your knees reach 90 degrees. Do three reps and then walk back down the stairs. Do three sets of stairs and squats for the first 3 days of your return to exercise.

GO FREE

Since you've lost some muscle but still have enough strength to stabilize what you have, use free weights instead of machines to work more muscle groups at once, Schafer says. If you feel a little flabby (your muscles might not be as tight now as they were before), do some extra sets of light, high-rep toning exercises for your arms and thighs: Holding a 5-pound dumbbell in each hand, with palms down, slowly raise your arms until they're parallel with the floor. Do three sets of 15 reps. For your thighs, do three sets of 15 lunges with a 5-pound dumbbell in each hand.

DO MUSIC INTERVALS

Intervals will crank up your rate of return by requiring your body to adapt to different speeds, explains Laura Keller, a physical therapist with the Stone Clinic in San Francisco. "You'll probably be returning at a slightly lower level of speed and endurance due to the 2-week break, and intervals help your heart retrain faster than running at one steady pace," says Jim Rutberg of Carmichael Training Systems in

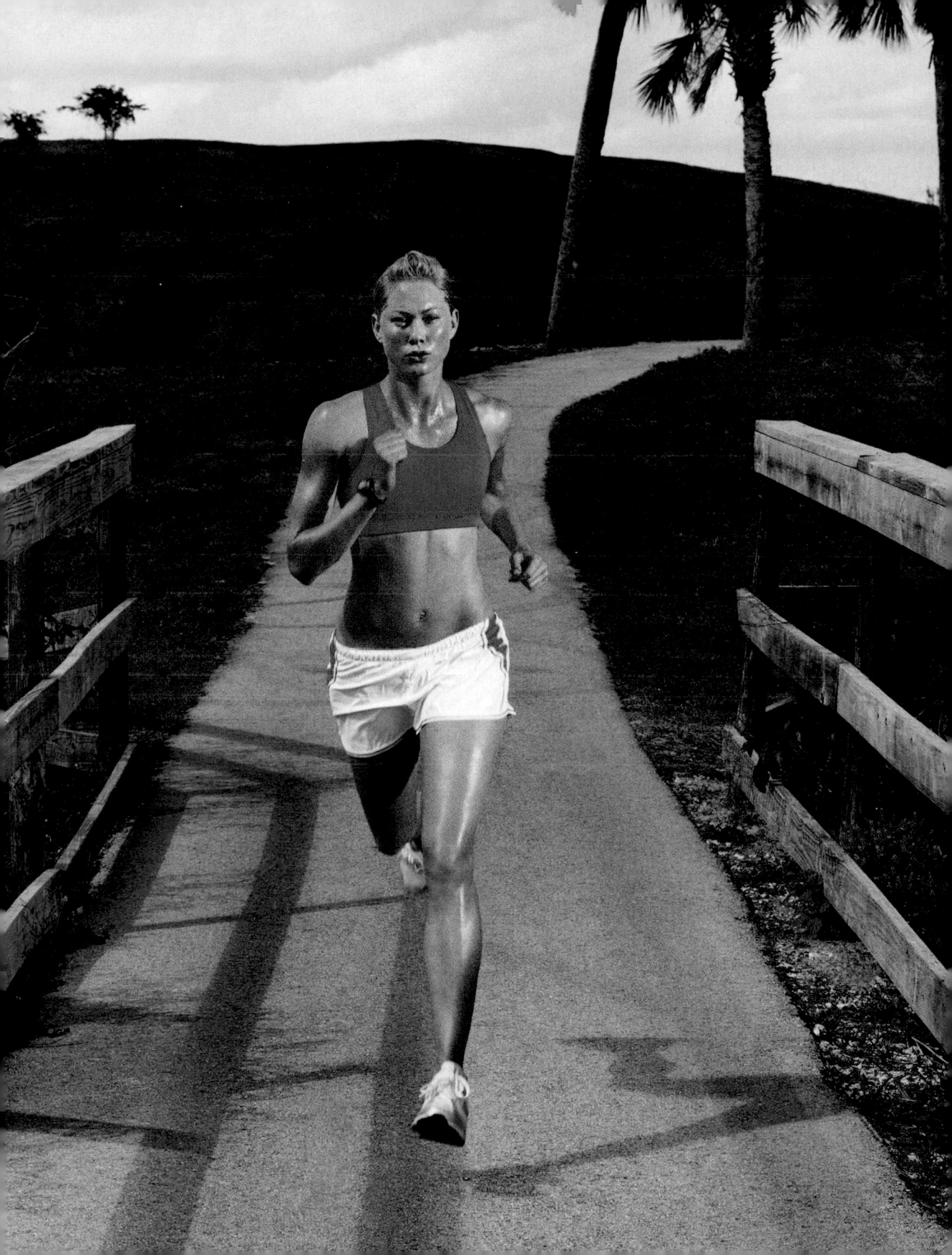

Colorado Springs, Colorado. Use your MP3 player for music tempos: After a 10-minute warmup jog, run fast for one song and at a slower pace for the next one. Continue this for at least five songs, or listen to a radio station for 30 to 60 minutes, running at a medium pace during songs and alternating sprinting and walking through commercials.

Your break: 2 months

Loss of muscle strength: 35 percent

Loss of aerobic endurance: 18 percent

Comeback time: 6 weeks

What happened: The extra project you took on led not only to stress acne and late-night Chow Ming dinners, but also to a significant loss of your fitness base. "Your muscles haven't been fatigued lately, so your first workout back may actually feel pretty good, but then your performance is going to go downhill fast," Rutberg says. "Plus, you've lost a considerable amount of your range of motion, so even doing a simple biceps curl can put you at risk for injury." And after 2 months off of cardiovascular workouts, getting back on the elliptical trainer for 45 minutes is going to feel like climbing the Statue of Liberty. "Your lungs are not as efficient at pumping oxygen to your blood, and your heart is not as efficient at pumping blood to your muscles," says Ann Trombley, an Olympic mountain biker and physical therapist in Boulder, Colorado. "Therefore your fuel supply—oxygen—is low. It's like running out of gas in your car; you're going to chug and sputter."

Get it back: You'll need to cut back on your old intensity and slowly build your fitness over the 6-week period, which is actually the length of a solid strength-building cycle. Modifying both your cardio and strength exercises will help you gradually ramp your routine up to where it was before you stopped working out. Schedule at least three workouts each week, and revise your old plan like this:

BREAK THE CYCLE

Sometimes your vacation from fitness was anything but a trip. Whether you were sidelined by a sprain, a scalpel, or a screaming "precious," here's what you should know about specific fitness breaks.

COMING BACK FROM AN INJURY: Severe ankle sprains, for example, can take 6 weeks or more to heal. But if there's only minimal swelling, and you're able to walk normally on the ankle, chances are it's mild and you'll be able to resume activity within a few days, says athletic trainer Mary Mundrane-Zweiacher. To loosen and strengthen an ankle that's been on the outs, trace the alphabet in the air with your toes. Next, place a towel on a wood or tile floor and scrunch it with your toes. For a fracture, you may be out 6 to 8 weeks and need up to a month more of rehab.

COMING BACK FROM SURGERY: If you've had an appendectomy, a hysterectomy, or anything else that's muddled your midsection, heed your doc's advice and sit tight for the allotted time

PLAY QUARTERS

And we don't mean at the local frat house. Do one-fourth the cardio you were doing before the break, which will help prevent overexertion yet still ease you back into shape, Keller says. "If you were previously cycling for 2 hours, ride for 30 to 45 minutes, three times a week, and increase by 15 minutes each week," she says. If you were jogging for 1 hour on the treadmill, cut your session back to 15 minutes, adding more minutes each week.

PUSH UP YOUR STRENGTH

Because your pectoral and arm muscles are weaker, you're at much greater risk for injuring them if you drop and give us military-style pushups, Mundrane-Zweiacher says. On your first day back, do as many modified pushups (with your knees on the floor) as you can. Do them three times a week, and when you can do 30, switch to military style. If you can't do 30, finish the set with modified pushups. This move builds muscle quickly in a safer way than the classic and uses nothing but your body weight; you're less likely to injure yourself doing a pushup than trying to maneuver weights.

GET WITH THE BAND

You're more likely to be sloppy and hurt yourself if you use free weights right away, Schafer says. "Resistance bands will help you quickly regain the strength you've lost without causing an injury, because they keep you in place much like machines do. But the resistance depends on how hard you pull, so they're gentler."

BE PARTIAL

The muscles on the insides of your knees might be weaker than the ones on the outsides, because your IT bands (the tendons on the outsides of your thighs) tighten with inactivity. As a result, you start using your muscles differently, according to Mundrane-Zweiacher. That puts you at risk for knee problems, and jumping back into regular squats could make

(usually around 6 weeks). "If you have abdominal surgery, you're out for the count, because anything you do, even walking with vigor, can put pressure on the abdomen," says Pamela Peeke, M.D., a nationally recognized fitness expert. Take it easy when you return to activity, and do gentle exercise like hatha yoga for the first few weeks. "But avoid ashtanga or vinyasa styles, which are too aggressive for your weakened state."

COMING BACK FROM DELIVERY: Pooches are cute—when they're on a leash. Even the most seasoned athletes with six-packs can get postpartum pooches, because a growing uterus can cause a diastasis, which is a separation of the abdominal muscles. "Some 98 percent of women who've had a child have a diastasis, and it can take up to 6 months for it to heal," says Julie Tupler, R.N., author of Lose Your Mummy Tummy. "Doing crunches post-pregnancy can actually make it worse, because you end up putting pressure on the wrong places." Try the seated Tupler technique: Sit in a chair and contract your transverse abdominus muscle by drawing your belly button toward your spine. Hold for a moment and then release. Work up to 100 reps, five times a day. It can take about 6 weeks to get your pre-baby fitness level back, but up to 6 months on average to return your abs and pelvic floor to normal.

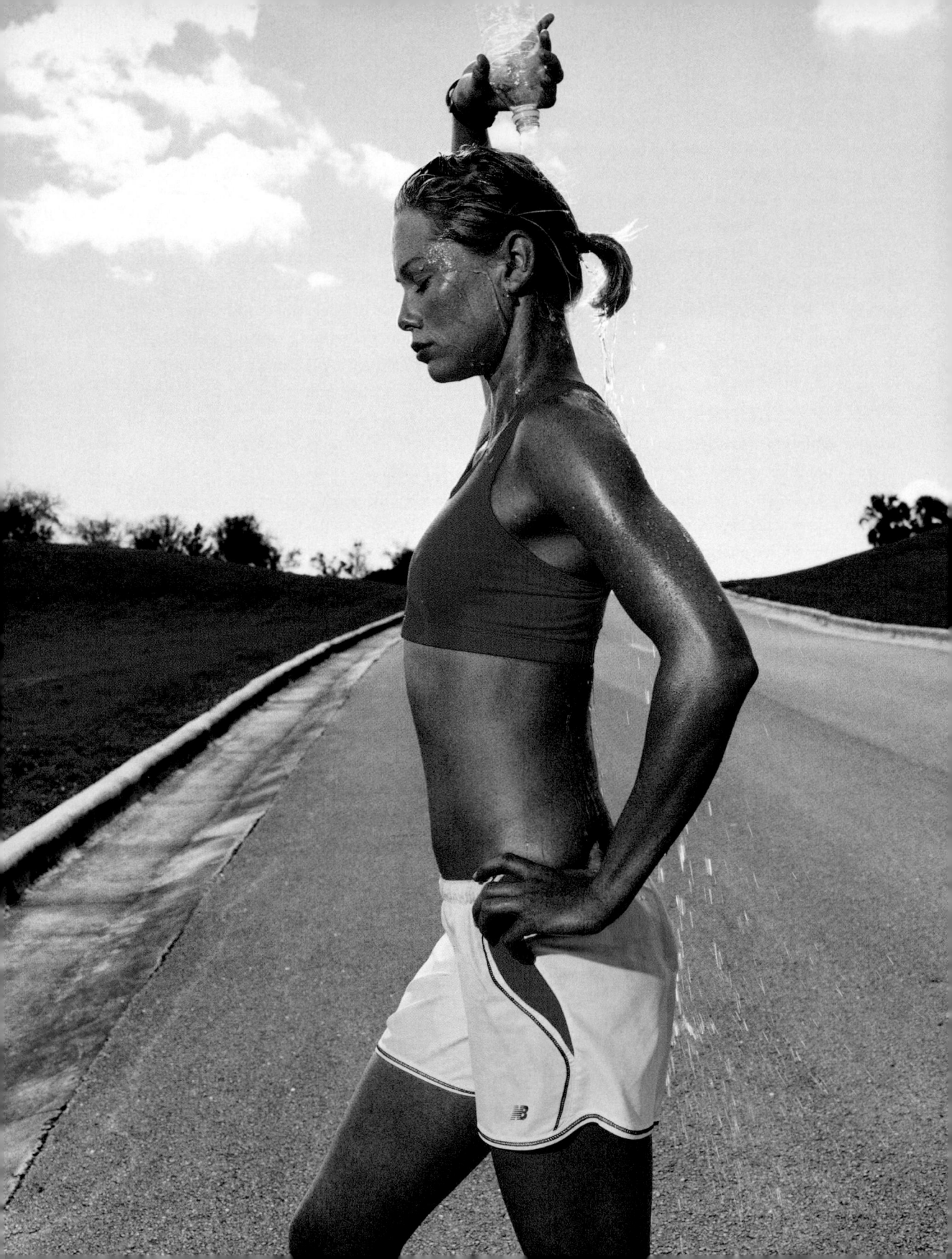

that risk higher. For the first 2 weeks, do partial squats by standing with your feet shoulder-width apart and bending your knees to 45 degrees.

Your break: 2 years

Loss of muscle strength: **Up to 50 percent**
Loss of aerobic endurance: **Up to 50 percent**
Comeback time: **12 weeks**

What happened: Seriously. What happened? Unfortunately, you could be half the woman you used to be, even if your jeans size has doubled. "After a 2-year hiatus from weight training, lifting a 10-pound dumbbell is going to feel like lifting a 30-pound one because your muscle fibers have shrunk," Trombley says. Your body will feel softer, and your butt could feel sore after climbing the two flights to your apartment.

Get it back: Considering you flexed your intelligence more than your muscles for 2 years (well, let's hope so), a 3-month retraining period really isn't that bad. Pamela Peeke, M.D., author of *Body for Life for Women*, recommends building onto your routine in a pyramid format to avoid overstressing yourself too quickly. For example, in strength training, start with a set of 15 reps. Add 2 pounds for the next set and cut it back to 12 reps. To ease into your cardio routine, crank the resistance on a bike up a level each week. One warning: If after a few weeks you feel like you've been hit by a bus, don't sweat it.

"You might feel exhausted, because your body's not used to building new muscle," Dr. Millar says. "But your energy level will improve after about a month."

GO HARD CORE

Your core is the center of your fitness universe, and at this point you'll need to rebuild it. Try Mundrane-Zweiacher's 90-90 holds. Lie on your back with your spine in a neutral (neither arched nor rounded) position, with your abs pulled tight. Next, lift your feet so that your knees and hips are both at a sharp 90 degrees. On day one, hold it for 10 seconds, then add 10 seconds each day until you reach 2 minutes.

WALK AWAY

You're more prone to shin splints and a sore back because of possible muscle imbalances, and walking is one of the gentlest ways to work those muscles evenly while easing your cardiovascular system back into shape, Keller says. Plus, a recent University of Texas at Austin study showed that walking for just 30 minutes relieves depression, providing the same pick-me-up some people seek in Krispy Kremes. Keller suggests doing 2-mile walks three times a week for 3 to 4 weeks. After a month of walking, alternate between walking and running for another month, which will help your body adjust more slowly to the demands of running. After 6 weeks of total exercise, start adding mileage to your runs and picking up the pace.

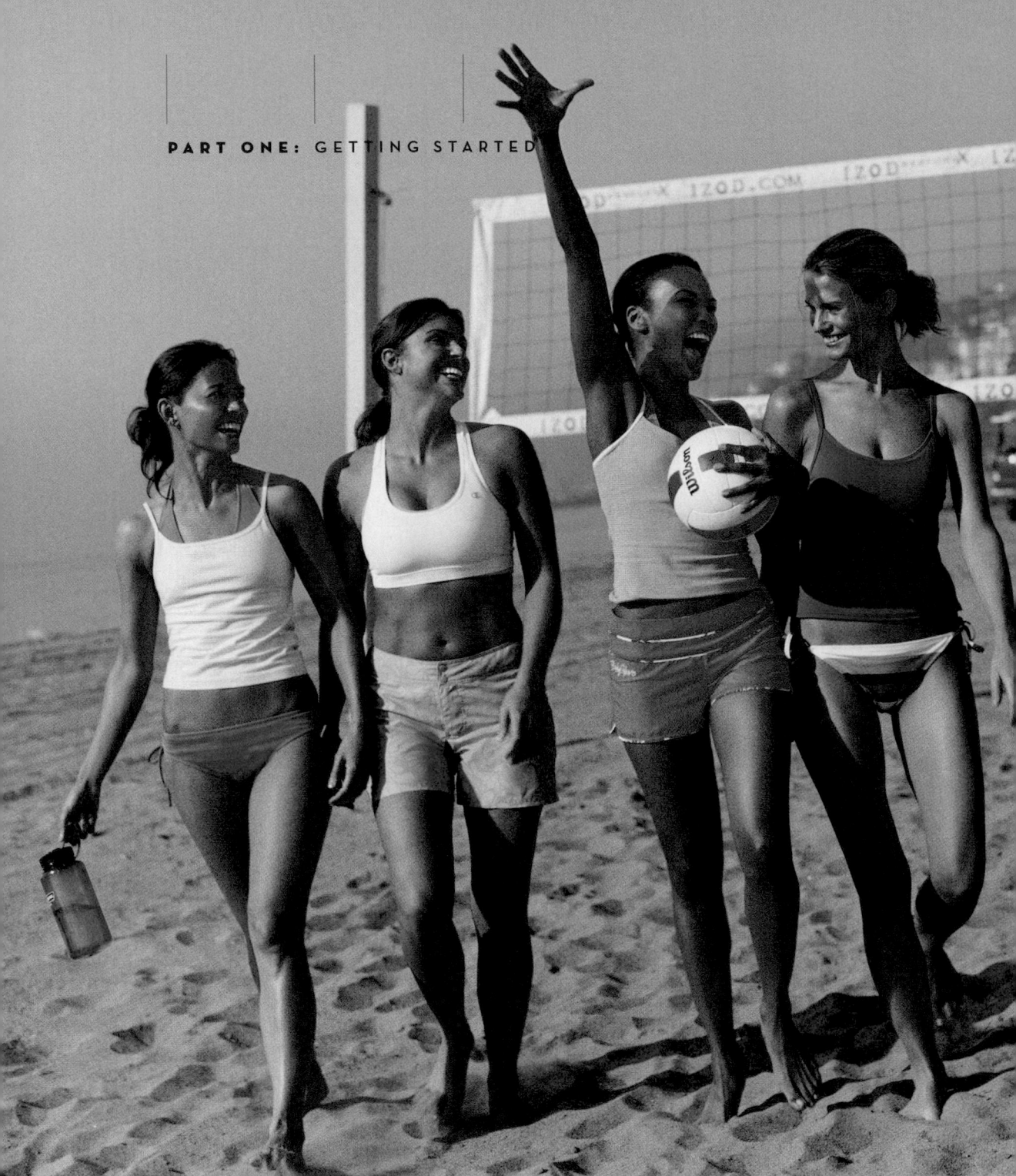

30

CHAPTER THREE

YOUR PERFECT WEIGHT:
GET THERE, STAY THERE

DETERMINE YOUR IDEAL SIZE WITH OUR BODY ANALYSIS GUIDE, THEN MAKE IT A REALITY WITH OUR THREE-STEP SYSTEM TAILOR-MADE FOR YOU.

BY JULIE UPTON, R.D.

OF ALL THE NUMBERS you carry around in your head—security codes, credit cards, gym-lock combinations—there's one series of digits that probably drives you crazy. Not because it's hard to remember—in fact, you could never forget it. This number represents your ever-elusive perfect weight. If you could only achieve it—and stay there—you're certain you'd be better in bed, more confident in meetings, sexier and sassier in jeans, and in every way 10 times happier than you are right this minute.

But what is this magical number, and how do you arrive at it?

Is it a reasonable weight that falls within the ranges provided on doctor-approved charts? Or is it a weight you dipped to once, 4 years ago, after living through a painful breakup and that killer intestinal thing? The first key to hitting your number is to make it a realistic one, based on your bone structure and body type. The good news is that once you determine the right number and set your mind to reach it, your body will help you get there, despite late-night cravings and sluggish treadmill sessions.

STEP 1
Do the Math

There's no single formula for predicting an exact, down-to-the-decimal weight for every woman alive, but there are certain guidelines you can use to set a realistic weight-loss goal. Here are four that can help you find your magic number.

A Your baseline

To start, let's go back to Nutrition 101. Take the number of inches you are over 5 feet and multiply that number by five. Add this to 100 for a rough initial estimate of what someone of your height should weigh. So if you're 5'7", multiply 7 by 5 and add 100. Your target weight is 135. But you still need to assess—and factor in—the other elements that contribute to your perfect weight.

B Your bone structure

Remember that phrase "you're just big-boned"? It seems like a euphemism for "fat" (see also "husky," "chunky," "pleasantly plump"), but the truth is that your frame—in effect, your bone structure—can run large or small, no matter how tall you are. Researchers now recognize that having a large frame can add up to 10 pounds of healthy, unavoidable weight to your body.

Okay, now take that baseline figure you arrived at in Step A and adjust accordingly—5 to 10 pounds more for a bigger frame, 5 to 10 pounds less for a smaller frame (see the chart below).

C Your overall body fat

One of the best indicators of whether you're at a healthy weight is how much of your bulk is fat. While between 20 and 31 percent is considered

MATCH YOUR WRIST TO YOUR HEIGHT
TO DETERMINE YOUR BONE STRUCTURE, MEASURE THE CIRCUMFERENCE OF YOUR WRIST

If you're under 5'2"

SMALL FRAME: wrist size under 5.5"

MEDIUM FRAME: wrist size under 6"

LARGE FRAME: wrist size under 6.25"

If you're between 5'2" and 5'5"

SMALL FRAME: wrist size 5.5" to 5.75"

MEDIUM FRAME: wrist size 6" to 6.25"

LARGE FRAME: wrist size 6.25" to 6.5"

If you're over 5'5"

SMALL FRAME: wrist size over 5.75"

MEDIUM FRAME: wrist size over 6.25"

LARGE FRAME: wrist size over 6.5"

a "normal" range for women, an ideal level for fitness (and looking fit) is around 21 percent. The best way to measure body fat is with calibration tools—either old-fashioned skin-pinching calipers or more sensitive bioelectric impedance analysis machines, which use electrical currents to measure body mass. Is your bioelectric impedance machine in the shop? You can get a good estimation of your fat and how much of it you need to lose by using the chart on page 35.

D Your belly fat

Now you want to figure out whether you're packing too much belly fat—dangerous because the same fat that gathers around your abdomen, called adipose fat, is also likely to be collecting around vital organs and preventing healthy bloodflow. And researchers at the New York Obesity Research Center at St. Luke's-Roosevelt Hospital found that waist size correlates better than overall body mass to risk factors for heart disease, such as high blood pressure, blood sugar, and cholesterol.

To calculate your waist size, wrap the tape measure around the top of your hip bones. Take the measurement at the end of a normal breath. Then place your index finger next to your belly button and, standing up straight, see how many inches of belly fat you can grasp between your index finger and thumb.

If your waist is over 33 inches and you can pinch 2 inches of fat, you need to lose at least 10 pounds from your current weight, no matter how you've scored in other tests. If you can pinch 1 inch, you need to lose at least 5 pounds.

PERFECT WEIGHT: Your "perfect weight" is between the figure you arrived at in Steps A and B and the amount of weight you need to lose as deter-

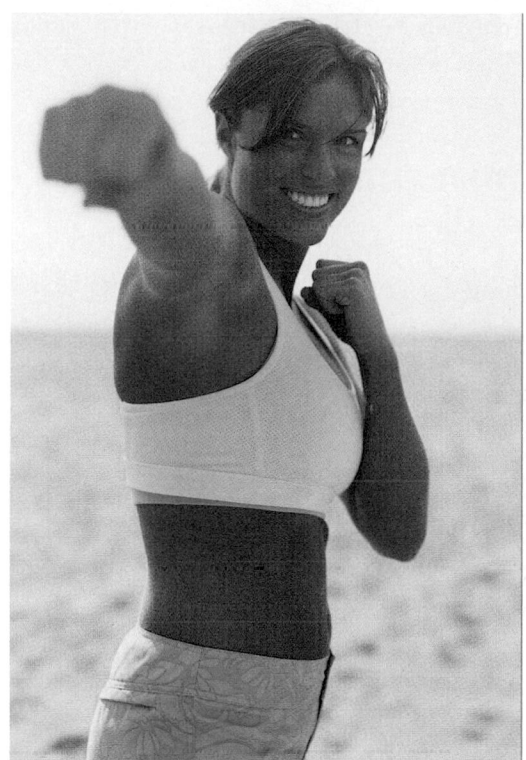

mined by the results of Steps C and D. You have the best understanding of what's realistic for you and how much your body can change, so don't let an overly ambitious goal ruin your day—or your healthy habits. Read ahead for our plan designed to burn off excess fat, build muscle, and get you to your perfect weight—and keep you there for good.

STEP 2 Get There

You know the drill: To lose weight, you have to consume fewer calories than you burn. And to do that, you need to know your metabolic rate—the amount of calories you burn throughout the day. "Most women have a metabolic rate of just under 1 calorie per minute, or about 1,440 calories per day," says David Nieman, Ph.D., a nutrition and exercise professor at Appalachian State University. Use this chart to determine your metabolic rate and daily calorie needs.

YOUR VITALS

A Your weight in pounds _____

B Multiply A by 11 to get your basic calorie needs (how much your body burns just by existing) _____

C Multiply B by 1.6 to estimate your resting metabolic rate (rate of calorie burn when you factor in your daily activities) _____

YOUR EXERCISE

D AEROBIC TRAINING

Multiply the number of minutes per week that you run, cycle, or play sports by 8 _____

E STRENGTH TRAINING

If you're doing a total-body exercise plan, add 600 to your answer from D. If you're doing three sets, add 840 to your answer from D.

F Divide that by 7 _____

YOUR CALORIE NEEDS

G Add C and F to get your daily calorie needs _____

H If you're happy with your weight, stop here. Otherwise, subtract 500 from G _____ This is your estimated daily calorie budget if you want to lose 1 pound per week. Subtract 1,000 to lose 2 pounds a week. Anything more and you'll lose more muscle than fat.

Based on your calorie and weight-loss goals, use the nutritional advice and the workouts in this guide to customize the perfect diet and exercise plan. You're on your way to your perfect weight!

STEP 3 Stay There

Losing weight is the easy part. But we all know that. Somehow, as soon as you've closed in on your magic number, it becomes harder and harder to stay there. And in fact, the wrong dieting habits can slow your metabolism, canceling out all your hard work. Well, no worries. Here's how to retool your eating behaviors and exercise routine to maintain your new, svelter self.

On a healthy weight-loss diet, about three-quarters of every pound you lose is fat and one-quarter is lean body mass. Lose too much too fast and you're more likely to have trouble keeping it off. "Depending on how rapidly you lose weight and on your diet and exercise patterns, your resting metabolic rate can decrease significantly during weight loss," says Chris Melby, Dr.P.H., a professor at Colorado State University. But even if you go at a safe, slow pound a week, your body still adapts to the loss—and makes it hard to stay slim. For every pound you lose, your total daily calories need to be reduced by about 10. Lose 10 pounds, and your body needs 100 fewer calories a day, on average, to sustain itself.

Getting more daily exercise is one way to help offset this drop in metabolic rate, but it still doesn't mean you can ignore what you eat. And beware of postworkout snacking: A study from the School of Human Kinetics at the University of Ottawa in Ontario found that a woman's appetite postexercise may drive her to eat as many calories as she burned during exercise. "Even if you exercise for an hour or more a day, our body is so fuel-efficient that you'll still have to watch what you eat. Exercise because it's good for your health, but watch your diet because it ultimately controls how lean you are," Dr. Nieman says.

TO FIND YOUR OVER-ALL BODY FAT...

A First determine your body mass index, a ratio of weight to height. It's tricky, so follow this example of a 145-pound, 26-year-old woman who's 5′10″ (70 inches).

Multiply your height in inches by your height in inches.
Example: 70 × 70 = 4,900

Divide your weight by that number.
Example: 145 / 4,900 = .029

Multiply that by 703 to find your BMI.
Example:
BMI = .029 × 703 = 20.39

YOUR BMI: _____

B Determine your body fat percentage.

Multiply your BMI by 1.20.
Example: 1.20 × 20.39 = 24.46

Then, multiply your age by .23.
Example: .23 × 26 = 5.98

Add those two numbers together.
Example: 24.46 + 5.98 = 30.44

Subtract 5.4 from that number to find your body fat percentage.
Example: 30.44 - 5.4 = 25.04

YOUR BODY FAT: _____%

C Use the chart on the right to determine how far over the goal you are (or aren't!). At 25 percent body fat, our sample woman is carrying 14 percent more fat than the ideal of 21 percent.

D Translate your body fat percentage into how much sheer fat you're carrying around by multiplying your body fat by your current weight.
Example: (145 × 25%) = 36.25, meaning 36.25 pounds of our 145-pound woman comes from fat.

YOUR WEIGHT FROM FAT:

_____

E Finally, multiply your percentage over goal from C by your total body fat in answer D. That's how many pounds of fat you should seek to lose.
Example: 36 × 14% = 5.14 pounds

YOUR WEIGHT-LOSS GOAL:
_____

BODY FAT PERCENTAGE

BODY FAT	PERCENT OVER GOAL
22	4
23	7
24	11
25	14
26	18
27	21
28	25
29	29
30	32
31	36
32	39
33	43
34	46
35	50
36	54
37	57
38	61
39	64
40	68
41	71
42	75
43	79
44	82

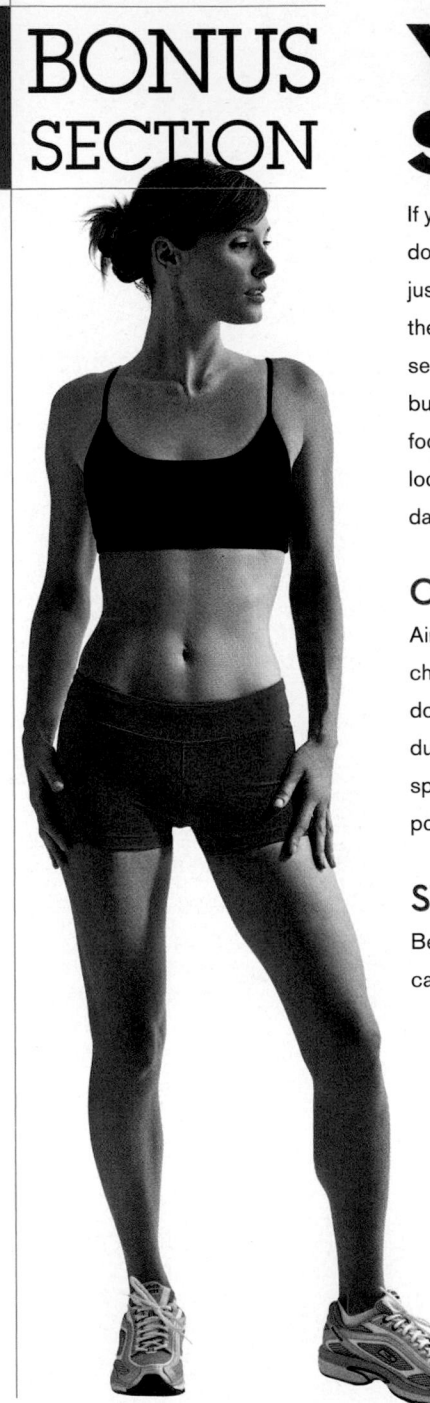

BONUS SECTION

YOUR WEEKLY SCHEDULE

If you are like us, you are more accountable when you write things down, whether it's a matter of remembering your cousin's birthday, or just getting in four runs per week. So we've made it easy for you. On these pages you can track your weekly cardio and strength-training sessions for a full 6-week program. (Be sure to check out the fat-burning workout plans in Part Three.) We've also provided a 2-week food log to help you jumpstart your diet. Keep in mind you are not locked into this schedule. You can rearrange the workouts to accommodate your life—just be sure that you get them all in each week.

CARDIO LOG

Aim to get at least 30 minutes of cardio 4 days per week. Feel free to choose the activities you like the best, but make sure to mix it up so you don't get in a running rut or bored with biking. Intervals are not required during every workout, but they do boost your fat burn, so we've included space for interval length and intensity to remind you to include some power sessions.

STRENGTH-TRAINING LOG

Begin each of your three weekly strengthening workouts with a 5-min cardio warmup and end each with 5-min cardio cooldown.

2-WEEK FOOD LOG

WEEK 1. Write down everything you eat and drink—yes, even the crackers and Cabernet you downed before dinner—but don't change a thing about your eating habits. At the end of the week you should have a realistic picture of your dietary strengths and weaknesses (red flag: adding a "midnight snack" section to this grid).

WEEK 2. Continue to track your eating, but start to integrate the meals and tips found in Part Two to help curb your cravings and reduce calorie intake.

CARDIO LOG

		WEEK 1	WEEK 2	WEEK 3	WEEK 4	WEEK 5	WEEK 6
DAY 1	Activity						
	Time						
	Intervals						
DAY 2	Activity						
	Time						
	Intervals						
DAY 3	Activity						
	Time						
	Intervals						
DAY 4	Activity						
	Time						
	Intervals						

TOTAL FITNESS GUIDE 2008

W|H

MONDAY ABS

	WEEK 1 Reps	WEEK 2 Reps	WEEK 3 Reps	WEEK 4 Reps	WEEK 5 Reps	WEEK 6 Reps
KNEE-DROP CRUNCH, p. 163						
SWISS BALL CRUNCH, p. 120						
PRONE KNEE DRIVES, p. 121						
DOUBLE-SIDE JACKKNIFE, p. 258						
DYNAMIC V-CRUNCH, p. 259						
RAISED HIP CRUNCH, p. 260						
SIDE DOUBLE CRUNCH, p. 260						

WEDNESDAY UPPER BODY

	WEEK 1 Weight/Reps	WEEK 2 Weight/Reps	WEEK 3 Weight/Reps	WEEK 4 Weight/Reps	WEEK 5 Weight/Reps	WEEK 6 Weight/Reps
DUMBBELL PULLOVER, p. 117						
HAMMER CURLS, p. 159						
CHEST PRESS, p. 206						
ONE-ARM ROW KICKBACK, p. 252						
LATERAL RAISE, p. 252						
WALKOVER PUSHUPS, p. 252						

FRIDAY LOWER BODY

	WEEK 1 Reps	WEEK 2 Reps	WEEK 3 Reps	WEEK 4 Reps	WEEK 5 Reps	WEEK 6 Reps
BRIDGE ABDUCTION, p. 242						
BALLET SQUAT p. 243						
SQUAT KICK p. 286						
GRASSHOPPER BEATS p. 287						
BACK LUNGE SERIES, Ch. 30						
HEEL RAISE SERIES, Ch. 30						
1¼ BARBELL SQUAT, p. 302						

FOOD LOG

WEEK 1	MON	TUES	WED	THURS	FRI	SAT	SUN
BREAKFAST							
LUNCH							
SNACKS							
DINNER							

WEEK 2	MON	TUES	WED	THURS	FRI	SAT	SUN
BREAKFAST							
LUNCH							
SNACKS							
DINNER							

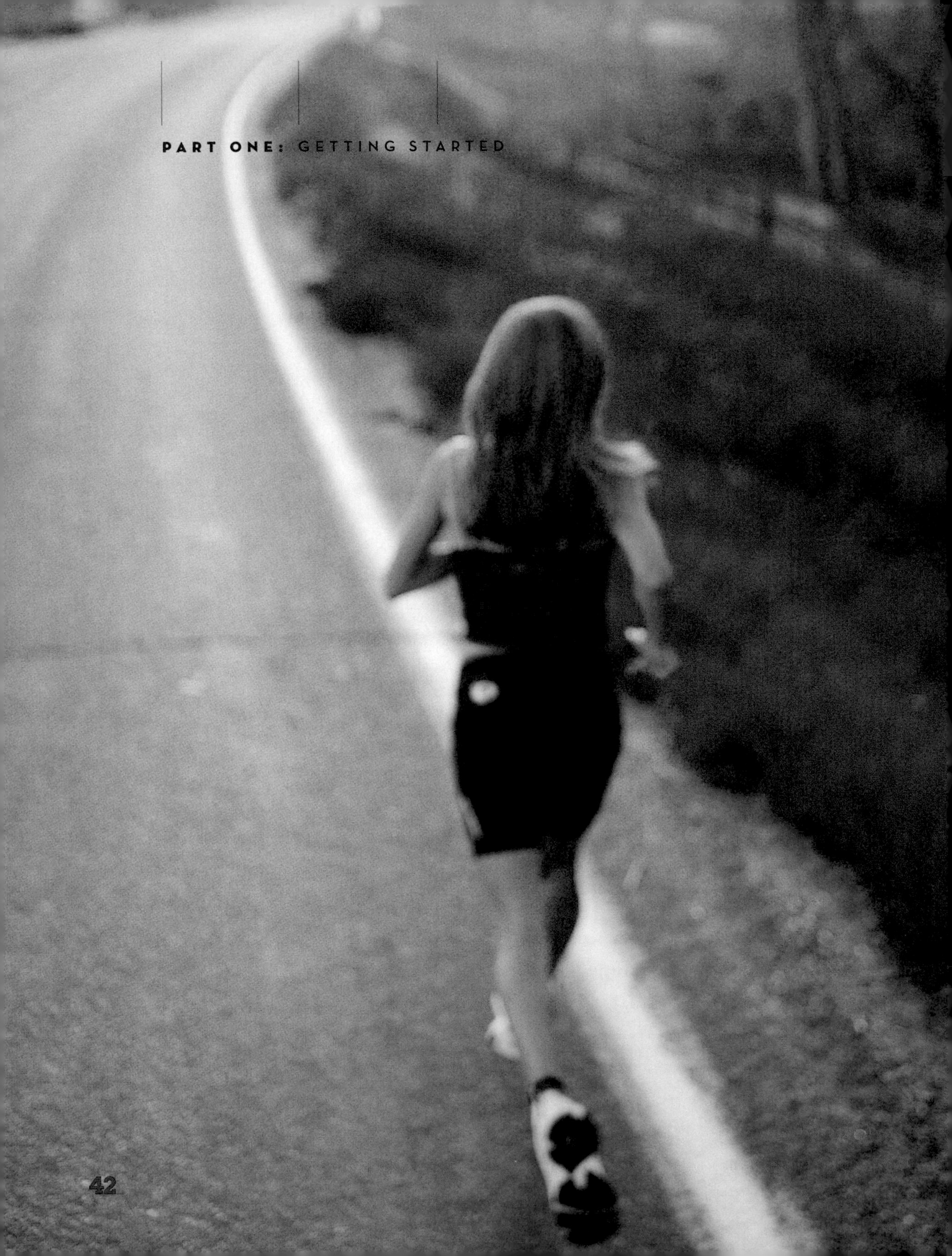

CHAPTER FOUR

STAY THE COURSE

KEEP ON THE STRAIGHT AND NARROW WITH THESE LUCKY 13 MOTIVATIONS.

BY KIMBERLY DAWN NEUMANN

13

BUY FISH, VEGGIES, and gym membership in attempt to make good on New Year's resolution to lose 12 pounds. Make healthy meals and work out five times a week for first 3 weeks. Then two times a week for a month. Then, oh, never. Sound familiar? Maintaining your diet and exercise enthusiasm can be the trickiest part of the weight-loss equation. But before you give in to the Twinkies demon perched on your shoulder, check out these proven motivation boosters.

READER POLL

THE TOP FIVE THINGS THAT MOTIVATE YOU TO LOSE WEIGHT, ACCORDING TO A POLL OF 700 *WH* READERS

1. Improving your health
2. Fitting into clothes better
3. Seeing photos of yourself when you're heavy
4. Seeing photos of yourself when you're slim
5. The upcoming bikini season

1. Have lots of sex First off, it's pretty damn fun. But it can also keep you on the slim track. Having an orgasm releases the same endorphins in your brain that eating chocolate does—without the calories. And research shows that the more weight you lose, the better your sex life gets: A Duke University study found that even a 10 percent reduction in weight (that's 15 pounds if you weigh 150) resulted in major improvements in all areas of the participants' sex lives, including arousal, feelings of attractiveness, and enjoyment of sexual activity (read: oodles of Os).

2. Make a promise It's really hard to blow off a commitment you've made to lots of people. For example, "joining an athletic event to raise money means if you default on your training, you're not just letting yourself down but also the charity and every-one who sponsored you," says New York City-based Dan Hamner, M.D., author of Peak Energy. Go to stepbystepfundraising.com and click on Athletic Events to find one near you. Choose something strenuous enough that you'll need to train seriously in advance. (Triathlon, anyone?) Some groups, including Team in Training for the Leukemia & Lymphoma Foundation (teamintraining.org), even provide free coaching for participants nationwide.

3. Enlist Fido Consider adopting a fuzzy friend if you don't have one already. Studies show that owning a dog can help you drop pounds. Why? Come rain, sleet, or snow, you've got to get your butt outside with pooch a few times a day (unless you really want urine-soaked carpets). What's more, most pet owners say they don't want to let down their exercise-starved doggy at walk time. It's another version of rule number 2.

4. Rock out A recent study by the North American Association for the Study of Obesity found that women are more likely to stick to an exercise program if they listen to music while working out. So thank God for jogtunes.com. The site lets you select your workout pace, then download playlists of songs with bpm (beats per minute) that match your heart rate. For example, if yours gets up to about 150 bpm when you exercise (the mid to upper target range for a healthy 30-year-old woman), songs like the Killers' "Mr. Brightside" are perfect.

5. Get out your sexiest skinny outfit You know that yogurt commercial where a woman takes a teeny-weeny yellow polka-dot bikini and hangs it on her wall to help motivate her to lose weight? She's one smart cookie. "I tell clients to take out an outfit they love and haven't been able to wear for a long time," says Christopher Warden, C.S.C.S., a personal trainer in New York City. "Just pulling it out of the closet serves as a visual reminder of the goal they're trying to accomplish."

6. Lift the weight you've lost A great way to keep yourself from sliding into what-the-hell eating mode when your weight loss plateaus: Use dumbbells that correspond to the number of pounds you've already dropped. You can't possibly forget how far you've come when you're straining to complete three sets of triceps kickbacks with a 10-pound weight. Feel how much you're struggling to lift? That used to be on your butt!

7. Get gabbing Reams of studies prove that support from other people can keep you motivated to lose weight. And a new study from the University of Kansas shows that dieters who get counseling over the phone lose just as much as those who get it face to face. So if you can't make that 5 p.m. Weight Watchers meeting, check out Bally's Built to Fit weight-loss and nutrition program at ballynutrition.com, which offers weekly 15-minute phone sessions starting at $1 per minute.

8. Call on your inner cheapskate You don't blow off the dentist, even though having your teeth drilled is about the most un-fun thing you can imagine. Why? Because you'll get charged whether you show or not. Consider buying a package of personal training sessions and scheduling all your appointments now. Ditto with yoga or dance classes: Buy a bunch in advance and sign up at the same time. Who would throw away workouts that are already paid for?

9. Become a class regular Join a group exercise class and make friends with your fellow regulars. Seeing your pals will inspire you to attend even when you feel like playing hooky. The guilt factor—always highly motivating—can help here too. After all, in a place where everybody knows your name, they'll also know when you've missed a workout.

10. Get rubbed A new study from Ohio State University shows that women who accept their bodies are more likely to have better eating habits. And decadent as it may sound, getting a massage can help with that. "Allowing themselves to be touched by another person—even when they aren't at their ideal weight—can help women become more comfortable with their bodies," says Mitch Klein, a licensed massage therapist in New York City.

11. Face your reflection When you feel fat you probably shun mirrors. Turns out you should do the opposite. A study in the International Journal of Eating Disorders found that mirror-exposure therapy—staring at your bod in the mirror and stifling the usual criticisms of your thighs—can improve body image, which, as we said in rule 10, can help keep you committed to healthy eating. Try it: Speak to your reflection without using any negatively charged words. For example, instead of "I have a huge butt," say, "My waist looks smaller thanks to my curves."

12. Chart your progress Weight loss is serious business. Treat it that way. Weigh yourself every morning—a study in the Annals of Behavior Medicine shows that people who do daily weigh-ins are more successful losers—and write the number down. (We like the Tanita HD-351 digital scale, which displays your current weight plus the number from your previous weigh-in; $64, amazon.com.) If you're even vaguely computer savvy, it's a snap to create a chart with a fever line that shows the pounds dropping away over time. When you get discouraged—say, you haven't lost a pound in a week—seeing your long-term progress will boost your motivation.

13. Score some free stuff There's no motivation like saving money. And since insurance providers want you to stay healthy so you don't develop expensive diseases like diabetes, some offer perks that make getting fit easier. Highmark Blue Cross Blue Shield, for example, gives its members discounts to certain gyms and free consultations with a dietitian. Check with your provider.

Need a Hand with Fat?

Here's who you're gonna call

BY VIRGINIA SOLE-SMITH

Certain things in life (bikini waxes, tax preparation, brain surgery) just go better when you hire a professional. If you've tried the motivation tricks in this story and still can't shed a pound, it may be time to call in the big guns. Here's who they are and what they can do for you.

DIET DOCTOR (BARIATRIC PHYSICIAN)

Who Is She? An M.D. who is certified by the American Board of Bariatric Medicine and trained to spot medical causes of weight gain.

Try Her If You're overweight enough that your "waist size is bigger than your bra size," says Mary Vernon, M.D., president of the American Society of Bariatric Physicians.

What Will She Do to Me? Ask for your health history and give you a physical exam, then run blood tests to see if your glucose, insulin levels, and thyroid are normal. Once she's pinpointed the cause of your weight problem (like a hormonal deficiency), she'll prescribe any necessary meds and work with you on a diet plan.

Best Weight-Loss Tip Kick processed carbs to the curb—they cause spikes in your blood sugar, which can lead to insulin resistance over time.

Cost From $200 to $400 for the initial evaluation, then $30 to $50 for weekly follow-ups, plus the cost of any meds.

How to Find HER Visit asbp.org and click on Locate a Doctor.

REGISTERED DIETITIAN (R.D.)

Who Is She? Someone with a bachelor's degree in nutrition or science who's passed a national certifying exam.

Try Her If You're confused about what kind of eating plan to follow.

What Will She Do to Me? Ask you to write down everything you put in your mouth, so she can find out what you're eating, when, where, and why. Then she'll create a meal plan and show you how to incorporate healthier foods into your diet, control portion sizes, and cut back on junk food. "We tailor everyone's program to her specific needs," says Dawn Jackson Blatner, R.D., a spokesperson for the American Dietetic Association.

Best Weight-Loss Tip Load at least half your plate with produce, a quarter with protein, and a quarter with grains (preferably whole), says Blatner.

Cost From $15 for 15 minutes with an R.D. at your local hospital to $95 to $250 for an hour with one in private practice.

How to Find Her Visit eatright.org and search for an R.D. certified in Adult Weight Management.

WEIGHT-LOSS PSYCHOLOGIST

Who Is She? Someone with a Ph.D. in clinical psychology who specializes in eating disorders and weight control.

Try Her If "You know what you're supposed to do to lose weight but just can't make yourself do it," says Ed Abramson, Ph.D., a professor emeritus of psychology at California State University in Chico.

What Will She Do to Me? Ask you to talk—a lot—to get to the root of your food issues and figure out if you're overeating because you're bored, depressed, angry, stressed, or all of the above.

Best Weight-Loss Tip Go for a walk. "If you're stressed or depressed, it's hard to make the effort to lose weight," Abramson says. "But even mild physical activity will lift your mood and give you energy to do more."

Cost About $100 per 50-minute session (covered if your insurance plan offers mental health benefits).

How to Find Her Call your insurance company or state psychological association and say you're looking for a licensed psychologist who specializes in weight loss.

WEIGHT-LOSS COACH

Who Is She? Anyone who calls herself a weight-loss coach. The best are certified by the International Coaching Federation, which requires at least 125 hours of training and a final exam.

Try Her If You need a kick in the pants to put down the Fritos and get off the couch.

What Will She Do to Me? Ask you to keep a food log to pinpoint which emotions are triggering you to down an entire box of doughnut holes and then teach you to counter the negative thoughts that led you to the cupboard. She'll also help you find ways to overcome each skip-the-gym obstacle—whether it's reworking your schedule or learning to say no to people who eat up too much of your time.

Best Weight-Loss Tip "Refuse to beat yourself up for overeating," says Brooke Castillo, a weight-loss coach in Shingle Springs, California. "That keeps you trapped in the negative thinking that made you eat in the first place."

Cost About $100 to $150 per session

How to Find Her Visit coachfederation.org and click on Find a Coach.

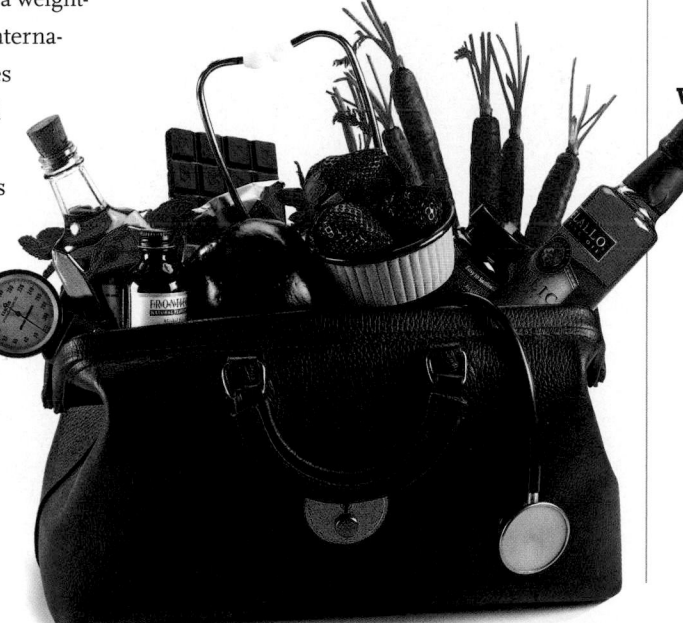

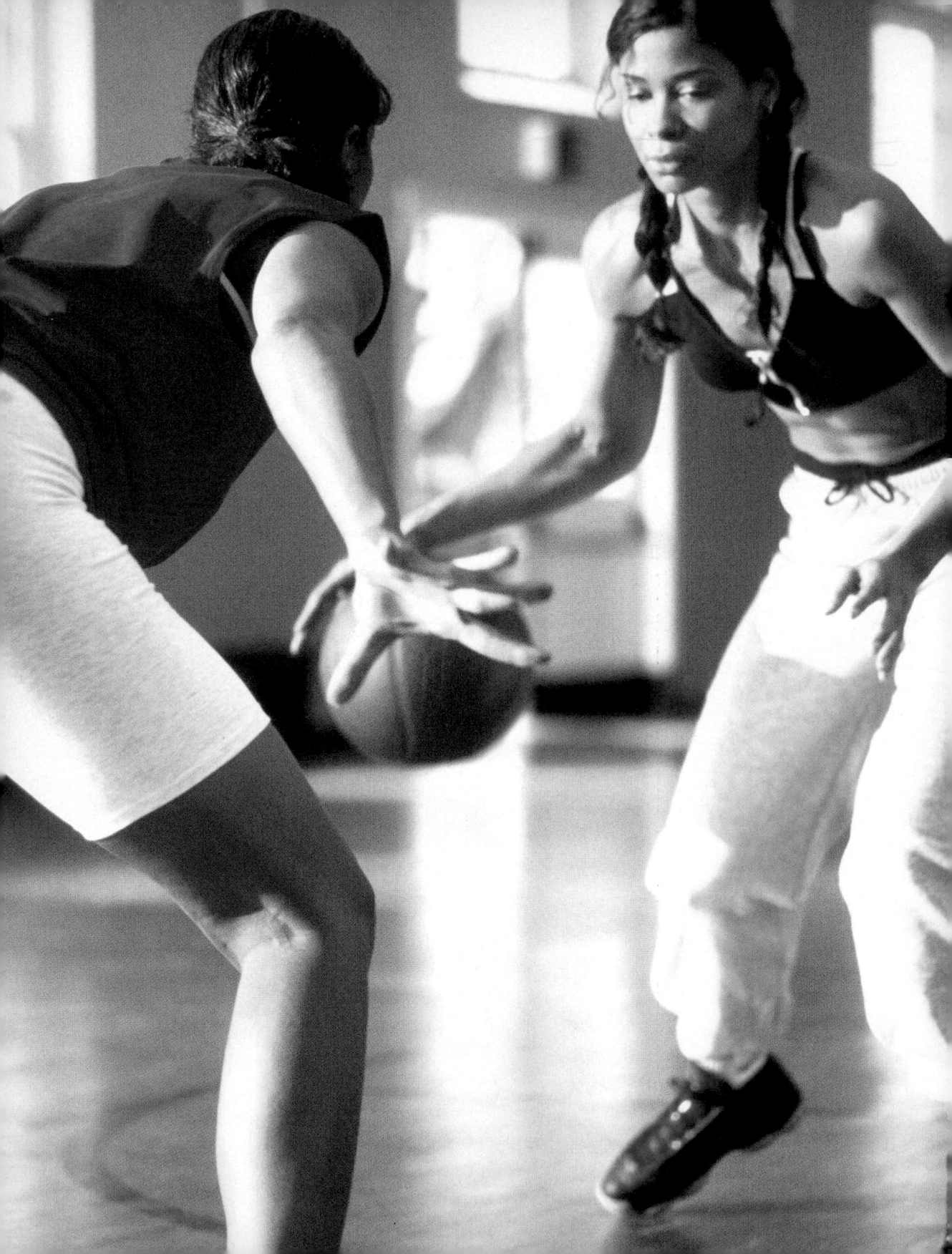

■ PART TWO

food for thought

Before you can lose that pooch or rock that workout, you have to eat. But wait a sec—put down that Frito! Instead reach for these tasty tidbits of information and you'll be upping your game without a morsel of regret.

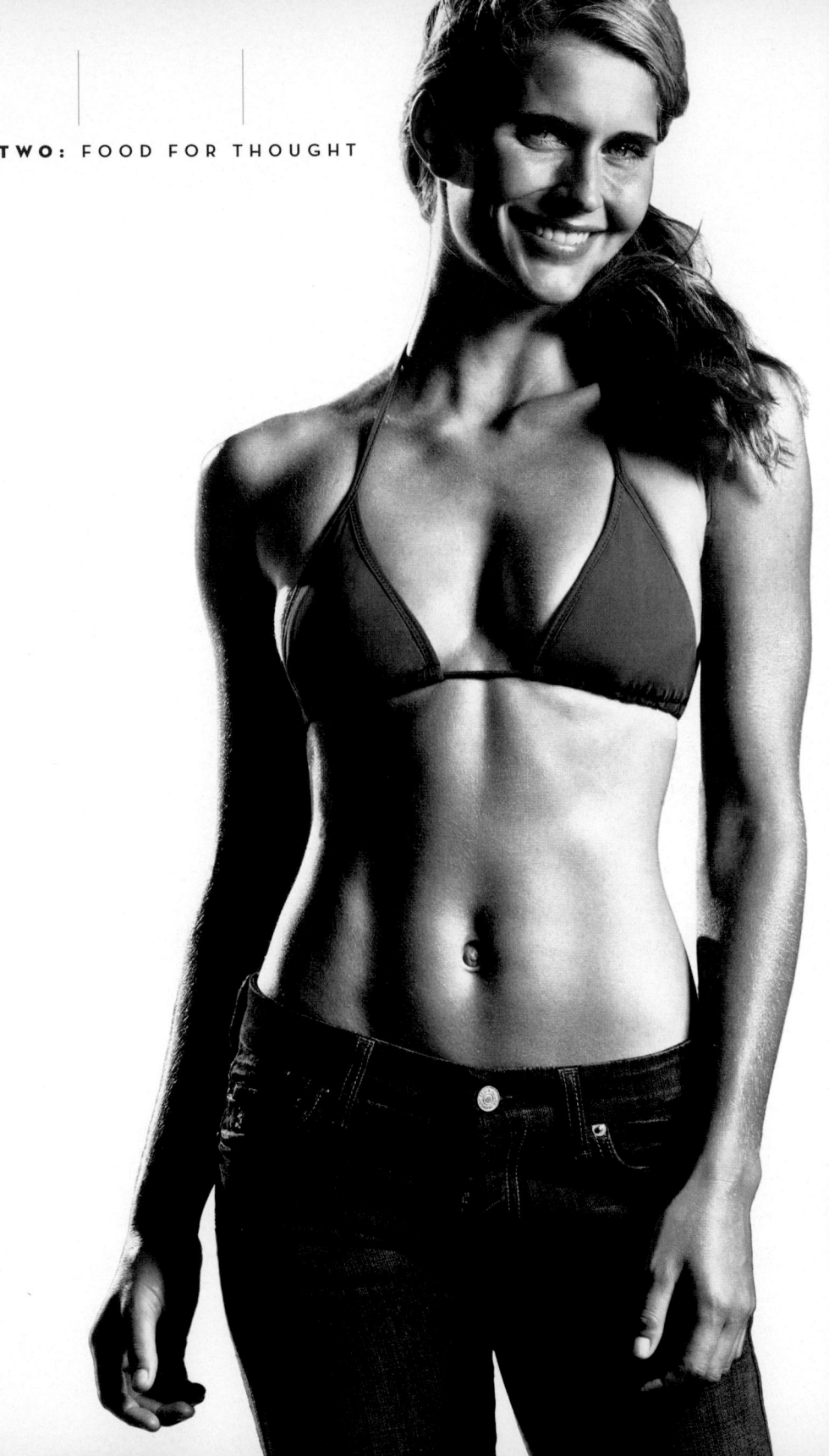

CHAPTER FIVE

THE 7-DAY BYE-BYE BELLY PLAN

IF ENERGY SLUMPS AND AFTERNOON CRAVINGS ARE MAKING YOUR JEANS FEEL SNUG, THEN BALANCING YOUR BLOOD SUGAR MAY BE THE KEY TO BEATING THEM. FIGHT YOUR FLAB AND SEND YOUR ENERGY SOARING WITH THIS 7-DAY EATING PLAN.

BY VIRGINIA SOLE-SMITH

STROLL THROUGH THE DIET BOOK SECTION at Barnes & Noble and you'd think that blood sugar was the secret to effortless weight loss: There's *The Sugar Solution, Sugar Busters!, Get the Sugar Out* (to name a few). Which made us wonder: What is blood sugar anyway? And how important is it, really, when you're trying to shed pounds? To find out, we consulted the experts, pored over the latest research, and cut through the, um, BS. We also partnered

WHAT THE HECK IS THE GLYCEMIC INDEX?

Many of the same fad diets that tell you to treat carbs the way Brad treated Jen also preach the glycemic index (GI), a system that assigns food a number per 50-gram serving based on how quickly you digest its carbohydrate content. For example, 50 grams of straight sugar has a GI of 100; 50 grams of apples has a GI of 55. The higher the GI number, the faster your blood sugar spikes and falls when you eat that food. (For a list of GI values, go to glycemicindex.com.)

Problem is, many people interpret the GI numbers incorrectly. "I'm not a fan of how the index gets used," says David L. Katz, M.D. "Carrots have a high GI [131]. But you find me the person who is overweight because she ate carrots and I'll quit my job and become a hula dancer." Carrots get a bad rap because the GI system is based on 50-gram servings, which in this case works out to 1.5 pounds. When that 50-gram bunch is broken down into real-life servings, carrots have a trim GI of 5.

Dr. Katz says: "If you stick to whole foods [grains, nuts, seeds, fruits, vegetables, and lean meats] that are still close to their state in nature, the glycemic load of your diet will be low without you having to worry about it."

with legendary chef Mollie Katzen, author of *The Moosewood Cookbook*, to give you a week's worth of delicious meals that will help you keep your blood sugar (and the number on your scale) under control. No bull.

BLOOD-SUGAR BASICS

Let's say you're having a tuna sandwich for lunch. As soon as you finish eating, your digestive system starts breaking down the carbs—the lettuce, tomato, and whole-wheat bread—into glucose. (In case you were dozing during Bio 101, glucose is a simple sugar found in plant and animal tissue.) Those glucose molecules race through your bloodstream, prompting insulin, a hormone made by your pancreas, to get in on the action. Think of insulin as your body's own personal UPS man (minus the foxy brown shorts): It scoops up the glucose in your blood and delivers it to sugar-hungry cells in your brain, muscles, and internal organs to use for energy. Insulin helps convert protein and fat into fuel too, but glucose is "your body's most useful form of energy," says David L. Katz, M.D., an associate professor at the Yale School of Public Health. "It's really the only fuel that brain cells and red blood cells use."

To get enough glucose, your body depends on carbs like the United States depends on foreign oil. That's why low-carb diets aren't a great idea for the long haul. "Although your body can process minimal energy from protein and fat, and your brain can use it in a real pinch—like to keep you alive in a famine—you don't want to count on them as your sole source," says Karen Chalmers, R.D., a dietitian and advanced practice diabetes specialist at Harvard's Joslin Diabetes Center.

"People who stay on low-carb diets long term find their thinking becomes fuzzy," because their noggins don't have enough fuel. According to the National Academy of Sciences, you need at least 130 grams of carbohydrates per day to keep you from feeling like a *Dumb and Dumber* extra.

So it's a good thing you're eating that tuna sandwich! Say you eat it at 1 p.m., and your insulin kicks into gear. In about 3 or 4 hours, the insulin has shuttled most of the glucose from your blood to your waiting cells. Your stomach starts to growl. If you don't eat anything by 5 or 6 p.m., you start to get really hungry—maybe even shaky, irritable, light-headed, or queasy. That's because your insulin has scraped up almost all the remaining glucose in your bloodstream, and your body's cells need more to keep chugging. Right now you probably have about 70 milligrams of sugar per deciliter of blood, versus a high of roughly 180 right after lunch (though numbers can vary widely depending on factors like your age, weight, overall health, and what you ate). Snack time!

You wander over to the office vending machine and buy a pack of Sno Balls. Hey, it happens. Minutes after you wolf them down, your blood sugar rockets up faster than it would take Borat to be ejected from high tea at Buckingham Palace. That sudden rush of glucose puts your pancreas into overdrive, inundating your body with insulin—which takes so much glucose out of your bloodstream at once that you crash, going from high to low blood sugar in as little as an hour. Result: You're crabby, jittery, starving, and craving more sweet treats to bring your energy—and your blood sugar—back up. "It's a vicious cycle," Dr. Katz says. And one guaranteed to add extra padding to your bod.

THE HEALTH CONNECTION

After a few years of eating a diet consistently high in Sno Balls and other refined carbs (think anything heavily processed or sugar laden that comes wrapped in plastic), your cells may start making like James Dean. They rebel against the blood sugar blitz by refusing to take any more glucose from your pushy insulin. That's a condition known as insulin resistance, also called prediabetes. So your pancreas, miffed, stops making enough insulin to get the job done.

But you're still downing Little Debbies, so the amount of glucose circulating in your blood begins to rise. The more pounds you pile on, the more your insulin starts to burn out and the higher your blood sugar gets—which can cause bigger problems than a bigger butt. We're talking the possibility of heart disease, stroke, and diabetes down the road. Reason: Excess blood sugar can increase the pressure your blood exerts on your organs, damaging them, says Walter Willett, M.D., chair of the nutrition department at Harvard University School of Medicine and coauthor of *Eat, Drink, and Weigh Less.*

Exactly how much glucose is unhealthy? Scientists are still trying to pin that down—it varies depending on your family history and other risk factors (see "Know Your BS" on page 54). But a 2006 study in the science journal *The Lancet* found that your risk for heart disease and stroke increases if your fasting blood sugar level (your blood sugar at its lowest, first thing in the morning before breakfast) is higher than 88 milligrams per deciliter (mg/dL). If it's between 100 and 125 mg/dL, you've got insulin resistance. About 9 percent of American women over age 20 do, according to the American Diabetes Association, though a third of

KNOW YOUR BS: HOW SWEET IS YOUR BLOOD?

CHECK ALL THE "TRUE" STATEMENTS THAT APPLY TO YOU.

❑ I am of African-American, Native American, Asian, or Hispanic descent. TRUE

❑ My body looks more like an apple than a pear. TRUE

❑ My waist measures 35 inches or more. TRUE

❑ More than 10 percent of my daily calories (three or more servings) come from simple sugars like baked goods, candy, or sweets. TRUE

❑ I eat fewer than three servings of whole grains per day. TRUE

❑ My triglyceride levels are above 150.* TRUE

❑ My blood pressure is above 130/80.* TRUE

❑ My body mass index is over 25 (to calculate it, go to womenshealthmag.com/toolbox). TRUE

❑ My mom, dad, or sibling has type 2 diabetes. TRUE

❑ My HDL (good cholesterol) is below 50 and my LDL (bad cholesterol)

is above 100, or my total cholesterol is above 200.* TRUE

❑ I eat less than 24 grams of fiber per day. TRUE

❑ I smoke. TRUE

*Your doctor should have these numbers on record if you don't know them offhand. Call her and ask.

0–4 TRUE Sugar Star You can't choose your family or your ethnicity, both of which can predispose you to high blood sugar levels (though researchers aren't sure why). But you're doing a great job on the factors you can control. Sweet!

5–8 TRUE Sugar Spiker You're chugging down the blood sugar highway to the danger zone. Chronic high blood glucose and sluggish or erratic insulin make it harder for you to lose weight and may increase your risk for heart disease. That's why

elevated triglyceride, cholesterol, or blood pressure levels should be as much of a wake-up call as a thickening waist or high BMI. Use our meal plan to get yourself back on track and make sure your doc is monitoring your heart health.

9–12 TRUE Sugarholic You're knee-deep in the vicious cycle of eating bad carbs, crashing, and eating some more. You're gaining weight (yet you never feel full), and your health is suffering. It's time to take charge of your eating habits—our plan can help—and ask your doctor for a fasting glucose test to find out if you're hyperglycemic or even diabetic. (Your fasting glucose levels, which are measured after 8 to 10 hours of not eating, are what doctors use to determine whether your blood sugar is too low or too high.) With a few doable lifestyle changes, you can undo the damage and drop the pounds.

them don't know it. It can make you feel cranky and exhausted—and if left untreated, can lead to type 2 diabetes, a serious condition where your body stops making enough insulin and which may require drugs for blood sugar management.

Okay, so high blood sugar is bad. But low blood sugar is no picnic either. If your glucose levels are consistently below 70 mg/dL, you have hypoglycemia, a condition that triggers feelings of nausea, dizziness, fatigue, and extreme hunger. Less than 1 percent of us have this problem, usually people who are genetically predisposed to it or on meds that can cause it. Though the long-term effects generally aren't as bad as for those with high blood sugar, ask your doc to test your glucose levels if you suspect you have either condition. She may recommend drugs or an eating regimen to keep you feeling steadier.

SUGAR BUSTING

Which brings us to our main point: When it comes to dieting—and staying healthy—getting blood sugar on your side is all about keeping it even-steven. That way it's available for the cells that need it but not taxing the rest of your body, and you don't have those panicky bring-on-the-doughnuts-now moments. All you have to do is eat the right foods at the right times.

Ideally, each meal will consist of 50 to 60 percent high-fiber carbs (like fruits, veggies, and whole grains), 15 to 20 percent protein (like lean meats and fish), and 20 to 30 percent healthy fat (like olive oil and nuts). You digest high-fiber carbs more slowly than refined ones, so your glucose levels will rise at a steady, leisurely pace and won't come careening down—they'll lower slowly over the course of 2 to 3 hours. Which is about

how often you should eat—every 3 of your waking hours—to keep your blood sugar at an optimal level. Sounds like you'll be shoveling in more than Takeru Kobayashi at a Nathan's hot dog–eating contest, but you won't: If you sleep 8 hours a night, you've got 16 hours in the day, so you should nosh about five times. Eat a small breakfast, lunch, and dinner and two snacks, and you're there.

Working out also helps keep you level. "Exercising lowers your blood sugar because your muscles burn glucose when you move," Dr. Willett explains. "It also reduces insulin resistance almost immediately." In fact, in a recent study in the journal *Metabolism,* 12 weeks of aerobic training improved insulin sensitivity by 23 percent in overweight teenage girls. And that was before they even started losing weight. Aim for at least 30 minutes of moderate cardio, 5 days a week.

So get moving! But make sure to grab a healthy-carb snack like a slice of whole-grain bread or a piece of fruit about 90 minutes before you lace up your sneakers, since the immediate drop in blood sugar you experience during exercise can cause you to crash midrun or be ravenous afterward. Also, having the right kind of fuel in your tank will help you work out better: In a recent study in the *International Journal of Sport Nutrition and Exercise Metabolism,* runners who breakfasted on All-Bran cereal and fruit ran 7 minutes longer than those who ate white toast, jam, and cornflakes.

The bottom line: While balanced blood sugar isn't a magic fat-busting bullet, it's a useful weapon in your dieting arsenal. It helps prevent cake cravings, keeps hunger levels down, and generally makes you feel better as you lose. Isn't that the sweetest thing.

BETTER BLOOD SUGAR: MEAL PLAN

To help you stabilize your blood sugar levels (and lose weight), Mollie Katzen, coauthor of *Eat, Drink, and Weigh Less* and a founding member of the Harvard School of Public Health Nutrition Round Table, created this 7-day, 1,600-calorie meal plan exclusively for *Women's Health.* Stay steady by eating within 2 hours of waking up and then every 3 hours or so after that. Do 30 minutes of moderate exercise on five of the days, and you can lose 1 to 2 pounds per week.

DAY 1

Breakfast (7 a.m.)

2-egg omelet with ½ oz grated Swiss cheese and scallions (cooked in 1 tsp butter or olive oil)

½ pink grapefruit

Coffee or tea with optional low-fat milk and 1 tsp sugar or honey, or noncaloric sweetener

Snack (10 a.m.)

1 apple

Lunch (1 p.m.)

1 4-inch whole-wheat pita filled with ⅓ c hummus, unlimited vegetables (lettuce, cucumbers, tomatoes, etc.)

5 olives (optional)

1 orange or 2 tangerines

Snack (4 p.m.)

6 pecan halves with 10 chocolate chips

8-oz glass low-fat or fat-free milk (optional)

Dinner (7 p.m.)

1 c broth-based soup (miso, vegetable, or chicken)

1 protein-of-choice (any palm-size serving of beef, chicken, salmon, shrimp, tempeh, or tofu, cooked as you like)

1 heaping c broccoli cooked with 1 tsp olive oil

1 fist-size sweet potato, dressed with lime juice

2 kiwis, sliced and sprinkled with 1 Tbsp toasted, unsweetened coconut

8-oz glass low-fat or fat-free milk (optional)

DAY 2

Breakfast

1 c cooked whole-grain cereal, such as oatmeal or Kashi breakfast pilaf, topped with ½ medium chopped apple (save the other half for your snack) and 1 Tbsp chopped walnuts

½ c low-fat milk

Coffee or tea with optional low-fat milk and 1 tsp sugar or honey, or noncaloric sweetener to taste

Snack

1 oz cheddar or string cheese

½ medium apple (leftover from breakfast)

Lunch

1 c broth-based soup

Salad with unlimited spinach and vegetables plus up to 3 Tbsp olive oil and vinegar dressing, topped with 1 palm-size protein-of-choice

1 orange or 2 tangerines

Snack

8 small whole-grain crackers (totaling 130 calories or fewer)

1 Tbsp nut butter

1 tsp low-sugar jam (optional)

Dinner

$1\frac{1}{2}$ c vegetarian chili

$\frac{3}{4}$ c bulgur or couscous, drizzled with 1 tsp olive oil and lemon

1 heaping c cooked green beans with 1 tsp olive oil

1 sliced peach (fresh or canned in water) with $\frac{1}{2}$ c plain low-fat yogurt

1 Tbsp dried cranberries

8-oz glass low-fat or fat-free milk (optional)

DAY 3

Breakfast

French toast (whisk together 1 egg and 1 Tbsp butter, coat 2 slices whole-wheat bread, and cook in 1 tsp butter or canola oil)

1 Tbsp real maple syrup

$\frac{1}{2}$ c blackberries (fresh or unsweetened frozen, defrosted)

Coffee or tea with optional low-fat milk and 1 tsp sugar or honey, or noncaloric sweetener to taste

Snack

10 almonds with 10 chocolate chips

Lunch

$\frac{1}{2}$ medium cantaloupe

1 c low-fat cottage cheese

1 Tbsp raisins

2 Tbsp granola

Snack

$\frac{1}{4}$ c fat-free bean dip (any kind)

Unlimited baby carrots, celery sticks, and other raw vegetables

Dinner

2 c cooked whole-grain pasta

Unlimited tomato sauce (any kind) mixed with up to

1 c cooked lean ground beef, turkey, or crumbled veggie burgers

Large green salad with 3 Tbsp olive oil and vinegar dressing

$\frac{1}{2}$ c low-sugar frozen yogurt with 1 Tbsp chocolate sprinkles

8-oz glass low-fat or fat-free milk (optional)

DAY 4

Breakfast

1 oz (about 1 slice) meat or soy-based Canadian bacon

Unlimited sliced or canned tomatoes

$\frac{1}{2}$ whole-wheat English muffin with 1 tsp butter or olive oil

Coffee or tea with optional low-fat milk and 1 tsp sugar or honey, or noncaloric sweetener to taste

Snack

1 apple

Lunch

1 c broth-based soup

Sandwich made with
2 slices whole-wheat bread,
2 tsp mayonnaise, 3 slices
avocado, unlimited lettuce,
onion, and tomato with 1 oz
sliced cheese or 2 oz lean
turkey

1 orange or 2 tangerines

Snack

6 walnut halves with 1 Tbsp
dried cranberries

8-oz glass low-fat or fat-
free milk (optional)

Dinner

1 c broth-based soup

1 palm-size serving protein-
of-choice

1 heaping c cooked
asparagus with 1 tsp olive
oil

1 heaping c cooked spring
vegetable (like butternut
squash)

$1/2$ c sliced fresh or canned
pineapple sprinkled with 1
Tbsp toasted, unsweetened
coconut

8-oz glass low-fat or fat-
free milk (optional)

DAY 5

Breakfast

1 c fresh or unsweetened
frozen strawberries

1 c cooked whole-grain
cereal, such as oatmeal or
Kashi breakfast pilaf

$1/2$ c low-fat milk

Coffee or tea with optional
low-fat milk and 1 tsp sugar
or honey, or noncaloric
sweetener to taste

Snack

10 almonds with 10
chocolate chips

Lunch

1 c broth-based soup

Large romaine and mixed
green salad with 1 hard-
boiled egg, $1/2$ c cooked
chickpeas or edamame, 2
Tbsp crumbled blue cheese
or $1/2$ 6-oz can tuna,
unlimited cherry tomatoes,
cucumbers, sliced bell
peppers, red onions or
scallions, and 3 Tbsp olive
oil and vinegar dressing

1 medium orange or
2 tangerines

Snack

6 oz plain low-fat yogurt
(add a little honey or
noncaloric sweetener)

1 kiwi, sliced

Dinner

1 very lean beef or turkey
burger ($1/4$ lb raw weight) or
up to 2 veggie burgers on 1
whole-grain bun, topped
with up to 1 Tbsp ketchup,
up to 1 Tbsp mayonnaise,
and unlimited mustard,
sauerkraut, pickles, lettuce,
tomato, onion, and tomato-
based salsa

1 heaping c cooked broccoli
with 1 tsp olive oil

1 c unsweetened
applesauce with cinnamon
topped with 1 Tbsp raisins
and 2 Tbsp plain or vanilla
low-fat yogurt

8-oz glass low-fat or fat-
free milk (optional)

DAY 6

Breakfast

2 slices French toast (whisk
together 1 egg and 1 Tbsp
butter, coat 2 slices whole-

wheat bread, and cook in
1 tsp butter or canola oil)

1 Tbsp real maple syrup

$\frac{1}{2}$ c fresh or unsweetened
frozen raspberries

Coffee or tea with optional
low-fat milk and 1 tsp sugar
or honey, or noncaloric
sweetener to taste

Snack

1 apple

Lunch

Nachos made with 15
tortilla chips, $\frac{1}{2}$ c fat-free
refried beans, 1 oz cheese,
and unlimited tomato-based
salsa

1 orange or 2 tangerines

Snack 10 almonds and
1 Tbsp raisins

8-oz glass low-fat or fat-free
milk (optional)

Dinner

Up to 12 oz miso soup

Up to 3 c stir-fried
vegetables in 1 to 2 Tbsp
light Asian-style sauce,
such as San-J teriyaki or
Szechuan sauce

$\frac{3}{4}$ c cooked brown rice

1 palm-size serving protein-
of-choice

$\frac{1}{2}$ c low-sugar frozen yogurt
with $\frac{1}{2}$ c fresh or
unsweetened frozen
strawberries

8-oz glass low-fat or fat-free
milk (optional)

DAY 7

Breakfast

$\frac{1}{2}$ pink grapefruit

2 scrambled eggs cooked in
1 tsp butter or olive oil

1 slice whole-wheat toast
with 1 tsp butter or olive oil

1 tsp low-sugar jam

Coffee or tea with optional
low-fat milk and 1 tsp sugar
or honey, or noncaloric
sweetener to taste

Snack

1 peach or 2 plums

Lunch

1 c broth-based soup

Sandwich made with 2
slices whole-wheat bread
and up to 2 Tbsp peanut or
other nut butter, $\frac{1}{2}$ sliced
banana, and 2 tsp honey

Unlimited baby carrots,
celery sticks, and red bell
pepper slices

Snack

1 oz cheddar or string
cheese

1 Tbsp dried cranberries

Dinner

1 c tomato-based soup, like
Imagine Foods organic
creamy tomato

Main course salad made
with unlimited salad greens,
cherry tomatoes, red onions
or scallions, cucumber, and
sliced bell peppers with 1
palm-size serving protein-
of-choice, $\frac{1}{2}$ c chickpeas or
edamame, and 3 Tbsp olive
oil and vinegar dressing

8 small whole-grain
crackers (totaling 130
calories or fewer)

$\frac{1}{2}$ c low-sugar frozen yogurt
with 1 sliced kiwi

8-oz glass low-fat or fat-free
milk (optional)

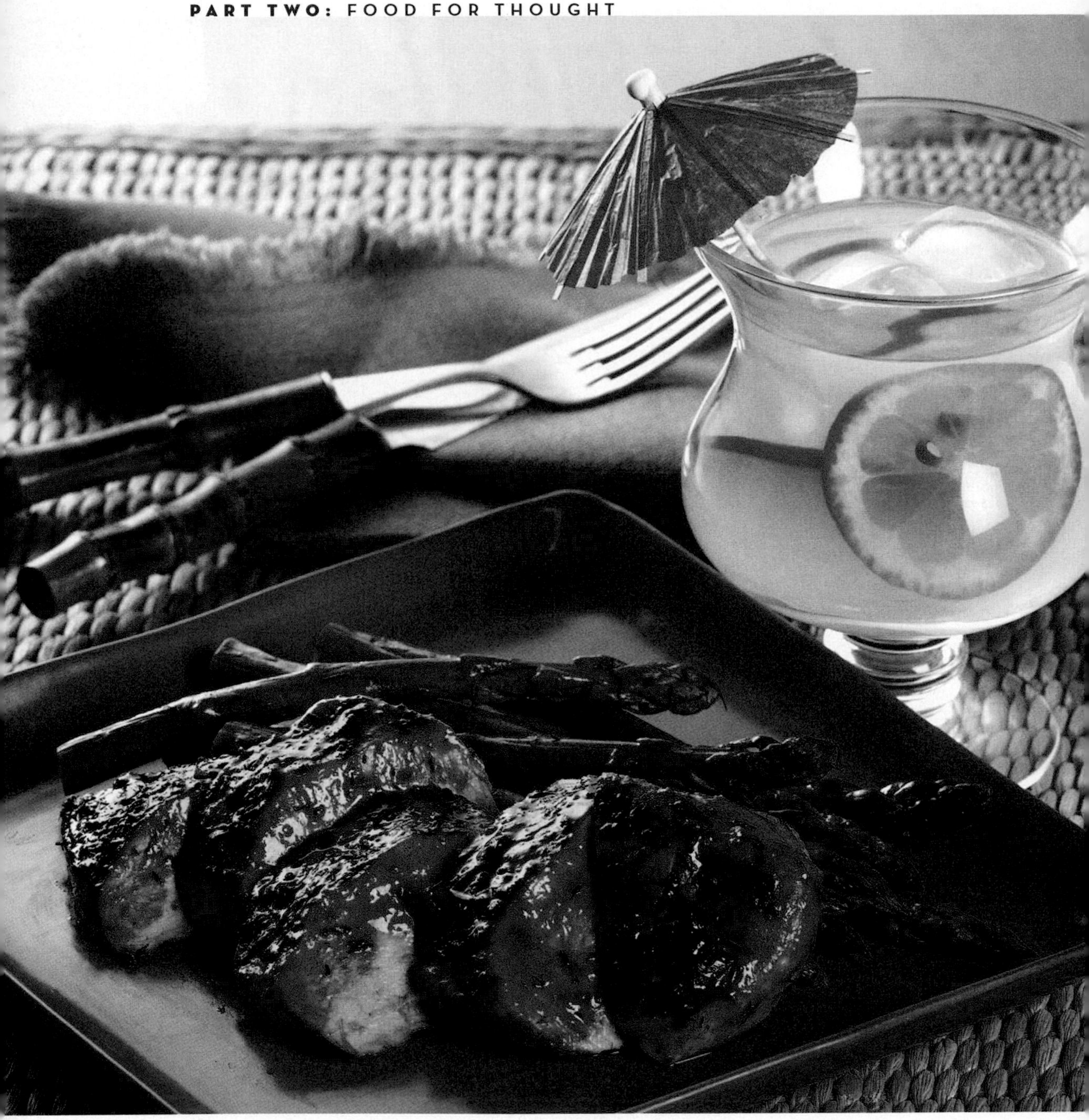

CHAPTER SIX

14 FAT-FIGHTING MEALS

GET MORE FROM YOUR MENU WITH THESE HEALTHY (AND DELICIOUS) MEALS.

YOU ALREADY KNOW the formula to weight loss: eat less, move more, and tame those glucose levels. But that doesn't mean you can't eat filling, great-tasting meals every day of the week. In fact, the key to building your best body is to stop thinking of food as the enemy and learn how to make your meals work for you. These 14 recipes are loaded with protein, whole grains, and fresh greens—all proven to keep your glucose levels steady and your cravings under wraps. So get cooking and start losing!

BARBEQUE CHICKEN PITA

- 1 Tbsp barbecue sauce
- ½ cup chopped precooked chicken
- 1 whole-wheat pita
- 1 cup chopped romaine lettuce
- 2 Tbsp diced cucumber
- 1 Tbsp low-fat ranch dressing

1. In microwavable dish, stir together barbecue sauce and chicken. Microwave for 30 seconds or until hot. Stuff chicken into each pita half.

2. In bowl, toss the lettuce and cucumber with the dressing, and stuff it all into the pita.

MAKES 2 SERVINGS

PER SERVING 162 cal, 12 g pro, 25 g carb, 2 g fat, ½ g sat fat, 28 mg chol, 3 g fiber, 660 mg sodium

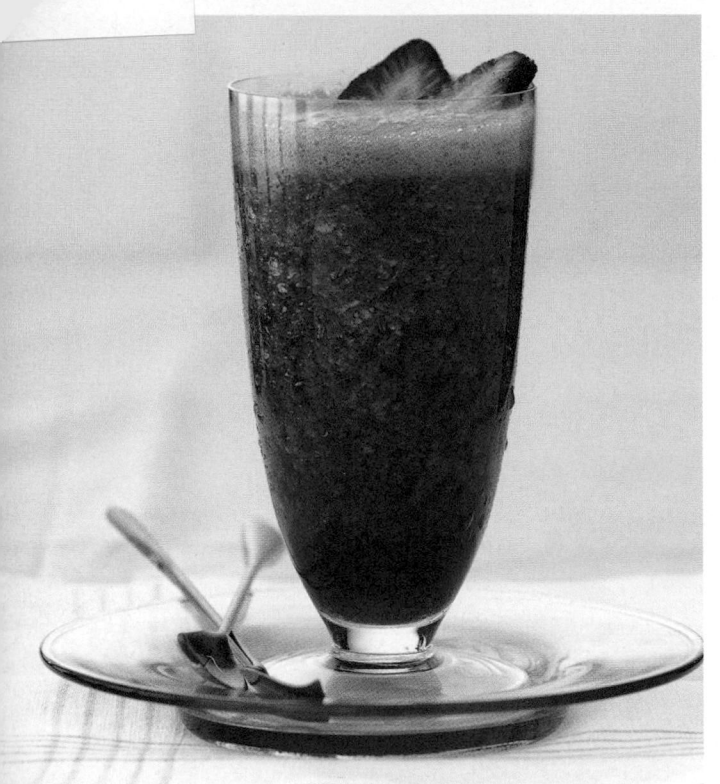

STRAWBERRY MELON SMOOTHIE

- ⅔ cup frozen unsweetened strawberries
- 1 medium banana
- ½ cup cubed honeydew melon
- ½ cup 1% milk
- 2 tsp vanilla whey powder
- 3 ice cubes, crushed

1. Blend ingredients for about 30 seconds until smooth.

MAKES 2 SERVINGS

PER SERVING 199 cal, 9 g pro, 39 g carb, 2 g sat fat, 4 g fiber, 117 mg sodium

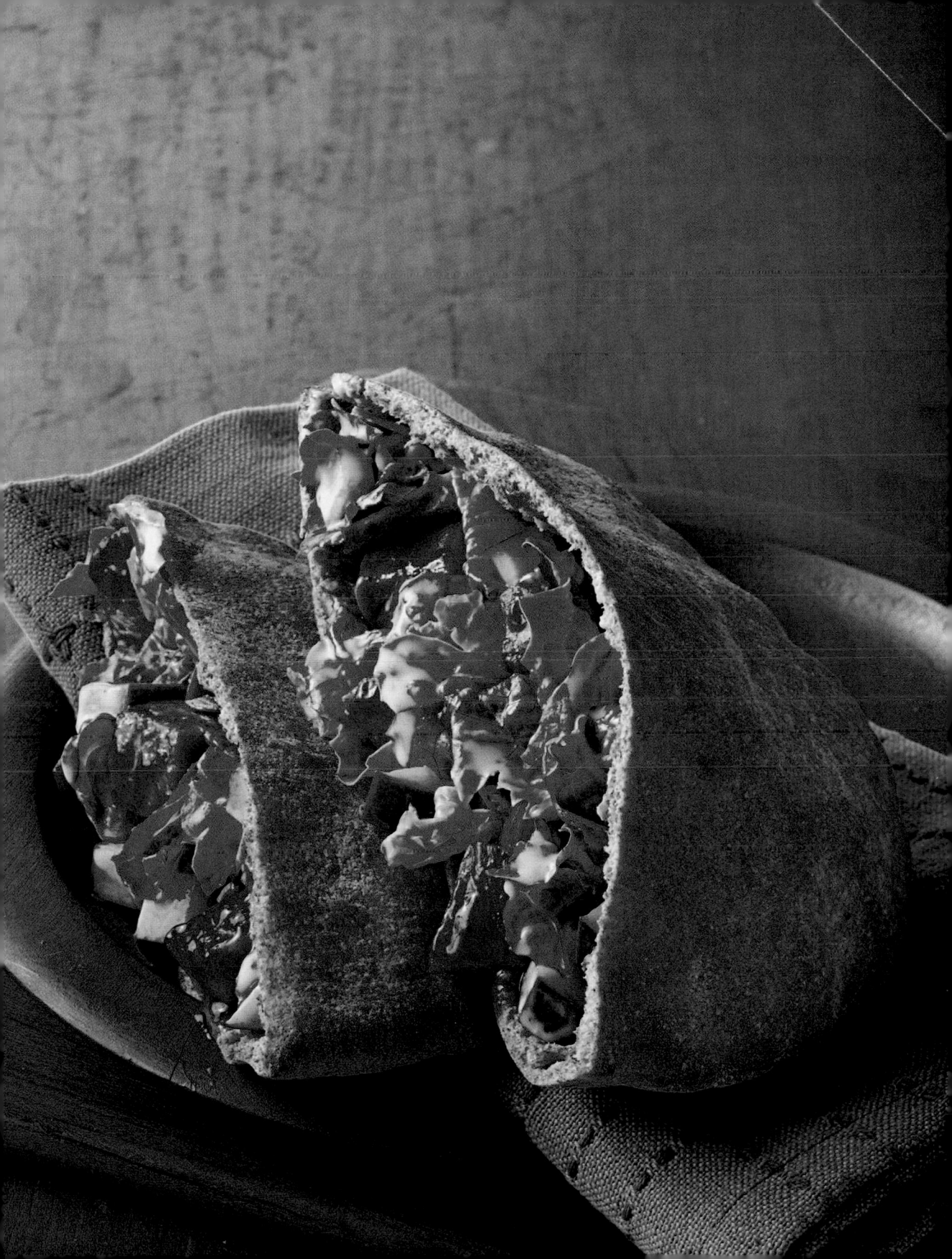

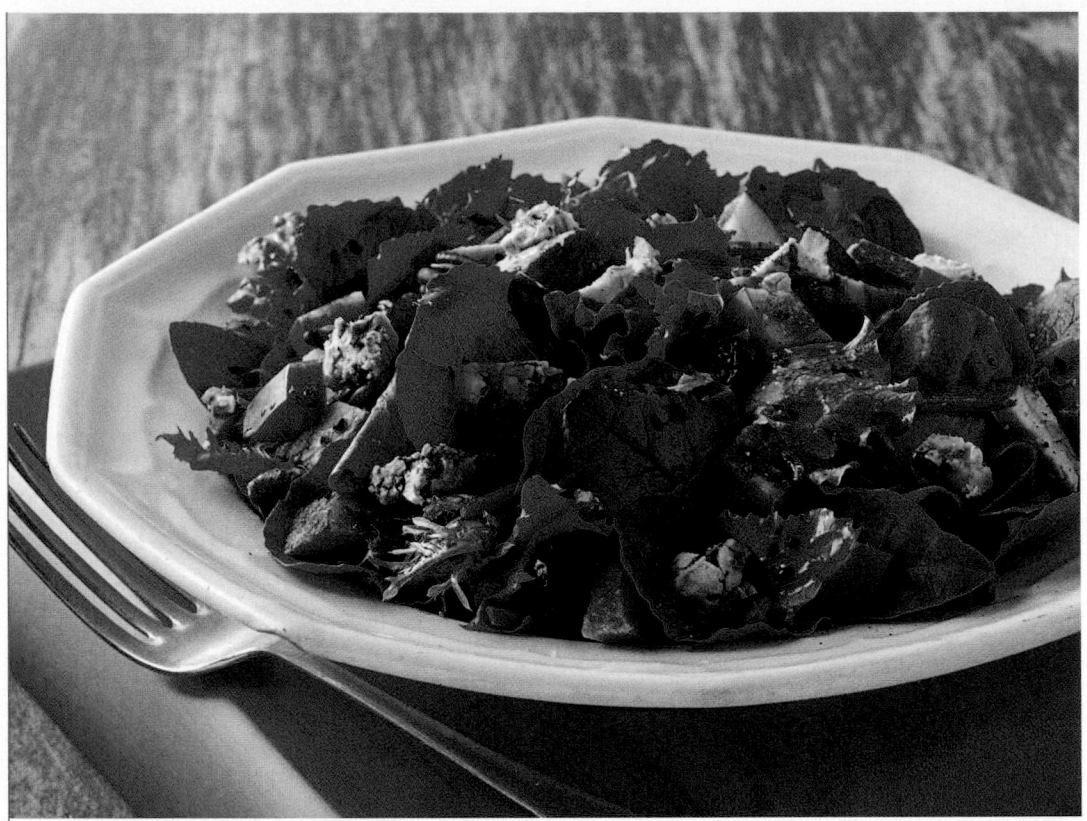

5-MINUTE MIXED GREEN SALAD

- 3 cups mixed greens
- 2 slices deli smoked-turkey slices, chopped
- ½ small Granny Smith apple, chopped
- 2 Tbsp grated carrot
- 1 Tbsp chopped pecans
- 1½ Tbsp Craisins (dried, sweetened cranberries)
- 1 Tbsp blue-cheese crumbles

1. Toss it all together and add dressing made by mixing 1½ teaspoons olive oil and 1 tablespoon balsamic vinegar.

MAKES 1 SERVING

PER SERVING 271 cal, 8 g pro, 28 g carb, 15 g fat, 3 g sat fat, 15 mg chol, 7 g fiber, 402 mg sodium

GRILLED BEEF AND ARUGULA SALAD

- 1 scallion, thinly sliced
- 2 Tbsp olive oil
- 2 Tbsp raspberry vinegar
- 1 Tbsp finely chopped parsley
- ½ tsp salt
- ¼ tsp freshly ground black pepper
- 4 ripe apricots, halved, pits removed
- 2 ¾" thick, or 4 oz, filets mignons
- 1 package (5 oz) baby arugula or spinach
- 3 Tbsp crumbled blue cheese (optional)

1. Prepare charcoal for grilling, preheat gas grill, or heat grill pan over medium heat.

2. In large bowl, whisk scallion, 1²/₃ tablespoon oil, vinegar, parsley, ¹/₄ teaspoon of the salt, and ¹/₈ teaspoon of the pepper and set aside.

3. Lightly brush cut surface of apricots with remaining oil. Season beef with remaining ¹/₄ teaspoon salt and ¹/₈ teaspoon pepper. Grill beef and apricots, cut side down. Cook apricots until soft, about 6 minutes. Turn beef midway, 8 minutes for medium-rare or longer for desired doneness. Remove from heat and let stand 5 minutes. Cut apricots into slices. Thinly slice beef against the grain.

4. In medium bowl, toss arugula with dressing to coat. Transfer to four serving plates. Top with slices of beef and 2 sliced apricot halves. Sprinkle with blue cheese, if desired.

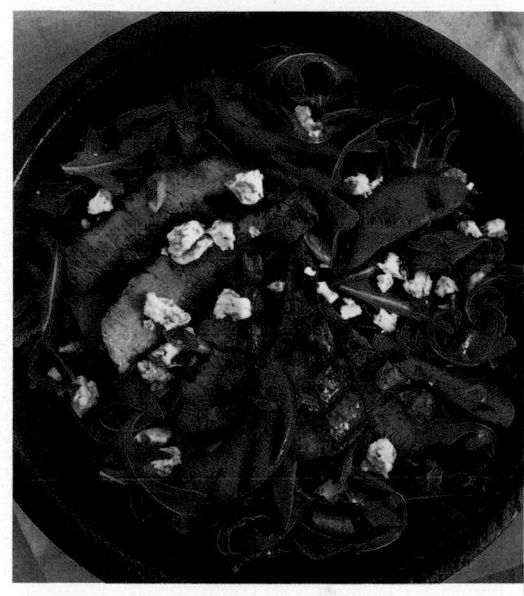

MAKES 4 SERVINGS

PER SERVING 184 cal, 13 g pro, 7 g carb, 12 g fat, 3 g sat fat, 35 mg chol, 1 g fiber, 332 mg sodium

W|H

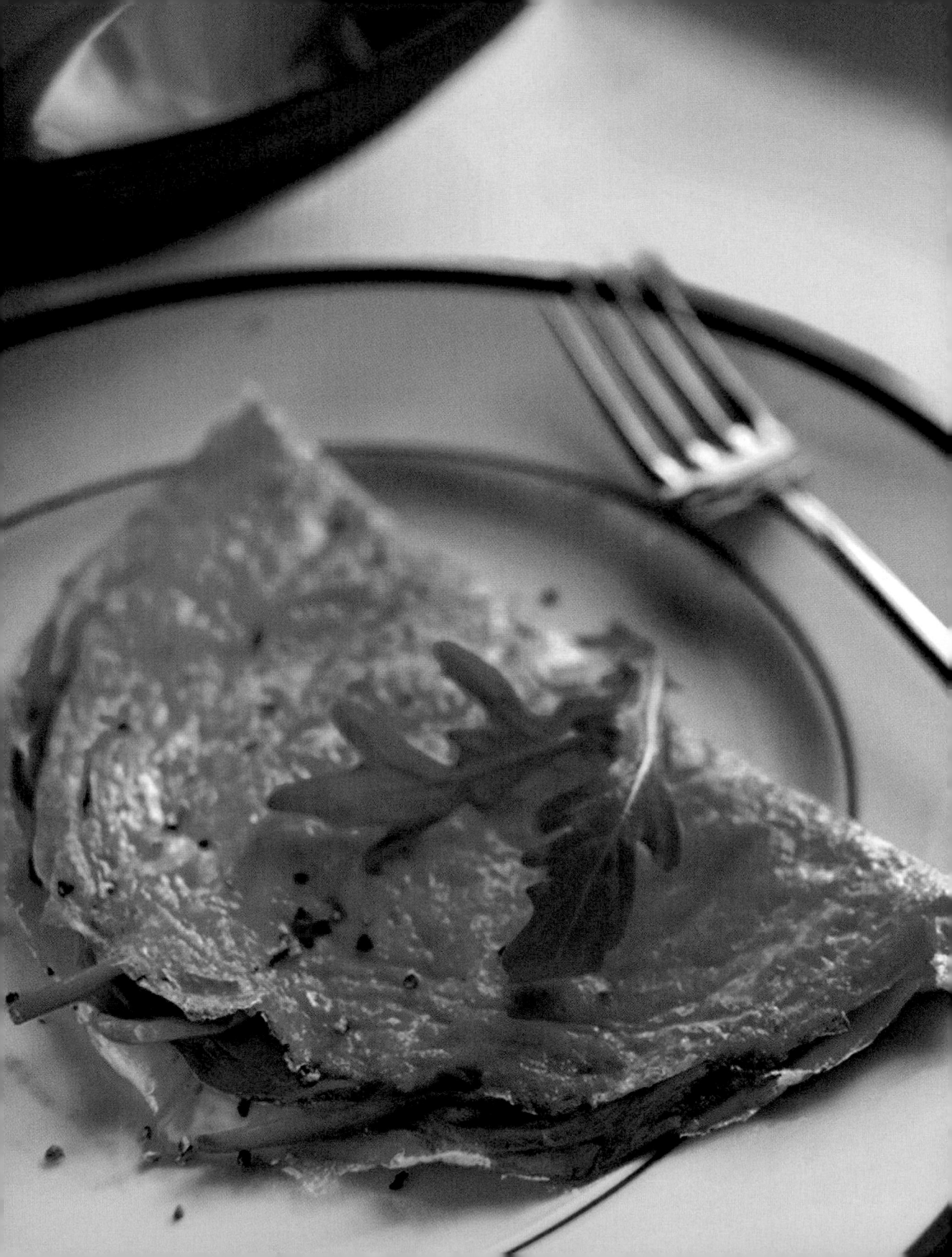

GREEN AND WHITE OMELET

2 eggs
1 Tbsp shredded part-skim
  mozzarella cheese
⅓ cup torn baby spinach leaves

1. Coat medium-size nonstick skillet with cooking spray over medium heat.

2. In bowl, beat eggs until blended. Add to pan, allowing them to cover bottom. When omelet begins to set, top one side with cheese and spinach.

3. Cook for 2 minutes. Carefully fold remaining half over filling. Flip and cook until egg is cooked through and lightly browned.

MAKES 1 SERVING

PER SERVING 168 cal, 14 g pro, 2 g carb, 0 g fiber, 11 g fat, 4 g sat fat, 428 mg chol, 197 mg sodium

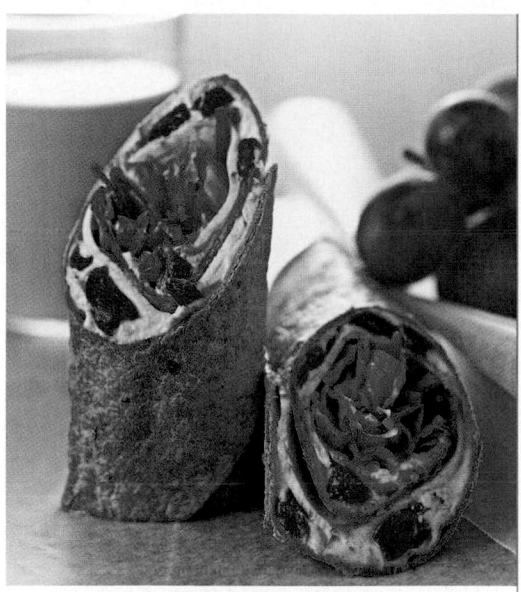

TASTY TURKEY WRAP

1 large whole wheat tortilla
2 Tbsp garlic-flavored hummus
¼ cup roasted red pepper strips
4 slices low-sodium, roast turkey breast
2 Tbsp chopped fresh mint leaves
¼ cup lettuce

1. Lay tortilla flat on large cutting board. Spoon hummus evenly over tortilla to within ½ inch of edge.

2. Lay peppers evenly over hummus and layer turkey slices. Sprinkle with mint and add lettuce leaves. Fold in sides, then roll to form wrap. Cut diagonally in half.

MAKES 1 SERVING

PER SERVING 323 cal, 35 g pro, 31 g carb, 7 g fat, 0.5 g sat fat, 61 mg chol, 4 g fiber, 543 mg sodium

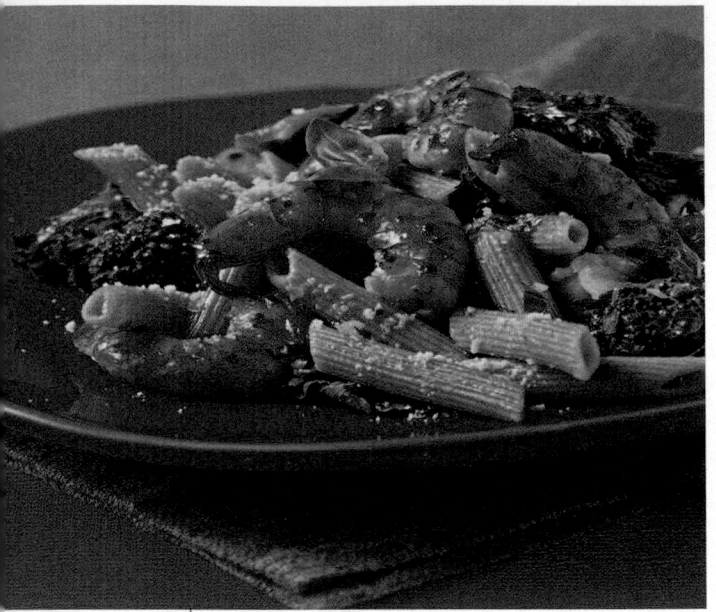

WHOLE WHEAT PENNE WITH SHRIMP

1. Bring 4 quarts of water to a boil in large pot over high heat. Add broccoli rabe and cook until crisp-tender, about 1½ minutes. Remove with slotted spoon or tongs and plunge into cold water. Drain and set aside.

2. In same water, prepare pasta per package directions.

3. Meanwhile, heat 2 tablespoons of the oil over medium heat in large, heavy-bottomed pan. Place shrimp in pan in single layer. Cook, stirring once or twice, until shrimp are pink and just cooked through, about 2 minutes. With slotted spoon or tongs, transfer shrimp to medium bowl and set aside.

4. Add remaining 2 tablespoons oil to pan and sauté garlic over medium heat 30 seconds. Add red-pepper flakes and broccoli rabe and sauté until soft but not soggy, about 2 minutes. Add shrimp, broth, and basil, and heat through, about 1 minute.

5. Drain pasta and transfer to large serving bowl. Toss with cheese. Add shrimp and broccoli rabe mixture and toss. Serve immediately.

1	bunch (about 1 lb) broccoli rabe or Broccolini, cut into 3" lengths
8	oz whole wheat penne
4	Tbsp olive oil
1	lb med uncooked shrimp, peeled and deveined
2	tsp minced garlic
¼-½	tsp red-pepper flakes
⅓	cup seafood broth or reduced-sodium chicken broth
½	cup chopped fresh basil
⅓	cup grated Parmesan cheese

MAKES 4 SERVINGS

PER SERVING 548 cal, 41 g pro, 48 g carb, 20 g fat, 3.5 g sat fat, 180 mg chol, 10 g fiber, 407 mg sodium

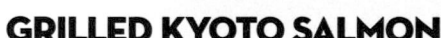

W|H

GRILLED KYOTO SALMON

⅓ cup low-sodium soy sauce

¼ cup orange juice concentrate

2 Tbsp olive oil

2 Tbsp tomato sauce

1 tsp lemon juice

½ tsp Dijon mustard

1 Tbsp green onion, minced

1 clove garlic, minced

½ tsp minced ginger

2 wild salmon steaks (4 to 5 oz each)

1. In a small bowl, mix all ingredients except salmon and transfer to a food-safe plastic bag. Add salmon and coat well. Marinate in refrigerator for at least 2 hours.

2. Grill salmon over high heat for 4 to 6 minutes per side or until slightly opaque throughout.

MAKES 2 SERVINGS

PER SERVING 269 cal, 31 g pro, 11 g carb, 11 g fat, 1 g sat fat, 0 g fiber, 300 mg sodium

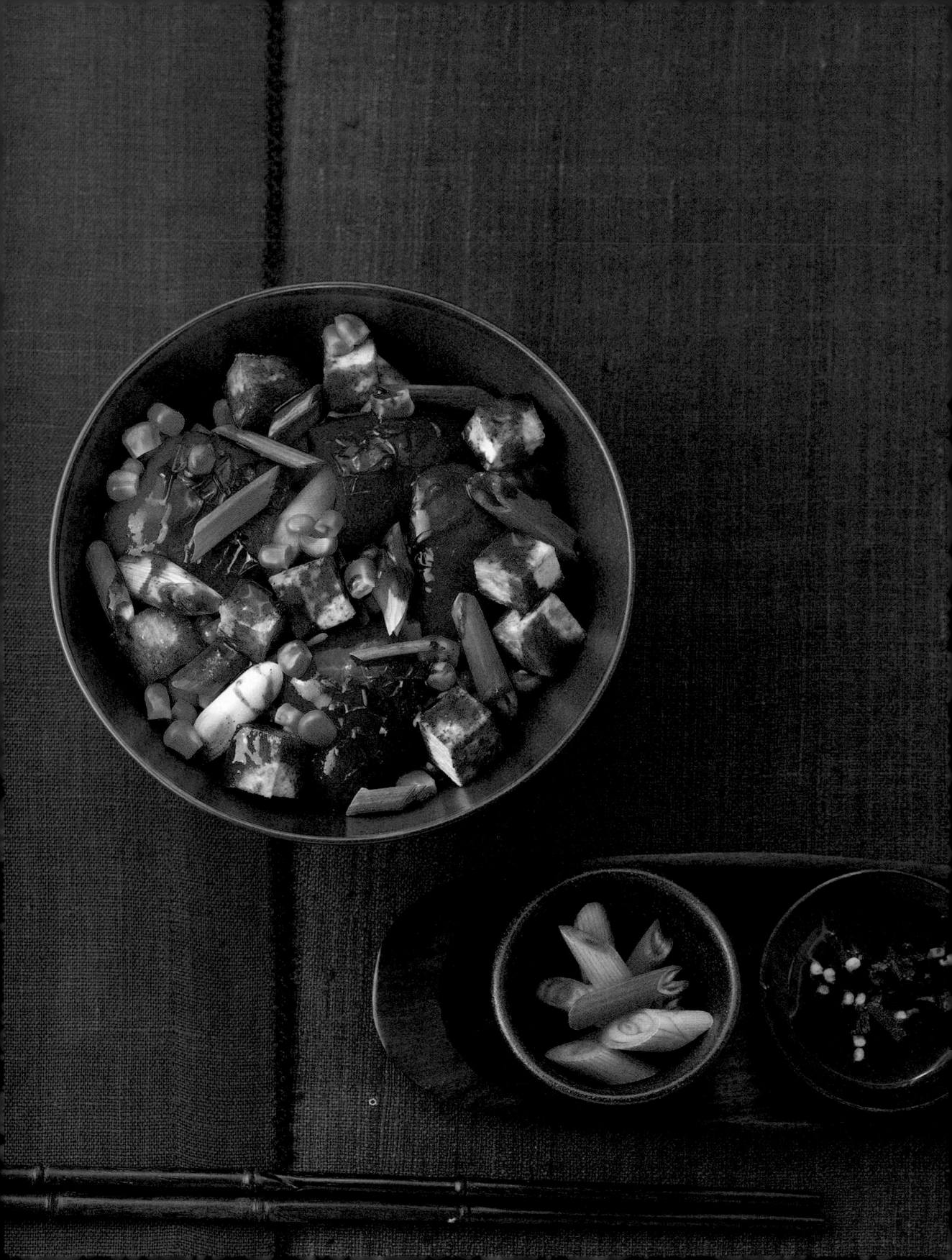

TOFU AND CORN WITH PEPPER STIR-FRY SAUCE

- 10 oz super-firm tofu, blotted dry
- 1 Tbsp soy sauce
- 2 Tbsp canola oil, divided
- 1 pint mini multicolored sweet peppers, trimmed, halved lengthwise
- ¼ cup classic stir-fry sauce
- 1 tsp grated garlic
- 1 tsp grated ginger
- 1 bunch scallions, trimmed
- 1 cup fresh corn kernels

1. Cut tofu into ½" cubes. Mix tofu and soy sauce in medium bowl.

2. Slice scallions into ½" diagonal pieces.

3. Heat wok or skillet over high heat. Add 1 Tbsp oil and tilt pan to coat. Add tofu; stir-fry until seared brown on all sides, 2 to 3 minutes. Transfer to side dish.

4. Add remaining 1 Tbsp oil to pan; add peppers; stir-fry until blistered and crisp tender, 2 to 3 minutes.

5. Return tofu to pan; add garlic and ginger; stir-fry 20 seconds. Add stir-fry sauce, scallions, and corn; stir-fry just to combine.

6. Transfer to serving dish.

MAKES 4 SERVINGS

PER SERVING 196 cal, 10 g pro, 19 g carb, 11 g fat, 1 g sat fat, 0 mg chol, 3 g fiber, 731 mg sodium

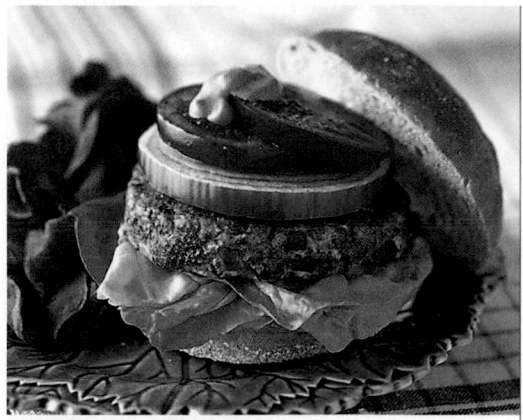

BAKED CHICKEN BURGER

- 1 lb ground chicken
- ½ cup chopped red bell pepper
- ¼ cup chopped green bell pepper
- ¼ cup chopped red onion
- ¼ cup chopped celery
- 2 Tbsp chopped parsley
- ½ tsp dried thyme
- 1 clove garlic, minced
- 1 Tbsp light soy sauce
- 1 cup soft bread crumbs

1. Preheat oven to 350°F.

2. Mix all ingredients together until just combined. Add black pepper to taste. Divide mixture to make four patties, and place on greased baking sheet.

3. Bake 12 to 15 minutes on each side, or until meat has reached 170°F. **TIP:** If you prefer, fry the patties in canola oil, 8 to 10 minutes per side.

MAKES 4 SERVINGS

PER SERVING 170 cal, 28 g pro, 9 g carb, 2 g fat, 0 g sat fat, 65 mg chol, 1 g fiber, 280 mg sodium

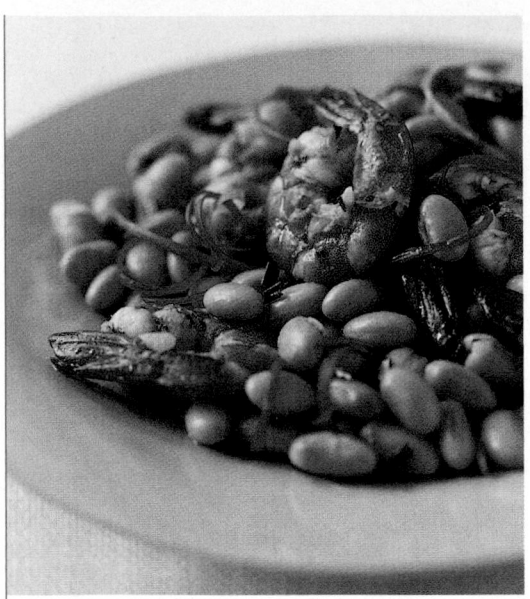

SHRIMP AND WHITE BEAN SALAD

2 Tbsp olive oil

2 cloves garlic, minced

½ tsp rosemary, crushed

6 oz shrimp

¼ cup chicken broth

1 can unsalted white beans, drained and rinsed

2 tsp lemon juice

1 scallion, thinly sliced, green parts only

1. In medium skillet, heat oil over medium-high heat. Add garlic and rosemary and cook until fragrant, about 1 minute. Add shrimp and stir-fry until pink and opaque. Add broth, cover, and lower heat. Simmer until shrimp are cooked through, about 4 minutes more.

2. Remove shrimp with slotted spoon, careful to let oil drain back into the skillet. In large bowl, toss with white beans and lemon juice until well mixed. Store in refrigerator until cool. Once cool, stir in scallions and serve.

MAKES 2 SERVINGS

PER SERVING 355 cal, 26 g pro, 25 g carb, 17 g fat, 2 g sat fat, 129 mg chol, 7 g fiber, 188 mg sodium

GRILLED FLANK STEAK WITH CHILE-TOMATO SALSA

- 2 Tbsp ground cumin
- 3 cloves garlic, minced
- 3 Tbsp lime juice
- 1 tsp coarsely ground black pepper
- ¾ tsp salt
- 1 beef flank steak or top round steak (1¼ lb), trimmed of all visible fat
- 1 large tomato, finely chopped
- 1 can (4.5 oz) mild green chiles, drained
- 3 scallions, thinly sliced

1. Coat grill rack with cooking spray. Preheat grill to medium-hot.

2. Place cumin in small skillet over medium heat and cook, stirring, 3 minutes or until fragrant and darker in color. Place in small bowl and let cool.

3. Remove 1 teaspoon toasted cumin and place in medium bowl. To small bowl, add garlic, 2 tablespoons of juice, pepper, and 1/2 teaspoon of salt and mix well. Place steak on prepared rack and rub cumin mixture over both sides of steak. Let stand at room temperature.

4. Meanwhile, in medium bowl with reserved cumin, combine tomato, chiles, scallions, remaining 1 tablespoon juice, and remaining 1/4 teaspoon salt. Let stand at room temperature.

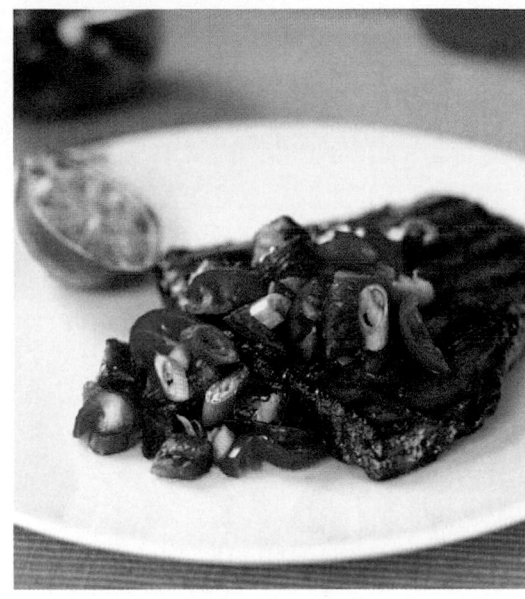

5. Grill steak 4 minutes per side or until an instant-read thermometer inserted in center registers 145°F for medium-rare.

6. Place steak on cutting board and let stand 5 minutes. Cut steak into thin slices and serve with salsa.

MAKES 4 SERVINGS

PER SERVING 269 cal, 33 g pro, 7 g carb, 11 g fat, 5 g sat fat, 58 mg chol, 2 g fiber, 605 mg sodium

W|H

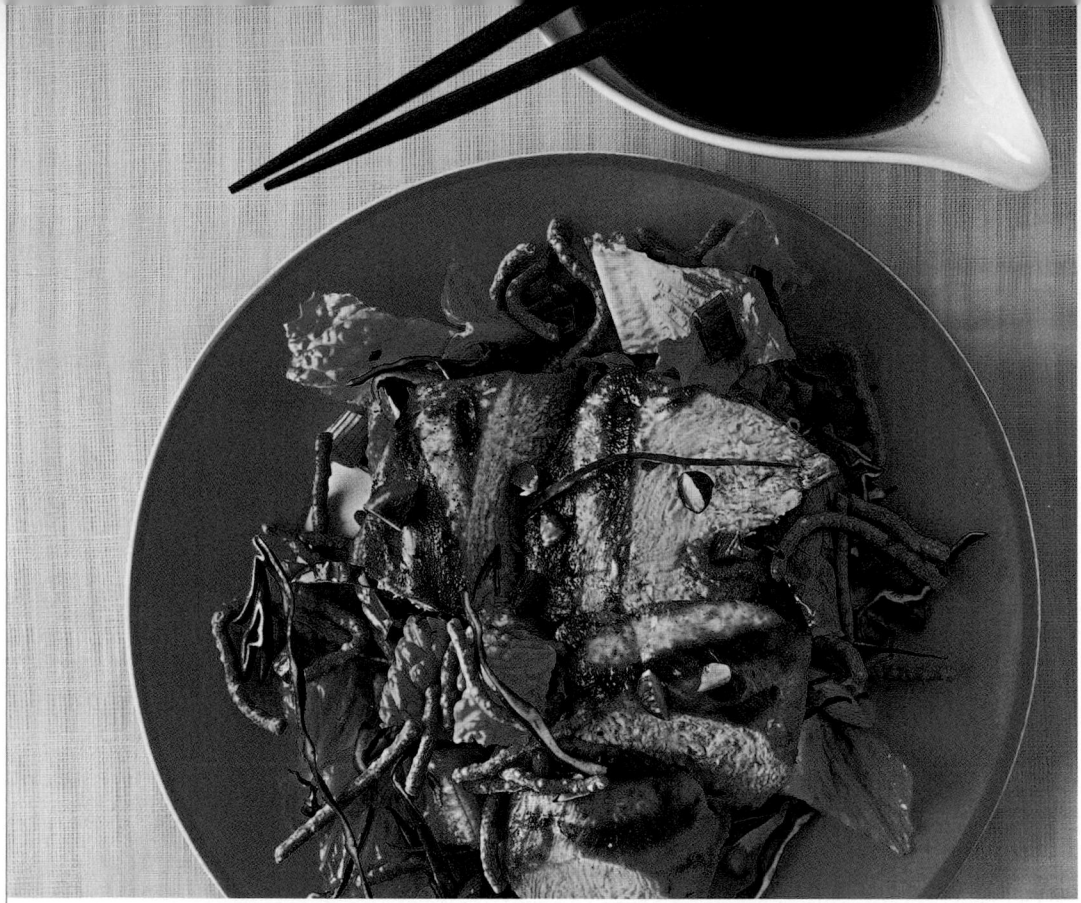

CHINESE CHICKEN SALAD WITH TOASTED ALMONDS

1 large head romaine lettuce, torn into bite-sized pieces

½ head red cabbage, shredded

8 scallions, sliced diagonally

½ cup chow mein noodles

1½ lb boneless, skinless chicken breast halves, grilled and sliced

½ cup chopped almonds, toasted

Dressing:

¼ cup vegetable oil

¼ cup rice wine vinegar

1 Tbsp reduced-sodium soy sauce

1 Tbsp toasted sesame oil

1 Tbsp sugar

¼ cup vegetable stock

1. In large bowl, combine lettuce, cabbage, scallions, noodles, and dressing. Top with chicken and almonds.

2. In small bowl, combine ingredients and mix well.

MAKES 8 SERVINGS

PER SERVING (salad) 252 cal, 24 g pro, 17 g carb, 10 g fat, 1.8 g sat fat, 50 mg chol, 4 g fiber, 171 mg sodium

PER SERVING (dressing) 99 cal, 1 g pro, 4 g carb, 9 g fat, 1.5 g sat fat, 0 mg chol, 0 g fiber, 75 mg sodium

JAMAICAN GRILLED CHICKEN

- ¼ cup jarred chutney
- 1 tsp Caribbean-style hot-pepper sauce
- 4 boneless, skinless chicken breasts (about 6 oz each)
- 2 Tbsp Jamaican jerk seasoning
- 1 lb fresh asparagus, trimmed

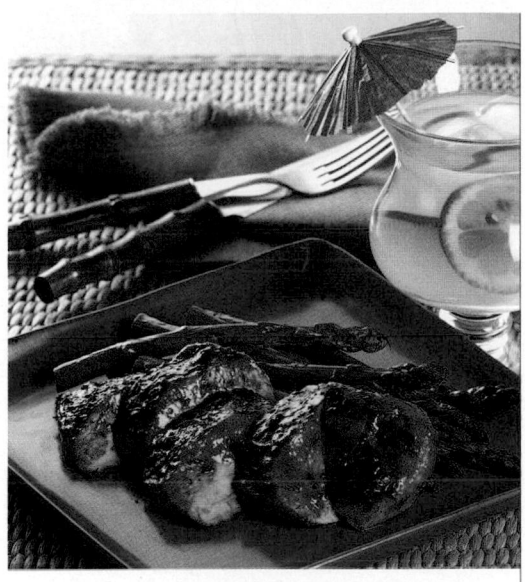

1. Preheat grill to medium-high. In small bowl, mix chutney and hot-pepper sauce and set aside. Rub chicken with jerk seasoning.

2. Grill breasts about 6 minutes per side, or until cooked through and no longer pink inside, brushing every few minutes with cutney mixture.

3. Meanwhile, grill asparagus about 6 minutes, turning occasionally. Remove chicken and asparagus from grill and arrange on platter to serve.

MAKES 4 SERVINGS

PER SERVING 200 cal, 35 g pro, 11 g carb, 2 g fat, 0.5 g sat fat, 80 mg chol, 3 g fiber, 550 mg sodium

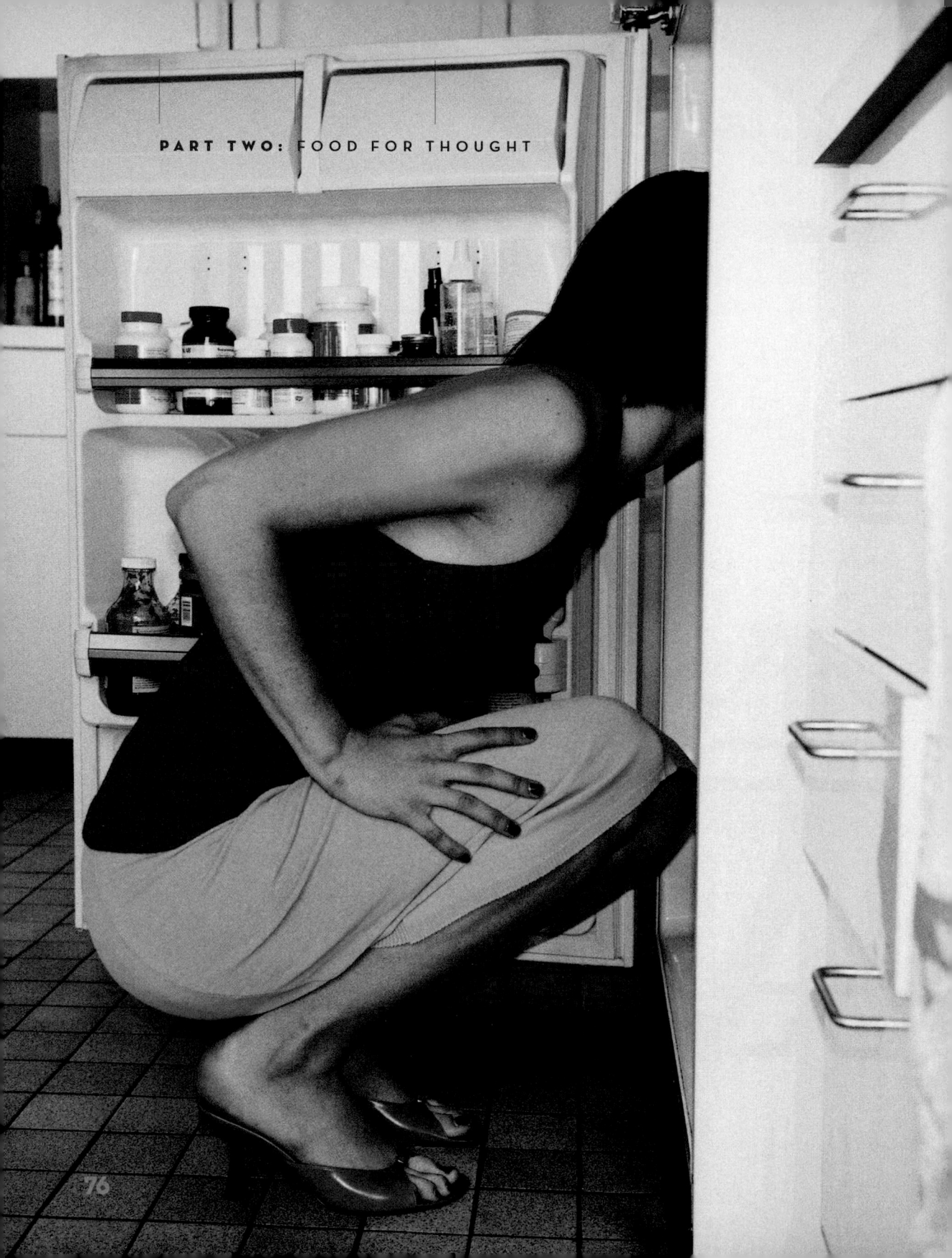

PART TWO: FOOD FOR THOUGHT

CHAPTER SEVEN

GET YOUR FILL

48 CURES FOR AN EMPTY STOMACH (AND 2 TO LOOK FORWARD TO)

BY MORGAN LORD

WHEN YOU'RE DIETING, a growling tummy is like a wedding toast: The longer it lasts, the more dangerous it gets. But your hormones, not your gut, are really to blame for most binges. Ghrelin, which makes you hungry, and leptin, your primary appetite suppressor, are eternally battling it out. Preventing these hormones from going haywire is the key to reining in calories without always feeling ravenous. So dig in—we're giving you 50 ways to fill up and conquer the growling beast that is your stomach.

1. **Pack a packet**

   Instant oatmeal beats out All Bran and Muesli for fullness factor. We love Quaker's Weight Control Maple and Brown Sugar—it tastes heavenly and has more fiber, protein, and whole grains than the regular variety.

2. **Find berry treasure**

   Raspberries are one of the most fiber-filled fruits, packing 8 grams into a cupful—a whopping 32 percent of your RDA. Add some to your cereal or yogurt.

3. **Can the juice**

   Whole fruit has a higher fiber content and makes you feel fuller than fruit juices, even those with pulp.

4. **Make a dinner date**

   A study found that women eat less than usual on dates (men tend to eat a lot more).

5. **But don't eat by candlelight**

   Dim light can trigger binge eating.

6. **Better yet, make it a blind date**

   It's worth a try—dine blindfolded and you'll eat 22 percent less food without missing it. Just watch out for the salad fork.

7. **Bulk up**

   Soluble fiber expands in your GI tract to make you feel full, so get your 25-gram RDA. That's a packet of oatmeal, two slices of whole-wheat bread, and 1 cup each of broccoli, edamame, and raw carrots.

8. **Ignore diet labels**

   One study found that after eating full-fat muffins, subjects were less hungry and ate less over the next 24 hours than after eating a fat-free version.

9. **Hold your breath**

   Just smelling a fresh-baked cupcake in the break room can induce the insulin secretion that makes you think you're hungry. Sight activates the appetite snowball too, so avert your eyes.

10. **Down a multivitamin**

    Research suggests that your body may compensate for a lack of nutrients by increasing your appetite so you'll eat more.

11. **Save your bread**

    Dodge the white wonder and go for whole wheat—it's 5.5 times more satisfying.

12. **Meet meat**

    One study found that people ate 441 fewer calories a day when following a 30 percent protein diet versus a 15 percent protein diet.

13. **Eat like a cow**

    Graze: Five evenly spaced, 350-calorie minimeals a day will regulate your appetite and ward off sugar cravings caused by skipping meals.

14. **Attempt ambidexterity**

    Switch your fork to your nondominant hand—you'll eat much more slowly. That gives you time to recognize your couldn't-eat-another-bite feeling when it first sets in.

15. **Skip soft drinks**

    High-fructose corn syrup, the main sweetener in soda, doesn't spur insulin production to make the body process calories, nor does it trigger leptin, the hormone that tamps down appetite.

16. **Trade your corkscrew for a bottle opener**

    Participants in one study ate more food while drinking wine than while drinking beer.

17. **Boost your bean count**

    The musical fruit's high fiber content causes glucose to be released slowly into the bloodstream, preventing the sudden slumps that cause hunger spikes. Add garbanzos or black beans to soup or salad.

18. Shape up

Wedge-shaped foods like pizza make it difficult to estimate proper portions. (No wonder the apple pie always goes so fast.)

19. Start with soup

Have a cup of soup, such as chicken noodle or vegetable, before your entrée—you'll feel fuller sooner and eat fewer calories overall.

20. But only one cup

Served buffet style, diners ate 73 percent more soup without realizing it or feeling any fuller.

21. Bag the dried fruit

Go for 2 cups of grapes over a quarter cup of raisins—both are 100 calories, but the grapes' water content feels more filling.

22. Dig pop culture

Because it's mostly air, popcorn is twice as filling as a candy bar or peanuts, with fewer calories. We like Pop Secret 100-calorie packs.

23. Slurp a smoothie

Make it with low-fat yogurt and loads of fruit for a satiety trifecta: protein (to decrease hunger), fiber (to fill you up without extra calories), and calcium (to help burn, not store, fat).

24. Whey your options

Boost that smoothie with 1 to 2 tablespoons of whey powder. New studies suggest that in addition to a protein punch, whey may affect the hormones that make you feel full. In one study, participants who ate a liquid meal made with whey ate significantly fewer calories 90 minutes later than their counterparts.

25. Go cuckoo for cocoa

Participants in one study were significantly

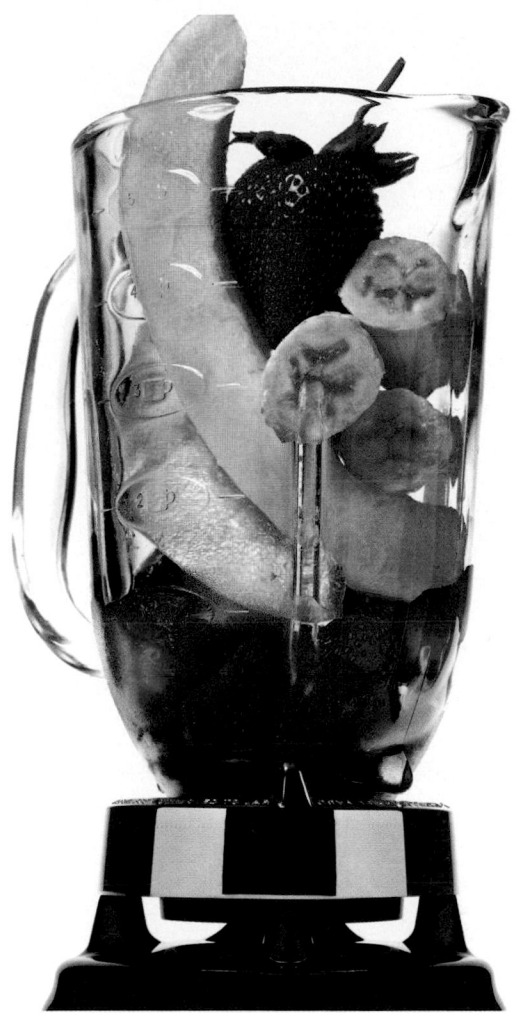

more satisfied 30 minutes after they drank low-fat chocolate milk than they were after they drank soda.

26. Crunch on raw carrots

Researchers in Ireland noted that carrots are more filling when they're uncooked. Bonus: A 1-cup serving has 3.6 grams of fiber.

27. Add avocado

Your body burns carbohydrates in an hour or

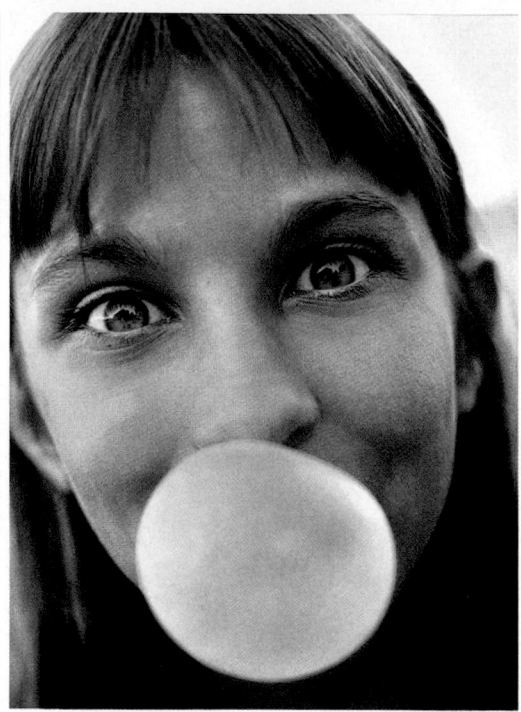

two, so toss a little healthy fat into the mix (avocado in salad, peanut butter on bread) to buy a few hours before the pangs hit.

28. Start a pack-a-day habit
Chewing gum (sugar-free or regular) suppresses your desire for sweets. (If you prefer potato chips, spit out the gum—it may make a salty craving worse.)

29. Get nutty
Nosh on pine nuts—they have the most protein of any nut or seed, and the pinolenic acid they contain stimulates two powerful hunger-suppressing hormones.

30. Listen to Norah Jones
Eating while listening to mellow music slows you down. It takes 20 minutes for your stomach to tell your brain it's full—that's the first seven tracks of "Come Away with Me."

31. Go beyond the pale
White pasta and other foods made with refined flour cause blood sugar to drop and leave you hungry again in no time. Choose whole-wheat pasta and you'll be satisfied almost twice as long.

32. Ride a roller-coaster
Nausea is responsible for a subsequent loss of appetite (bring your own barf bag).

33. Get hitched
A study found that happy marriages lower the risk of metabolic syndrome, which could lead to overeating. Women in consistently dissatisfying marriages were about 3 times more likely to develop metabolic syndrome. Widows carried nearly 6 times the risk.

34. Find a new china pattern
Research shows that blue is a natural appetite suppressant, so using blue plates, napkins, or placemats may make you eat more slowly and realize when you're full.

35. Re-paint your dining room beige
Red, yellow, and orange hues stimulate appetite and make you eat more.

36. Be antisocial
On average, people who eat with one other person consume about 35 percent more than when they dine alone; at a table of four, that figure rises to 75 percent more; if you're in a party of eight you'll nearly double your intake.

37. Enjoy your salad days
According to one study, women who ate a 100-calorie salad before dinner consumed 12 percent fewer calories during the meal without trying to diet or limit their intake. The fiber in the greens probably helped.

38. **Choose surf over turf**

Fish is more satisfying, per calorie, than lean beef or chicken, according to Dr. Susanna Holt's Satiety Index, a ranking of different foods' ability to satisfy hunger.

39. **Live in your own private Idaho**

If you need starches, yams and white potatoes (with skin) are seven times more filling than a croissant. Sorry, French fries don't count.

40. **Practice patience**

Before you go for seconds, wait 20 minutes. Once the leptin kicks in, you might find you're already full.

41. **Declare yourself perfect**

Accept your body and, according to a study at Ohio State University, you're more likely to eat healthily—and not for emotional reasons.

42. **Request a doggy bag**

Wrap up half your meal to go before you take the first bite and you're likely to eat less. Study participants who were offered a portion and a half of a food consumed 43 percent more of it and ate 25 percent more calories in the meal overall.

43. **Have a seaweed spritzer**

When you mix agar-agar, a fiber-rich thickening agent derived from seaweed, with fruit juice, it soaks up the liquid, making you feel full. Pick it up at Whole Foods Market.

44. **Make some miso**

When your metabolism is dragging and your energy dips, you crave foods and drinks that give you a quick lift. New research reveals that protein-rich miso soup boosts metabolism.

45. **Count sheep**

Sleep-deprivation leads to lower leptin levels and higher ghrelin levels, boosting your appe-

tite. Try to get at least 7 hours tonight.

46. **Have a cocktail with lunch**

Fruit cocktail, that is. Mixed fruit can curb a sweet tooth, and it has plenty of fiber, which helps regulate your blood sugar.

47. **Eject the junk**

Science has proven that a food's tasty appearance can trump feelings of fullness. Ask the waiter to remove your plate before you scarf the rest of those fluffy mashed potatoes.

48. **Turn up the heat**

Temperature is a satiety signal, and the cooler a room, the more people tend to eat—which is why restaurants often keep thermostats low.

And, in the not too distant future...

49. **Chew on this**

London researchers found that moderate doses of the "feeling full" hormone pancreatic polypeptide reduces the amount of food eaten by 15 to 20 percent. They're working on a chewing gum, but a finished product is still a good 5 years down the line.

50. **Pop a pill**

Italian scientists looking to make a more absorbent diaper lining ended up creating a cellulose pill that expands in your stomach to ward off hunger pangs for up to 7 hours.

Sources: The American Journal of Clinical Nutrition, Appetite, Archives of Internal Medicine, Behavioral Neuroscience, British Journal of Nutrition, European Journal of Clinical Nutrition, Holt's Satiety Index, International Journal of Obesity, Journal of Personality and Social Psychology, Journal of the American Dietetic Association, *Michigan State University, National Cancer Institute*, Obesity Research, *Ohio State University*, Physiology & Behavior, *U.S. Dept. of Agriculture, University of Illinois at Urbana-Champaign*.

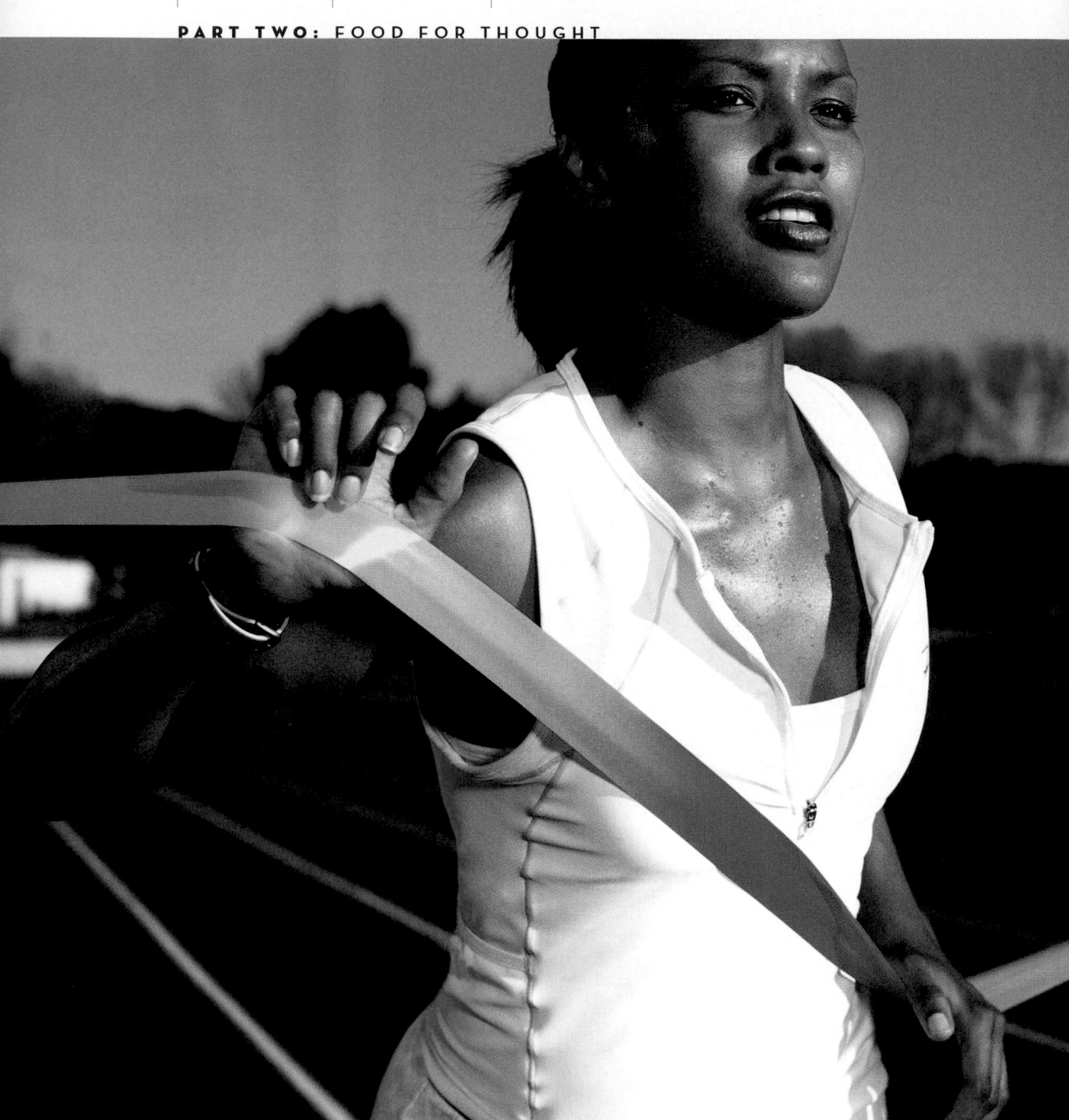

CHAPTER EIGHT

THE DEADLINE DIET

WANT TO TRASH THAT MUFFIN TOP PRONTO? DONE! JUST FOLLOW OUR EXPERT-APPROVED PLAN.

SO YOUR TRIP TO MEXICO is a month away and you've got to fit into that itty-bitty red bikini you bought in a size too small (hey, we all do it). You know starving yourself isn't healthy or smart—one sip of strawberry daiquiri and those pounds you lost will reappear faster than it takes Britney Spears to check in and out of rehab. Emergency liposuction? Also not an option. That's where we come in. This eating plan will help you hit your deadline—whether it's 1 week, 1 month, or 3 months away—without wrecking your health or driving you insane. You'll fit into that purple taffeta bridesmaid's dress in no time (lucky you!).

Week 1 Booty Boot Camp

Only 7 days between now and your high school reunion? Follow this 1,400-calorie plan and you can expect to lose between 2 and 4 pounds, even with an occasional night-time treat. If you've got a month or two (or three) before the big day, use this regimen for the first week. The meals and snacks are designed to kick-start your fat-burning engine with the perfect balance of lean protein, healthy fats, and complex carbs.

MEAL PLAN WEEK 1

	DAY 1	DAY 2	DAY 3
BREAKFAST	½ cup steel-cut oatmeal with ¼ cup skim milk, 1 cup mixed berries, and 1 Tbsp chopped pecans	**Strawberry Melon Smoothie (p. 62)**, reserve half for snack 3	1 cup whole grain cereal with ½ cup skim milk and ½ cup strawberries
SNACK	½ cup low-fat cottage cheese sprinkled with cinnamon	10 raw almonds	15 baby carrots with 2 Tbsp roasted red pepper hummus
LUNCH	4 oz grilled chicken, 3 cup mixed greens, ¼ cup sliced avocado, ½ cup sliced orange, and ½ cup hearts of palm with 2 tsp olive oil and 1 Tbsp lemon juice	1½ cup low-sodium minestrone soup; 1 oz mozzarella with tomato and basil on ½ whole grain roll	3 or 4 turkey meatballs (4 oz) with ½ cup marinara sauce and 2 Tbsp grated Parmesan; 2 cup steamed broccoli and carrots
SNACK	¾ cup edamame (in shells)	1 medium apple and 1 Tbsp natural peanut butter	1 granola bar
DINNER	4 oz grilled salmon marinated in 2 Tbsp balsamic vinegar and 1 tsp honey; 2 cups steamed spinach; 1 small baked sweet potato	1 cup miso soup; 1 tuna-avocado roll; 1 cup mixed greens with 2 Tbsp low-fat ginger dressing; 3 or 4 pieces tuna or salmon sashimi (if you use soy sauce, make it low sodium)	4 oz grilled chicken with 2 Tbsp low-sodium teriyaki sauce; 5 spears asparagus sautéed in 2 tsp sesame oil and sprinkled with 1 tsp sesame seeds; ½ cup steamed brown rice
SNACK	1 cup low-sugar hot cocoa	Strawberry Melon Smoothie leftovers	3 cups light popcorn

DAY 4	DAY 5	DAY 6	DAY 7
2 hard-boiled eggs with 2 slices tomato; ½ grapefruit; 1 cup low-fat soy or skim milk	1 whole grain English muffin with 1 Tbsp natural peanut butter; 1 medium banana	½ cup whole grain or bran cereal with ¾ cup plain fat-free yogurt and ¾ cup fresh berries	**Green and White Omelet (p. 67)**
1 cup apple with 2 Tbsp low-fat cheese spread	20 green grapes	1 Tbsp hummus and 3 whole grain crackers	1 cup fresh fruit salad (like banana, berries, and cantaloupe) with 2 Tbsp granola
Tasty Turkey Wrap (p. 67)	1 veggie burger with 2 Tbsp guacamole and 2 Tbsp salsa in 1 whole wheat pita; 2 cups mesclun salad and ½ cup grape tomatoes with 2 tsp olive oil and 1 tsp red wine vinegar	**5-Minute Mixed Green Salad (p. 64)**	TexMex salad: 2 cup mixed greens topped with 4 oz grilled chicken, 2 Tbsp salsa, 2 Tbsp shredded low-fat cheese, and ⅓ cup black beans
¾ cup plain low-fat yogurt with 1 tsp honey	Turkey and cheese roll-ups: 2 oz sliced turkey and 1 oz low-fat cheese	3 graham cracker squares with 1 Tbsp light cream cheese and 2 tsp jam	2 small oatmeal raisin cookies
3 oz extra-lean top sirloin steak; 2 cups grilled bell pepper and zucchini with 2 tsp olive oil	**Grilled Kyoto Salmon (p. 69)**; ½ cup whole wheat couscous; 1½ cup steamed broccoli	4 oz chicken roasted with fresh lemon and garlic; 2 cups spinach, tomato, and fresh garlic sautéed in 2 tsp olive oil and topped with 2 Tbsp grated Parmesan; 3 fingerling potatoes roasted with garlic, rosemary, and 1 tsp olive oil	6 oz tofu and 1½ cups mixed vegetables of your choice (such as snow peas, broccoli, and carrots) stir-fried in 2 Tbsp low-sodium teriyaki sauce and 2 tsp canola oil; ½ cup brown rice
Skip it.	1 cup pineapple or mango	½ cup low-fat vanilla or chocolate frozen yogurt with ½ c strawberries	Skip it.

W|H

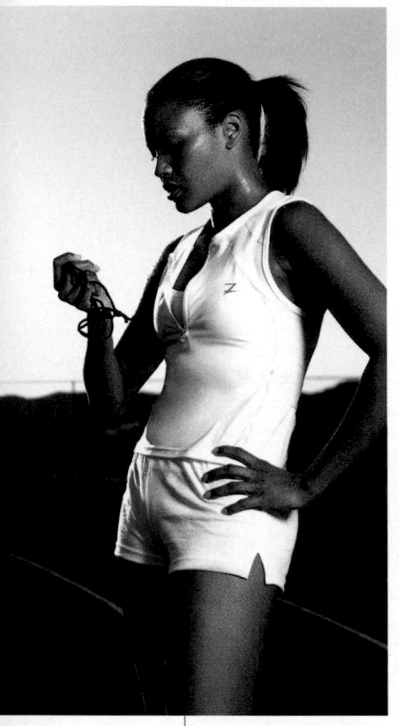

Weeks 2 to 4
Smart and Steady

Congrats! You've muscled through the toughest part of the plan, and your metabolism is hotter than Clive Owen on a summer day in Dubai. In this >>

MEAL PLAN WEEK 2

	DAY 1	DAY 2	DAY 3
BREAKFAST	2 multigrain waffles with 1½ Tbsp natural almond butter and ½ cup fresh strawberries	Omelet: 1 egg and 3 egg whites, ½ cup mushrooms and to-mato, and 2 Tbsp low-fat cheddar; 1 slice multigrain bread	1 cup whole-grain cereal with ½ cup skim milk and ½ cup strawberries
SNACK	10 raw almonds	1 cup fruit salad sprinkled with 1 Tbsp chopped pecans	8-oz skim latte
LUNCH	4 oz grilled salmon; 2 cups mixed greens with ¼ cup chopped baby tomatoes and ¼ cup artichoke hearts with 1 tsp olive oil and 1 tsp fresh lemon juice	**Barbeque Chicken Pita (p. 62)**	1 cup low-sodium lentil soup; 3 oz sliced turkey with lettuce, tomato, and Dijon mustard in 1 small whole wheat pita
SNACK	¾ cup plain low-fat yogurt with 1 tsp honey	1 granola bar	1½ cups celery and baby carrots with ½ cup low-fat cottage cheese
DINNER	4 oz cod baked with 2 Tbsp fresh lemon juice, 1 Tbsp capers, and 1 tsp fresh dill; ½ cup whole wheat couscous with 1 Tbsp toasted almonds and 1 Tbsp golden raisins; 1½ cups steamed broccoli	**Baked Chicken Burger (p. 71)** with ⅓ cup mushrooms sautéed in 1 tsp butter; 2 cups steamed green beans; 1 cup sweet potato "fries" (sprinkled with salt and pepper, brushed with 2 tsp olive oil, and baked at 425°F for 30 min)	4-oz grilled tuna steak marinated in 2 Tbsp low-sodium teriyaki sauce and 1 tsp minced garlic; 2 cups equal parts roasted corn, tomato, and snap peas with 2 tsp olive oil and 2 tsp lime juice
SNACK	1 cup low-sugar hot cocoa	Skip it.	2 small squares (1 oz) dark chocolate, 2 Hershey's Minia-tures or 4 Kisses

DAY 4	DAY 5	DAY 6	DAY 7
1 slice multigrain toast with 1 slice (1 oz) reduced-fat cheddar and 2 slices tomato; 1 cup melon; 1 cup low-fat soy or skim milk	½ cup steel-cut oatmeal with ¼ cup skim milk, ¼ cup apple, and 1 Tbsp chopped walnuts, sprinkled with cinnamon	1 egg and 2 egg whites scrambled with ½ cup broccoli and mushrooms; 2 pieces turkey bacon; 1 cup melon; 1 cup low-fat soy or skim milk	2 4-inch whole grain pancakes with 1 cup fresh berries, ½ cup plain low-fat yogurt, and 2 tsp honey
½ cup apple with 1 low-fat string cheese	½ cup low-fat cottage cheese sprinkled with cinnamon	3 whole grain crackers with 1 Tbsp low-fat soft cheese	8-oz skim latte
4 oz grilled shrimp with 2 cups fresh spinach and ½ cup roasted red bell pepper (brushed with 1 tsp olive oil and cooked in broiler for 10 to 12 min) topped with 2 Tbsp grated Parmesan, 2 tsp olive oil, and 2 tsp fresh lemon juice; 1 small whole wheat pita	**Tofu and Corn with Pepper Stir-Fry Sauce (p. 71)** 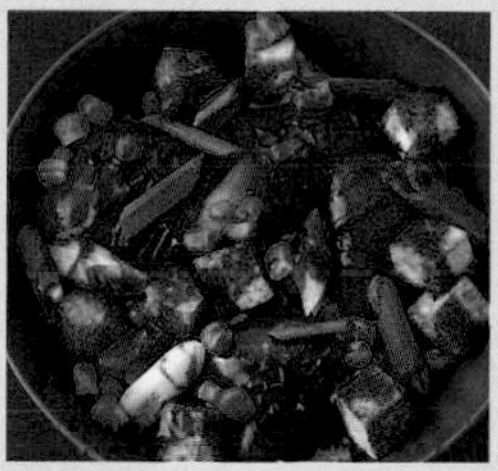 	4 oz grilled chicken breast with ½ cup couscous; 5 grilled spears asparagus	1 cup vegetable soup; 2 cups mixed greens and ½ cup tomato and cucumber with 2 tsp olive oil and 1 tsp fresh lemon juice; 2 whole grain crackers
¾ cup edamame (in shells)	4 graham cracker squares with 1 Tbsp light cream cheese and 2 tsp jam	4 oz low-fat vanilla or chocolate pudding with 1 Tbsp chopped walnuts	3 cups light popcorn
4 oz grilled chicken; 1½ cup arugula, ¼ cup red onion, ¼ cup baby tomatoes, 2 Tbsp olives, and 2 Tbsp low-fat feta with 1 Tbsp balsamic vinaigrette; ½ cup wild rice	4 oz grilled salmon marinated with 2 Tbsp balsamic vinegar and 1 tsp honey; 1 cup steamed spinach; 1½ cup roasted butternut squash (roasted at 400°F for 45 min)	4 oz grilled shrimp baked with ¾ cup tomato-basil sauce; ½ cup whole wheat penne pasta; 2 cups mixed greens and ½ cup baby tomatoes and cucumber with 2 tsp olive oil and 1 Tbsp balsamic vinegar	Fajitas: 4 oz grilled chicken, 1 cup grilled bell pepper and onion, 2 Tbsp low-fat cheddar, 2 Tbsp salsa, and 1 Tbsp low-fat sour cream in 2 small whole wheat tortillas
Skip it.	½ cup lemon sorbet (like Sharon's or Edy's) with ½ cup fresh berries	1 cup mango	¾ cup mango with 1 Tbsp shaved coconut

W|H

>> phase, you should continue losing about 1 to 3 pounds per week, for a total loss of up to 10 pounds for the month. The calorie count is still about 1,400, but you can lighten the workout load and incorporate more complex carbs to make the plan easier to sustain over the long haul. Still, if you exercise more or find that you're ravenous, you may require extra food to keep your body fueled in the upcoming weeks. Increase your daily intake by 100 calories by eating another snack (like a 6-ounce fat-free yogurt, an apple with 2 teaspoons of peanut butter, or an evening goody on days >>

MEAL PLAN WEEK 3

	DAY 1	DAY 2	DAY 3
BREAKFAST	1 slice multigrain bread with 1 Tbsp low-fat cream cheese, 1 tsp raspberry or apricot preserves, and 2 tsp ground flaxseed; ½ grapefruit	¾ cup plain low-fat yogurt with 1 cup papaya, ½ cup banana, and ¼ cup raisin-almond granola	1 cup whole grain cereal with ½ cup skim milk and ½ cup banana
SNACK	1 cup fruit salad sprinkled with 1 Tbsp chopped pecans	10 raw almonds	½ cup grapes and 1 oz low-fat cheddar
LUNCH	4 oz turkey with mustard, lettuce, and tomato on 1 slice whole grain bread; ½ cup lentil salad (¼ cup canned lentils and ¼ cup bell pepper and red onion with 1 tsp olive oil and 1 tsp red wine vinegar)	1 cup vegetarian chili; 10 mini whole grain crackers	2 slices whole grain bread with 2 Tbsp natural almond butter and 1 Tbsp all-fruit preserves
SNACK	¾ cup plain fat-free yogurt with 1 tsp honey	1 granola bar	1½ cup celery and baby carrots with ⅓ cup low-fat cottage cheese
DINNER	**Grilled Flank Steak with Chile-Tomato Salsa (p. 73)**; 1 small baked potato with 2 Tbsp plain low-fat yogurt and 1 Tbsp chives; 1½ cups mushrooms, tomato, and zucchini with 1 tsp olive oil and 2 tsp red wine vinegar	4 oz Italian chicken or turkey sausage grilled or pan-cooked with ½ cup marinara sauce and ½ cup bell pepper (any kind); ¾ cup whole wheat linguine; 2 cups arugula with ¼ cup red onion and 2 Tbsp shaved Pecorino Romano cheese, with 1 tsp olive oil and 1 tsp fresh lemon juice	1 cup miso soup; ⅔ cup edamame (in shells); 1 6-piece California roll; 3 or 4 pieces tuna or salmon sashimi
SNACK	2 small squares (1 oz) dark chocolate or 4 Hershey's Kisses	Skip it.	Skip it.

DAY 4	DAY 5	DAY 6	DAY 7
½ cup steel-cut oatmeal with ¼ cup skim milk, ¼ cup apple, and 1 Tbsp chopped walnuts, sprinkled wlth cinnamon	2 poached or scrambled eggs with 1 slice rye toast and 1 tsp butter; 1 cup fresh fruit salad	2 multigrain waffles with 1 cup fresh berries and 1 Tbsp light maple syrup	1 whole wheat tortilla with 1 egg and 2 egg whites scrambled with 2 Tbsp salsa and 1 Tbsp shredded low-fat cheddar; ½ cup strawberries and banana
8-oz skim latte	½ cup low-fat cottage cheese sprinkled with cinnamon	1 low-fat string cheese	½ cup low-fat cottage cheese
3 oz grilled extra-lean sirloin steak over 2 cups baby spinach, ¼ cup strawberries, 1 Tbsp toasted almonds, and 1 oz goat cheese with 1 tsp olive oil and 2 tsp balsamic vinegar	4 oz grilled chicken and 1 oz low-fat provolone cheese with lettuce and tomato in 1 whole wheat wrap	4 oz chunk light tuna with 1 Tbsp light mayonnaise; 3 cups mixed greens with ½ cup tomato, red onion, and carrots; 3 whole grain crackers	1 slice (3 to 4 oz) veggie pizza; 2 cups mixed greens and ½ cup tomato and cucumber with 1 tsp olive oil and 2 tsp balsamic vinegar
2 whole wheat fig cookies	1 serving soy chips with 2 Tbsp hummus	1 cup apple with 1½ Tbsp natural peanut butter	¼ cup trail mix (mixed raw almonds and cashews with dried cranberries or raisins); 1 clementine
4 oz tofu and 2½ cups snow peas, broccoli, water chestnuts, and carrots stir-fried in 2 Tbsp low-sodium teriyaki sauce and 2 tsp canola oil; ½ cup brown rice	4-oz chicken breast stuffed with ¼ cup diced apple and 2 Tbsp low-fat goat cheese, baked at 425°F for 20 to 25 min; 1 cup steamed green beans with 1 Tbsp slivered almonds; ¾ cup mashed sweet potato with 1 tsp honey and sprinkle of cinnamon	3 oz extra-lean grilled top sirloin or filet mignon; bruschetta (1 oz whole wheat baguette topped with ½ cup diced tomato, 2 tsp chopped basil, 1 tsp olive oil, 1 tsp balsamic vinegar, and ¼ tsp minced garlic); 1½ cups spinach sautéed with ½ tsp minced garlic and 2 tsp olive oil	**Jamaican Grilled Chicken (p. 75)**; ½ cup quinoa with 2 tsp pine nuts; 1 cup broccoli 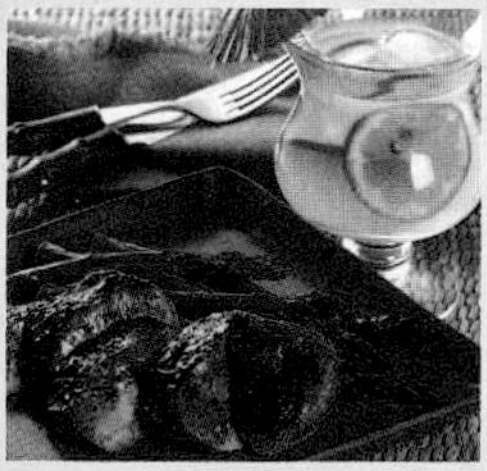
1 apple, cored, filled with 1 Tbsp each raisins and walnuts, baked 20 min at 350°F	4 oz low-fat vanilla or chocolate pudding	Skip it.	1 cup mixed berries with 2 Tbsp light whipped topping and 1 tsp cocoa powder

W|H

>> when one's not provided), adding about 2 ounces to your protein portion at lunch or dinner, or upping a carb serving from ½ to ¾ cup. If you're still starving after a few days, allow yourself another 100 calories. Since everyone's needs are different, you have to figure out what's right for your body. But don't top 2,000 calories (and eat that much only if you're working out at a high intensity for an hour or more, 4 to 6 days a week) or the number on the scale won't fall fast enough. You are on a deadline, after all!

MEAL PLAN WEEK 4

	DAY 1	DAY 2	DAY 3
BREAKFAST	2 multigrain waffles with 1 Tbsp natural almond butter; ¼ cup strawberries	2 hard-boiled eggs with 3 slices tomato; ½ grapefruit; 1 cup low-fat soy or skim milk	1 whole grain English muffin (like Thomas' Light) with 1 Tbsp natural peanut butter; 1 medium banana
SNACK	½ cup apple with 2 Tbsp low-fat cheese spread	¼ cup raw mixed nuts	½ cup low-fat cottage cheese sprinkled with cinnamon
LUNCH	1 veggie burger with 2 Tbsp guacamole and 2 Tbsp salsa; 2 cups mixed greens, ¼ cup chopped baby tomatoes, and ¼ cup artichoke hearts with 2 tsp olive oil and 1 tsp fresh lemon juice	4 oz grilled salmon; 2 cups mixed greens, 2 Tbsp capers, ¼ cup red bell pepper, and ¼ cup cucumber with 1 tsp olive oil and 1 tsp lemon juice; ½ cup wild rice with 2 Tbsp chopped scallion and dried cranberries	**Shrimp and White Bean Salad (p. 72)**
SNACK	6 oz low-fat soy or skim milk; 10 pecans	1 cup fruit salad with 2 Tbsp granola	2 small oatmeal raisin cookies
DINNER	3 or 4 turkey meatballs (4 oz) with ½ cup marinara sauce; ¾ cup whole wheat penne pasta; 1½ cups spinach sautéed in 1 tsp olive oil with ½ tsp chopped garlic	**Grilled Beef and Arugula Salad (p. 65)**	4 oz grilled tuna steak marinated in 2 Tbsp low-sodium teriyaki sauce and 1 tsp minced garlic; 2 cups equal parts roasted corn, tomato, and snap peas with 2 tsp olive oil and 2 tsp lime juice
SNACK	Skip it.	1 cup pineapple or ½ cup mango	Skip it.

DAY 4	DAY 5	DAY 6	DAY 7
¾ cup plain low-fat yogurt with 1 cup papaya and banana and ¼ cup raisin-almond granola	Smoothie: ¾ cup plain fat-free yogurt, ½ cup frozen mixed berries, ½ medium banana, and 2 Tbsp ground flaxseed	1 egg and 2 egg whites scrambled with ½ cup diced broccoli and mushrooms; 2 pieces turkey bacon; 1 cup melon	½ cup steel-cut oatmeal with ¼ cup skim milk, ¼ cup apple, and 1 Tbsp chopped walnuts, sprinkled with cinnamon
3 whole grain crackers with 2 Tbsp hummus	½ cup low-fat cottage cheese sprinkled with cinnamon	1 low-fat string cheese and 1 small apple	1 cup fresh fruit salad with 1 Tbsp granola
1 cup vegetable soup; 1 oz mozzarella with tomato and basil on 1 slice whole grain ciabatta bread	4 oz grilled shrimp; 2 cups fresh spinach, ¼ cup artichoke hearts, ¼ cup roasted red bell pepper, and 2 Tbsp grated Parmesan; 1 small whole wheat pita	4 oz turkey burger, ¼ cup onion sautéed in ½ tsp olive oil, and 2 Tbsp blue cheese on 2 slices whole grain bread	**Chinese Chicken Salad with Toasted Almonds (p. 74)**; 1-oz whole-grain roll 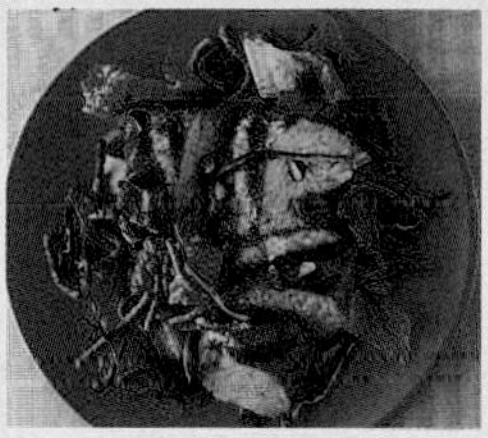
8-oz skim latte	1½ cups celery and baby carrots with ¼ cup hummus	4 graham cracker squares with 2 Tbsp light cream cheese and 2 tsp jam	¾ cup plain low-fat yogurt with 1 tsp honey
4 oz tofu and 2½ cups snow peas, broccoli, water chestnuts, and carrots stir-fried in 2 Tbsp low-sodium teriyaki sauce and 2 tsp canola oil; ½ cup brown rice	**Whole Wheat Penne with Shrimp (p. 68)** 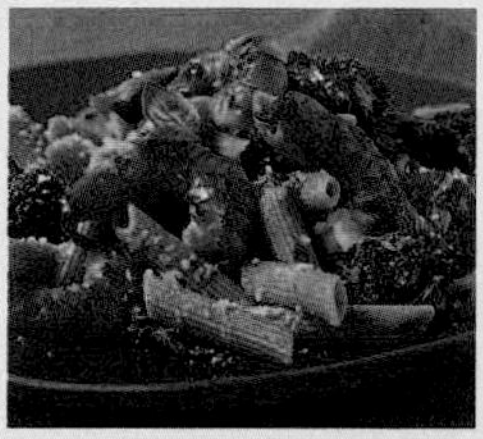	4 oz chicken roasted with ½ tsp rosemary, ½ tsp minced garlic, and 1 cup beets; 2 cups arugula with red onion, 1 Tbsp shaved Parmesan, and 1 tsp olive oil	4 oz cod baked with ½ cup diced fennel, olives, and orange; ½ cup quinoa with 2 tsp toasted pine nuts; 1 cup steamed broccoli
Skip it.	2 small squares (1 oz) dark chocolate	½ cup low-fat ice cream	1 cup mixed berries with 2 Tbsp light whipped topping

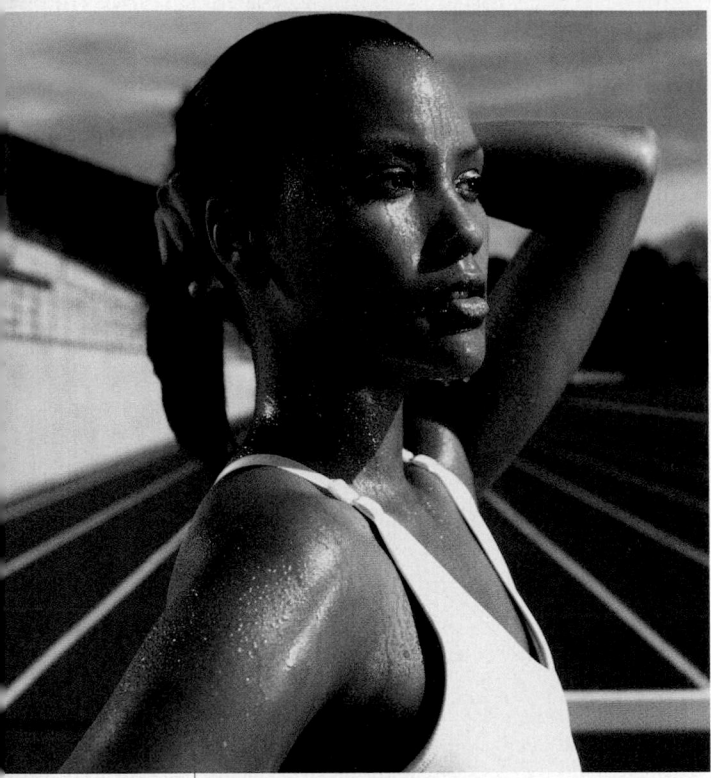

Months 2 and 3
Mix It Up and Meet Your Goal

YOU'VE MADE IT A MONTH! If you have 2 more to go before your deadline, it'll be a piece of cake. Stick to the basic plan for weeks 2 to 4 but use our swap list to keep things interesting. If you get sick of strawberries in your cereal, top your Total with a sliced banana instead. Or skip the salmon and sauté some scallops. We provide the serving-size equivalents, so all you have to do is pick your faves from the list, swap 'em with similar foods in the meal plan, and dig in!

SWAP LIST
Months 2 to 4

Fruit Swap
- 1 cup blackberries, raspberries, or strawberries
- ¾ cup blueberries
- 2 Tbsp dried fruit, like cranberries or raisins
- 1 cup melon, papaya, pineapple, or watermelon
- ½ cup mango
- 2 small apricots or clementines
- 1 kiwi
- ½ grapefruit
- 1 cup green or red grapes
- 1 medium apple, banana, nectarine, orange, peach, or plum

Vegetable Swap
- 1 cup raw or ½ cup cooked vegetables like bell peppers, broccoli, carrots, cauliflower, celery, green beans, snap peas, tomatoes, or zucchini (most veggies except starchy ones like corn, potatoes, and squash, which count as carbs)
- 3 cup arugula, mixed greens, spinach, or any type of lettuce
- 5 or 6 spears asparagus
- 1 medium artichoke

Carb Swap
- ½ cup cooked basmati, brown, jasmine, or wild rice
- 1 cup cooked grits, oatmeal, or other whole grain hot cereal
- ½ cup cooked barley, buckwheat kasha, bulgur (cracked wheat), couscous, millet, or quinoa
- ½ cup cooked pasta (whole wheat is always best), like angel hair, bow-tie, fettuccine, penne, or spaghetti
- 1 cup whole grain, high-fiber cold cereal
- 1 small (3-oz) sweet potato or regular potato
- ½ cup mashed potato or sweet potato

Protein Swap
- 4 oz seafood like calamari, crab, cod, halibut, lobster, orange roughy, salmon, scallops, sea bass, shrimp,

- sole, swordfish, tilapia, or tuna steak
- 4 oz skinless chicken or turkey breast, or ground chicken or turkey
- 3 oz buffalo, ham, pork, or extra-lean red meat
- 4 oz seitan, tempeh, tofu, or other vegetable-based protein
- ½ cup beans like black, cannellini, garbanzo, kidney, or navy
- 2 eggs or 1 whole egg plus 2 egg whites

Fat Swap
- 2 Tbsp mayonnaise
- 2 Tbsp canola, flaxseed, grapeseed, or olive oil
- 10 (about ¼ cup) raw almonds, cashews, pecans, or walnuts
- 1 Tbsp natural almond, cashew, or peanut butter

Dairy Swap
- 6 oz low-fat or fat-free yogurt (aim for plain to cut down on added sugar)
- 8 oz 1% or skim milk, or low-fat soy or rice milk

- 1 oz low-fat or reduced-fat cheese like cheddar, feta, or goat
- 1 low-fat string cheese
- 2 wedges (2 Tbsp) of spreadable cheese or 1 circle (1 Tbsp) of Bonne Bell
- ½ cup low-fat cottage cheese

Treat Swap
If there's something you love that's not on this list, eat it! Just make sure to keep the calories to 130 or less.
- 2 small squares (1 oz) dark chocolate, 2 Hershey's Kisses, or 1 mini peppermint patty
- ½ cup low-fat frozen yogurt, low-fat ice cream, or sorbet
- 1 single-serve low-fat pudding or 1 fudge pop
- 8 whole grain crackers
- 2 small cookies
- 15 baked tortilla chips with ⅓ cup salsa
- 3 or 4 bites of your favorite dessert when eating out
- 5 oz red or white wine
- 12 oz light beer
- 1½ oz hard liquor

THE HOME STRETCH

When your deadline's a few days away, use these four tricks to look even more svelte in your teeny bikini.

3 days before: Cut the carbs (except fruits and nonstarchy veggies). You'll shed any extra water you may have been holding onto, which can knock the scale down a notch or two. Skip excess salt too (it has the same water-retaining effect). Limit your daily sodium intake to 2,300 milligrams.

2 days before: Hit snooze. The amount of sleep you get affects the function of ghrelin and leptin—hormones that regulate your appetite and metabolism. Skimping on shut-eye can cause the hormone levels to fluctuate, which makes you hungry (especially for sugary, carb-heavy foods) and less able to tell when you're full. Aim for at least 7 hours of sleep a night and you won't be as likely to give in to that cheese fry hankering.

Pass on the gas. Steer clear of cruciferous vegetables like broccoli, cabbage, and Brussels sprouts—they're high in fiber and hard to digest, which means they make you bloated and, well, flatulent. They also contain sulfur, so when you let one rip, it's stinkier than a port-o-potty at Lollapalooza.

1 day before: Say sayonara to soda. When you drink carbonated beverages, you consume extra air, which makes your paunch puff up right after you've finished that Diet Dr. Pepper. So ditch the soda and seltzer and down water instead.

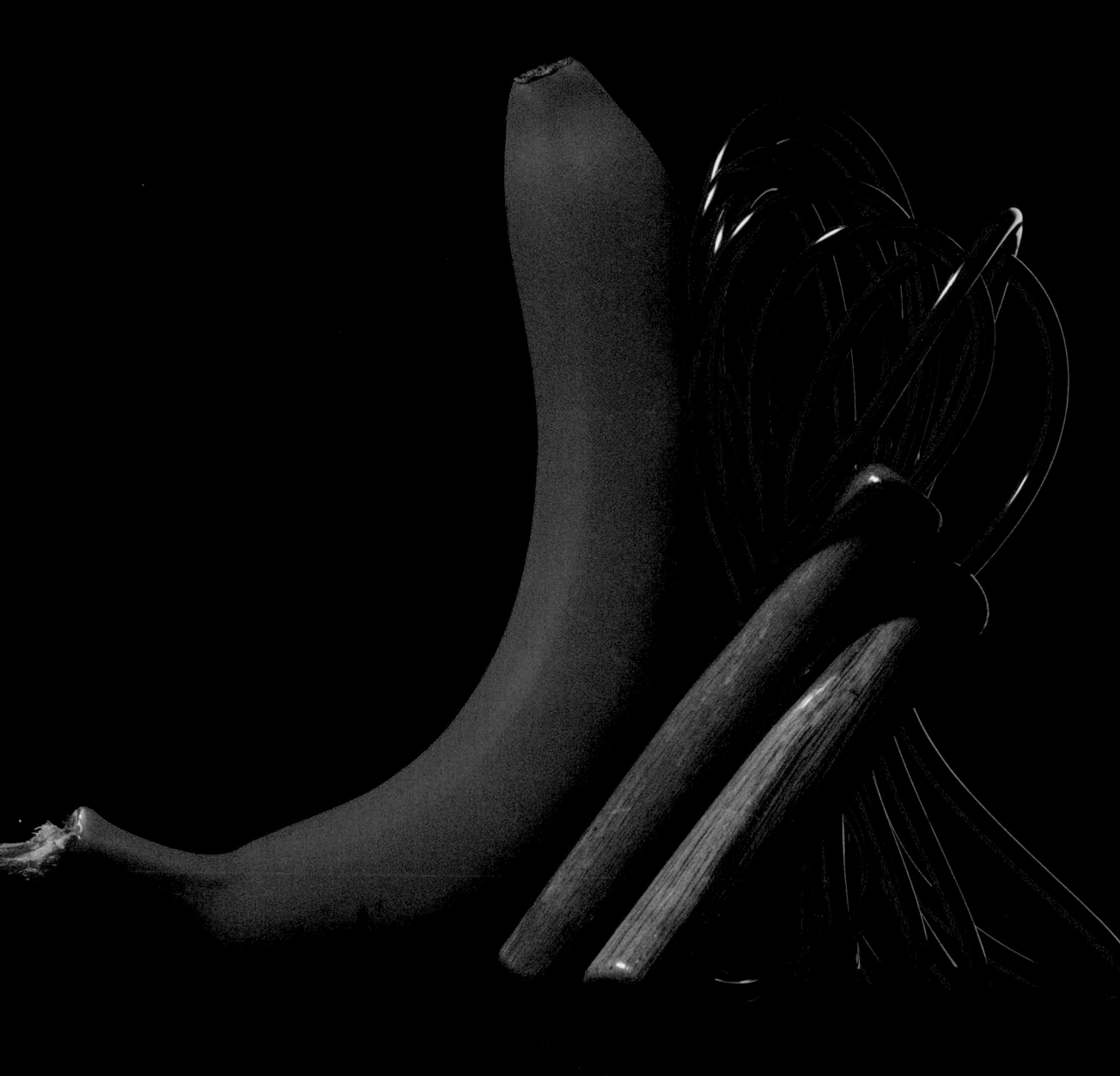

CHAPTER NINE

FUEL YOUR WORKOUT

POWER UP YOUR WORKOUT WITH THE 19 BEST FITNESS FOODS FOR WOMEN.

BY MAUREEN CALLAHAN, R.D.

CHOOSING A BAGEL over a peanut butter sandwich isn't the kind of life-altering decision that, say, changing your e-mail address is. But your pick could have heavy fitness repercussions. Grab a lame prerun snack and you'll be dragging to the finish. Reach for the wrong food when you put down those weights and next time you pump iron, you could be crashing harder than a disgraced beauty queen after an all-nighter. The simple truth is what you eat influences your performance in key ways. That's why we pored over a stack of scientific studies and picked the brains of a half dozen experts—top-notch researchers, coaches, and sports nutritionists—to single out the top 19 foods for any activity, from yoga to running to rock climbing. Stock your pantry with these staples to perform and feel your absolute best.

AVOCADOS

The cholesterol-lowering monounsaturated fat in these green health bombs can help keep your body strong and pain free. University of Buffalo researchers found that competitive women runners who ate less than 20 percent fat were more likely to suffer injuries than those who consumed at least 31 percent. Peter J. Horvath, Ph.D., a professor at the university, speculates that the problem is linked to extreme low-fat diets, which weaken muscles and joints. "A few slices of avocado a day are a great way to boost fat for women who are fat shy," says Leslie Bonci, R.D., director of sports nutrition at the University of Pittsburgh Medical Center.

BAGELS, WHOLE GRAIN

Never mind Dr. Atkins—carbs are the optimal workout food. "Not the simple ones, because they wind you up and drop you down," says Jackie Berning, Ph.D., R.D., a nutrition professor at the University of Colorado at Colorado Springs and counselor to sports teams. "You want complex carbohydrates in their natural package, aka whole grains." A whole grain bagel is an ideal presweat-session pick: You'll digest it slowly because of all the fiber, which will deliver a steady flow of energy over time rather than one big burst.

BANANAS

Thanks to bananas' high potassium content, peeling one is a speedy solution to that stitch in your side. While a lack of sodium is the main culprit behind muscle cramps, studies show potassium plays a supporting role: You need it to replace sweat losses and help with fluid absorption. Bananas are also packed with energizing carbohydrates. One medium-size fruit has 400 milligrams of potassium and as many carbs (29 grams) as two slices of whole wheat bread.

BERRIES

U.S.D.A. researchers recently placed fresh berries on their list of the 20 foods richest in antioxidants. Just a handful of blueberries, raspberries, or blackberries is an excellent source of these potent nutrients, which protect muscles from free radical damage that might be caused by exercise. Shop for berries by the shade of their skin: The deeper the color, the healthier the fruit.

CARROTS, BABY

Close your eyes and they almost taste like crunchy candy. Carrots pack complex carbs that provide energy to muscles and potassium to control blood pressure and muscle contractions, Bonci says. And a half cup has just 35 calories.

CEREAL, WHOLE GRAIN— WITH FAT-FREE MILK

Looking for something to nosh before you hit the gym? Raid your cereal stash. The healthiest brands contain endurance-boosting complex carbs and muscle-building protein. Sixty minutes before a workout, fuel up with a 200-calorie snack: $3/4$ cup of whole grain cereal with 4 ounces of fat-free milk.

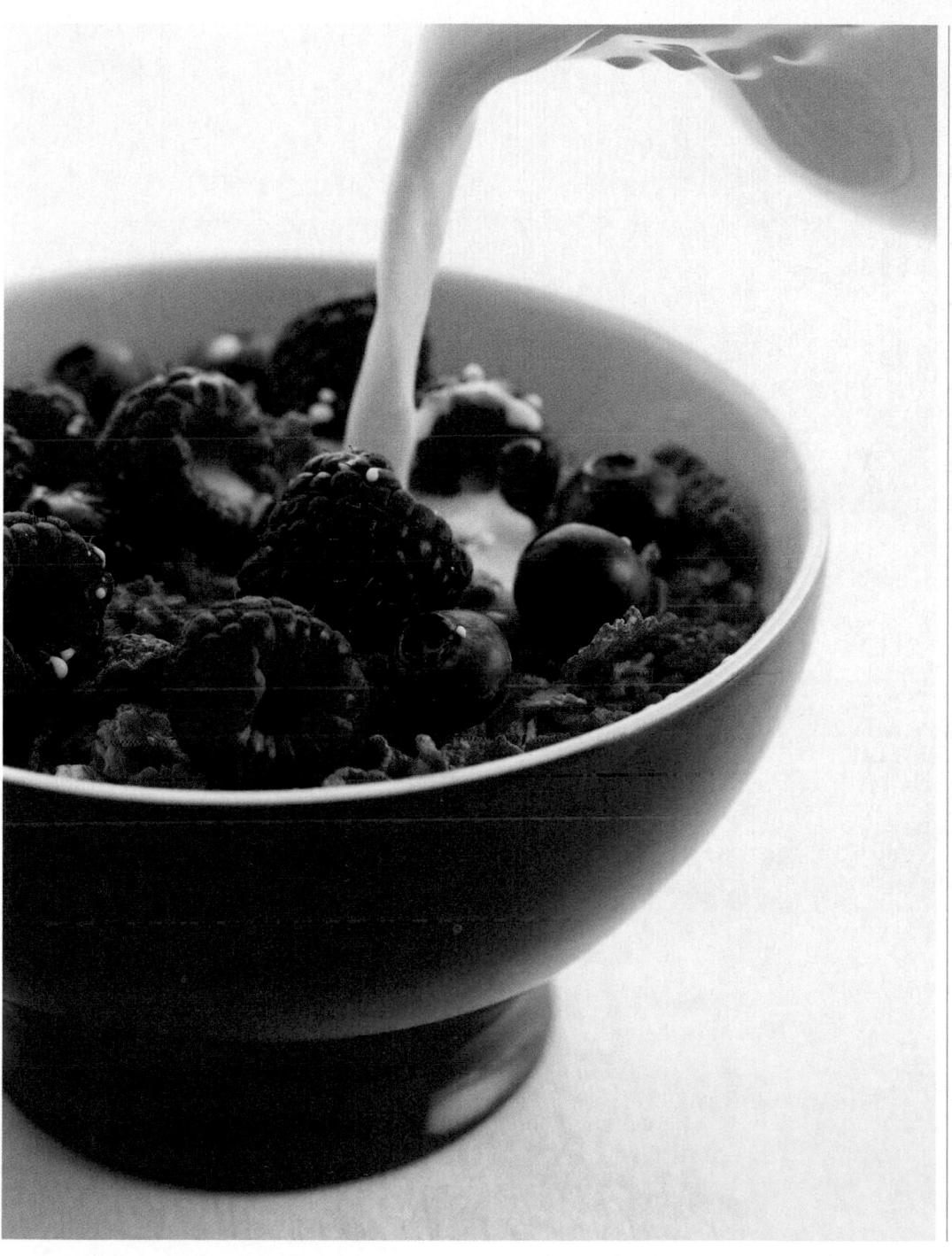

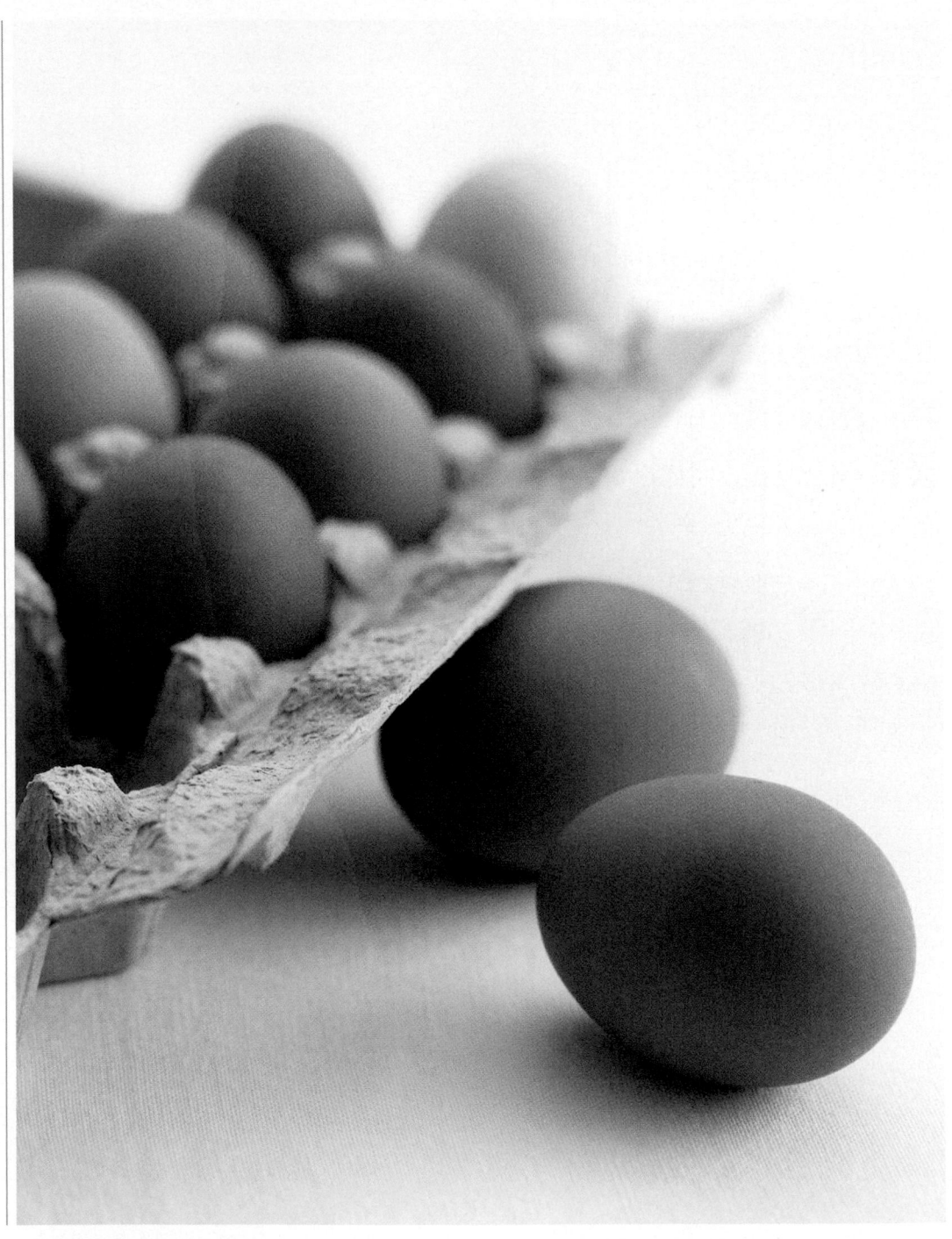

"When you eat something before exercising, you have more energy, so you can work out harder and perhaps longer. And you'll be less likely to overeat afterward," Bonci says.

CHICKEN THIGHS

Skimp on iron and zinc and your energy will flag. Cooking up some juicy chicken thighs or turkey drumsticks is the best way to get more of both. "Dark-meat poultry is significantly lower in fat than red meat yet has all the iron, zinc, and B vitamins that women need in their diets," says Seattle sports nutritionist Susan Kleiner, Ph.D., author of *Power Eating*.

CHOCOLATE MILK, LOW FAT

There's way more to milk than just calcium. In fact, it's a damn near perfect food, giving you a lot of valuable energy while keeping your calorie count low, Kleiner says. The chocolate kind is loaded with calcium, vitamins, and minerals just like the plain stuff, but new studies confirm that milk with a touch of cocoa is as powerful as commercial recovery drinks at replenishing and repairing muscles.

COTTAGE CHEESE, LOW FAT

Despite its frumpy image, this diet staple packs 14 grams of protein per half-cup serving, along with 75 milligrams of calcium and 5 grams of carbohydrates. That protein is crucial to healing the microscopic muscle tears that occur during exercise, says Amy Jamieson-Petonic, R.D., health education manager at Cleveland's Fairview Hospital.

CRANBERRIES, DRIED

This packable fruit delivers a generous pre- or post-workout blast of carbohydrates (25 grams per $1/4$ cup). Plus, cranberries have proanthocyanins, compounds that help prevent and fight urinary tract infections. Running to the bathroom every 5 minutes definitely isn't the kind of workout you need.

EGGS

Don't skip the yolk. One egg a day supplies about 215 milligrams of cholesterol—not enough to push you over the 300-milligram daily cholesterol limit recommended by the American Heart Association. Plus, the yolk is a good source of iron, and it's loaded with lecithin, which is critical for brain health, Kleiner says. What does brain power have to do with exercise? Try doing a sun salutation without it.

FLAXSEED, GROUND

"Flaxseed is full of fibers called lignans that promote gut health," Kleiner says. Since flax lignans contain both soluble and insoluble fiber, they keep you regular. "When you're trying to do an endurance sport, it can be disruptive to have digestive problems," she notes. A daily dose of 1 to 2 tablespoons of ground flaxseed tossed in your cereal nets you fiber without fuss.

HUMMUS

Complex carbohydrates, protein, and unsaturated fats—all the right elements to fuel activity—meet in one healthy little 70-calorie, 3-tablespoon package. Plus, hummus is often made with olive oil, which contains oleic acid—a fat that helps cripple the gene responsible for 20 to 30 percent of breast cancers, according to Northwestern University researchers.

ORANGES

"They're portable. They're a fruit you can get year-round. And they're a rich source of vitamin C," Bonci says, "which helps repair muscle tissue."

SHAKE IT, BABY

Blend these ingredients for the perfect pre- or postworkout mix of protein, vitamin C, and carbs, says Leslie Bonci, R.D. This may be the next best thing to an orange push-up pop.

1/2 medium banana

6 oz low-fat vanilla yogurt

4 oz orange juice

4 oz water

1 oz (2-Tbsp scoop) whey protein powder

PER SERVING: 370 calories, 2.5 g fat (1.5 g saturated), 160 mg sodium, 52 g carbohydrates, 2 g fiber, 35 g protein

One orange has all the C a woman needs each day—close to 75 milligrams. Vitamin C is also key for making collagen, a tissue that helps keep bones strong.

PEANUTS

No wonder Mr. Peanut never stops tap-dancing. Female soccer players kicked and sprinted just as well in the final minutes of a game as they did at the start when they added 2 ounces of peanuts a day to their regular diet, Horvath says. The extra fat may help improve endurance by giving muscles energy to burn up front so they can spare muscle glycogen stores later.

POTATOES, BAKED

Sweat like a pig? Four shakes of salt (about 1,100 milligrams of sodium) and a small baked potato is the perfect recipe for electrolyte replacement. "The electrolytes, sodium and potassium, help maintain fluid balance in and around cells and make sure muscles contract as they need to," Bonci says.

SALMON

Great for heart health, but here's an added twist: New studies are suggesting that monounsaturated fats and omega-3 fats might help lessen abdominal fat. It's too soon to understand the link, but "this could be particularly good for women working to tone their core," Kleiner says.

WHEY PROTEIN

"Whey protein contains the ideal assortment of amino acids to repair and build muscle," Kleiner says. Plus, it's digested fast, so it gets to muscles quickly. Stir a scoop into a smoothie for a delicious boost before or after your next workout.

YOGURT

Immune-strengthening probiotics are a fabulous feature, but the best thing about yogurt is that it will spike your energy without making your stomach gurgle in yoga class. "It's liquidy in consistency and because you can digest it quickly, it's easy on the gut," Bonci says.

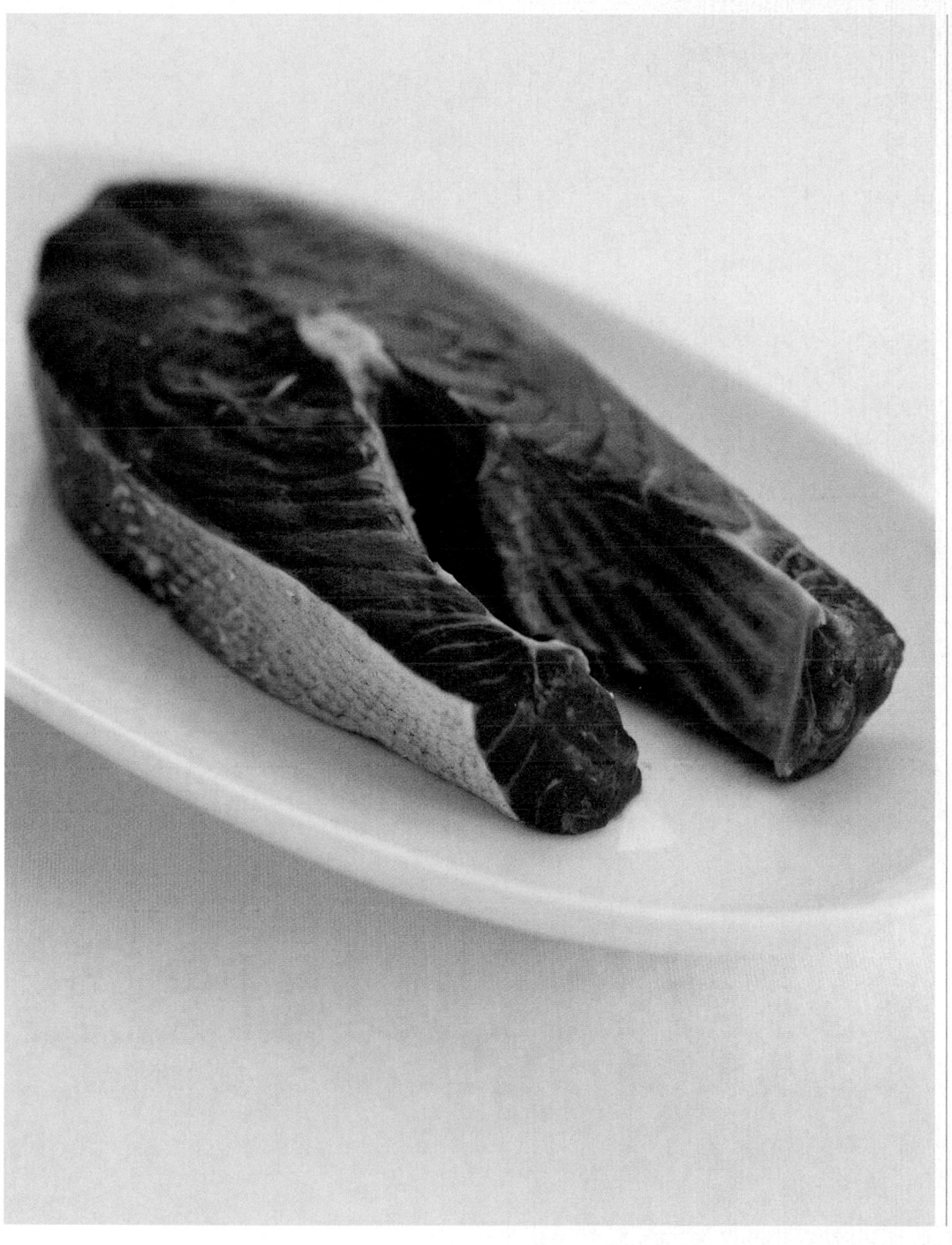

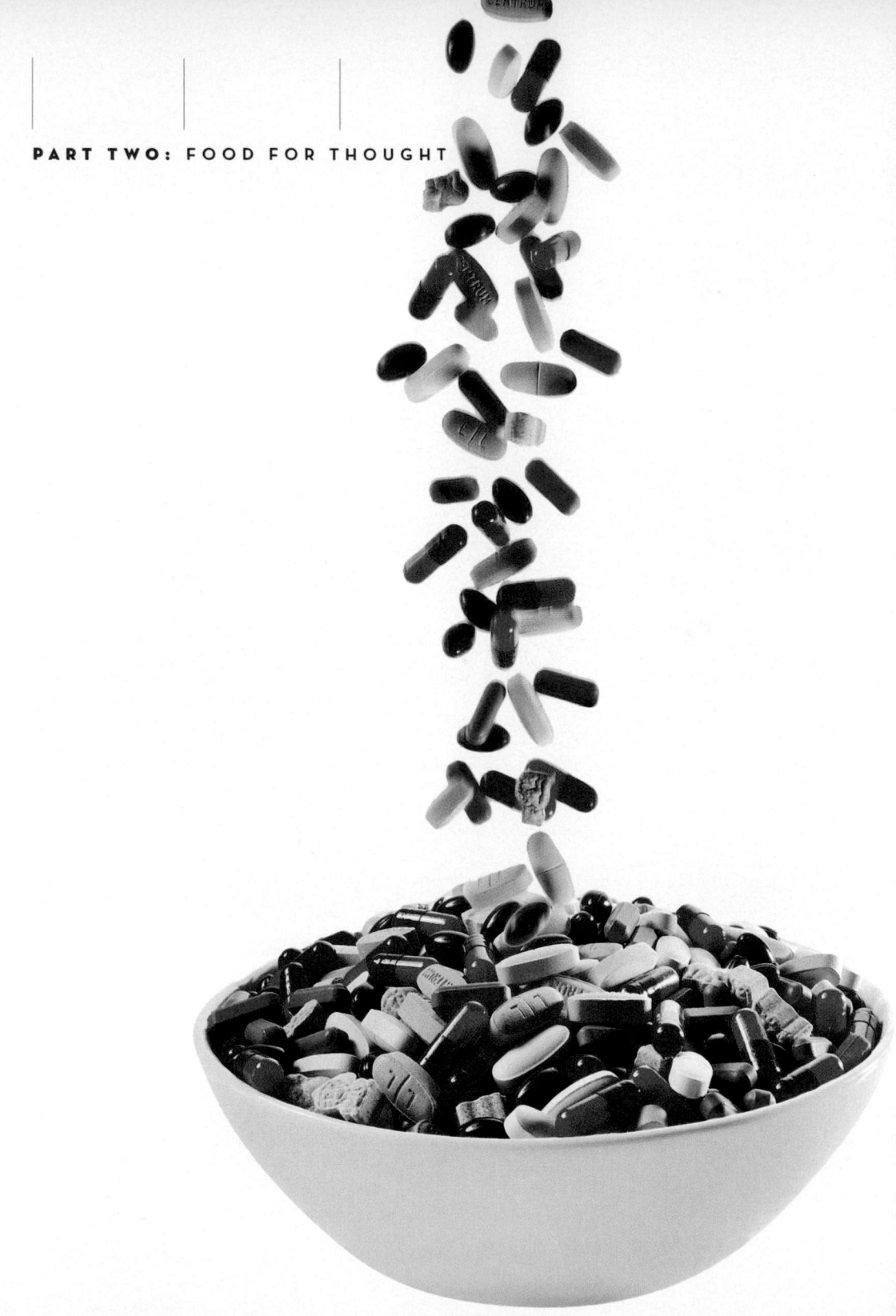

CHAPTER TEN

MULTIPLE CHOICE

THE FORMULA MOST MULTIVITAMINS ARE BASED ON IS WAY OUT OF DATE. HERE'S WHAT YOUR BODY NEEDS NOW.

BY RICHARD LALIBERTE

A MULTIVITAMIN IS YOUR DIETARY BACKUP, your edible wingman, your nutritional safety net on the off chance you swap your Special K for Cap'n Crunch or order the fries instead of the salad. So it makes sense that the more ingredients listed on the label, the more confident you feel you're getting all the nourishment you need for unbreakable bones, calorie-melting muscles, unstoppable energy, and hair that reflects more light than a disco ball.

But of course it's not that simple. Most multis are packed with far more vitamins, minerals, herbs, and who knows what other plant and animal substances (bee pollen, pine bark, chasteberry...) than the FDA recommends, sometimes in dangerously high quantities. Yet in spite of

ADD-ONS
FIT INTO THESE CATEGORIES? THEN YOU NEED SOME NUTRITIONAL EXTRAS

If You're . . . an Avid Athlete or If You're . . . Pregnant

You need more . . . iron. Intense exercisers (women who train for a sport for at least an hour daily) need 30 percent more iron than average, according to the National Institutes of Health. When you're pregnant, Baby gloms on to some of your iron stores, and increased blood volume and blood loss during delivery take their toll, too. WH pick: Floradix Iron + Herbs Extract (10 mg iron, 10 mg vitamin C). The dose is lower than many iron supplements, so you're less likely to hit the 45-mg upper limit, and the vitamin C helps you absorb it. Take with a meal, but avoid washing down with milk—calcium can stop iron absorption.

If You're . . . Breastfeeding

You need more . . . zinc. Feeding Junior can sap your zinc stores, especially if you're a vegetarian. Ask your doctor before taking. WH pick: Zand Lemon Zinc HerbaLozenge (5 mg). Your multi delivers most of what you need, but this low-dose lozenge provides extra insurance.

Take at the same time as your multivitamin to ensure a balancing hit of copper, which zinc can otherwise deplete.

If You're . . . a Vegetarian

You need more . . . vitamin B_{12}. Natural B_{12} comes only from animal foods like meat and fish, so vegetarians tend not to get enough. B_{12} is so safe that no upper limit has been established. WH pick: Country Life Vitamin B_{12} (500 mcg). While more than 8,000 percent above the DV (and still safe), the dose is nonetheless low for a B_{12} supplement, so you won't get more than you need. Take with a glass of water after dinner. You also need more . . . iron. WH pick: Floradix Iron + Herbs Extract (10 mg iron, 10 mg vitamin C). Take with a meal but not with milk—calcium prevents iron absorption.

If You're . . . a Vegan

You need more . . . vitamin A. Eggs and milk are typical sources, so vegans are the rare people who may need more A. Still, toxicity dangers such as nerve damage and birth defects make food a better choice than a supplement on top of a multivitamin. WH pick: a cup of carrot juice daily. Drink with dinner or shortly after to allow fat in food to boost absorption. Or snack on a cup of baby carrots.

all that's in them, studies show they still come up surprisingly short on a few key nutrients. Even more problematic, many experts believe the FDA recommendations themselves are outdated and in desperate need of readjustment. Our goal: to sort out the debate over supplements and find a simple solution that will keep your body going strong and looking gorgeous day in and day out.

OLD RULES, NEW FOOD

Doubt about the benefits of multivitamins surfaced late last year, when a National Institutes of Health review panel scrutinized studies on the disease-fighting capabilities of multis and raised some red flags. "One of the things we were concerned about is what happens when you take a supplement on top of what you get in food, some of which is already fortified with extra nutrients," says panelist Diane Birt, Ph.D., director of the Center for Research on Botanical Dietary Supplements at Iowa State University.

From antioxidant-laced jelly beans to cereals spiked with vitamins A to Z, the nutrient density of packaged foods has rocketed over the past few decades. Meanwhile, the government's recommended Daily Values (DVs)—which most multis and other supplements base their formulas on—haven't budged since they were set in 1968 by the National Academy of Sciences (NAS). It's no wonder health officials worry we're getting too much of a good thing.

On the bright side, thanks to years of research, more accurate recommendations do exist. Developed by the Institute of Medicine (a branch of the NAS) from 1997 to 2005, they're called Dietary Reference Intakes (DRIs). DRIs are closer to the mark because they take age and gender into account, and they recommend different levels for people with different concerns (like pregnancy and breastfeeding).

But don't expect to see these better benchmarks on labels anytime soon. The FDA requires supplement companies to use the DVs because they act as a nutritional (albeit outdated) average for everyone and allow shoppers to compare products easily. Less-than-perfect multivitamins are the result.

The obvious solution is to update the DVs based on the DRIs, but getting everyone to agree on how to do that isn't so simple. "People want a single number on labels, but whose should it be—women's or men's—and for what age group?" says Suzanne Murphy, Ph.D., R.D., a professor at the University of Hawaii who sits on a DRI planning committee at the NAS. Until the government brings DVs into the 21st century, it's up to consumers to read labels and know what works for them.

GIVE A LITTLE, TAKE A LITTLE

Several large-scale studies have made it clear that our well-intentioned attempts to eat the best of everything have begun to backfire. For example, women who take a multivitamin and eat fortified foods are often getting too much vitamin A. Many of us look for 100 percent of the DV for A in our multi because it's frequently praised for having immune-boosting antioxidant powers. But if you take that multi at breakfast with a bowl of fortified cereal and milk, you're likely to ingest more than your daily vitamin A requirement before you step out the door. Even small excesses of A have been linked to an increased risk of birth defects, liver problems, and nervous system disorders, as well as long-term bone damage that can eventually lead to hip fractures.

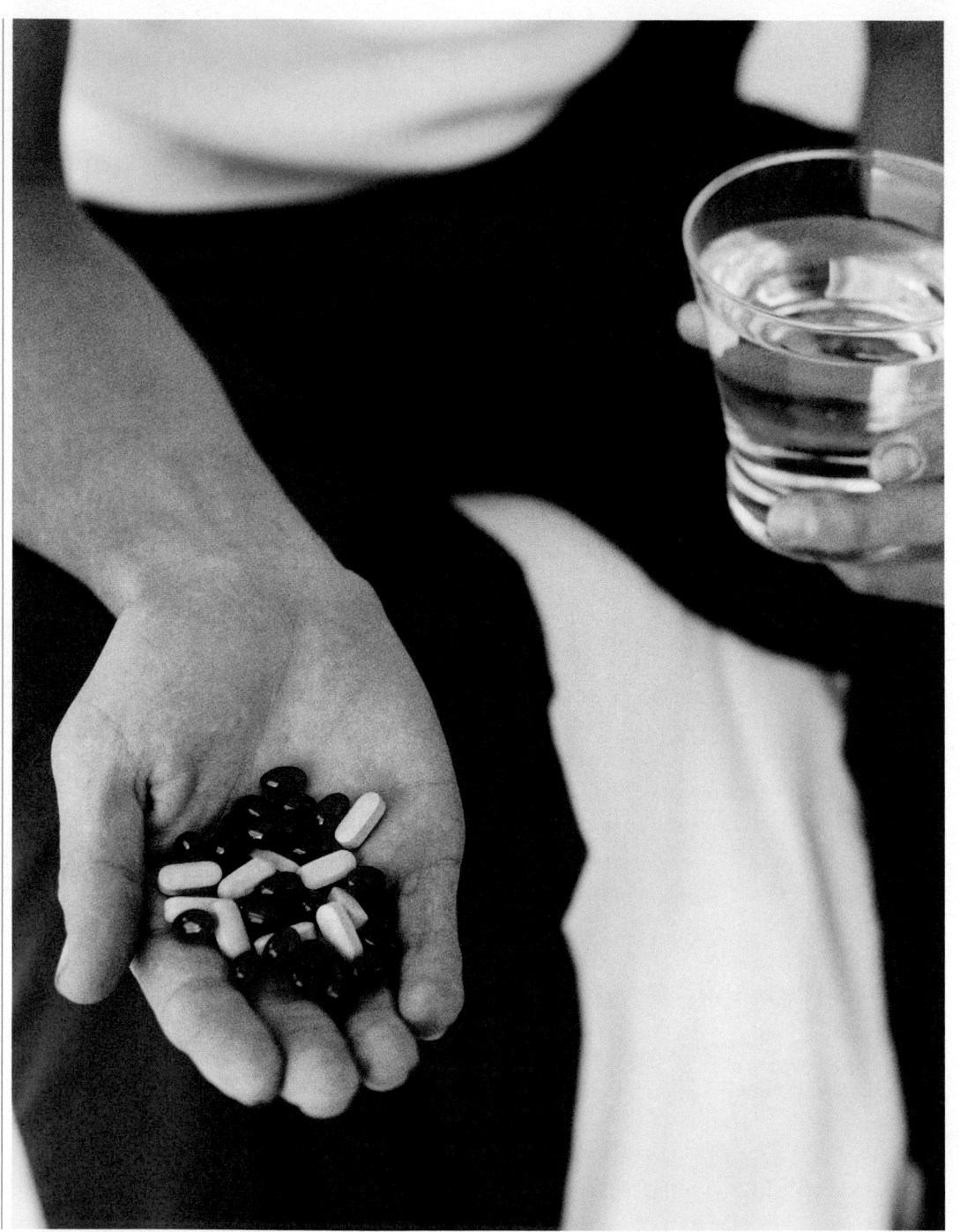

Yet regardless of how many fortified PowerBars you devour on top of your multivitamin, you're probably still not hitting the DRI for some other important nutrients. For example, 78 percent of women don't get enough calcium, and 50 percent need more vitamin D. That's partly because we tend to shy away from foods that contain both, namely dairy products, which we fear are fattening. But it's also because many multis don't contain much of these particular vitamins and minerals, so they fail to make up the difference.

What's a health-conscious girl to do? "Your best option is to take a multivitamin that doesn't deliver too much of the nutrients that are easy to come by—especially if they may be harmful [in large amounts]—and take additional vitamins and minerals to fill in gaps not covered by either your diet or the multivitamin," says Brent Bauer, M.D., director of the Complementary and Integrative Medicine Program at the Mayo Clinic. With the multitude of options out there (and knowing that the DV isn't really all that much help), how can you figure out which multivitamin is best for you? The good news is that you don't have to—we did all the work. See our pick for the best multi on page 108 and find out how to make it even better.

For more details on the best vitamins for your body, check out our supplement finder at womenshealthmag.com/vitamin.

TOTAL FITNESS GUIDE 2008

W|H

BONUS SECTION

THE BEST SUPPLEMENTS FOR WOMEN

What exactly should be in a multi, and which brands really deliver? We scoured the research to find optimal doses, then turned to Consumer Lab.com, a Web site that independently analyzes dietary supplements, to compare the quality of various options. *WH* pick for best multi: One-A-Day Women's. This classic brand's formulation adheres to the updated DRIs more closely than most other multis. It's right on the mark for most nutrients, gives you more of the ones you're missing (calcium, vitamins K and D), and provides less of the one you're likely to overdo (vitamin A).

But even the best multis can't stuff everything in (unless you want to choke down a pill the size of an egg), so you'll need to take additional supplements for some vitamins and minerals. Here's exactly what's in a One-A-Day Women's. We've listed our choices for best brands.

Add-Ons: One pill can't do it all. Maximize your multi with these top picks

Vitamin A 2,500 IU (50 percent DV), 20 percent as beta-carotene. The 100 percent DV of 5,000 IU is too much for women with relatively healthy diets, which is why One-A-Day Women's cut that amount in half. Most multis pack in too much A—typical doses range from 3,500 to 5,000 IU—and some provide even more. Part of One-A-Day's vitamin A comes

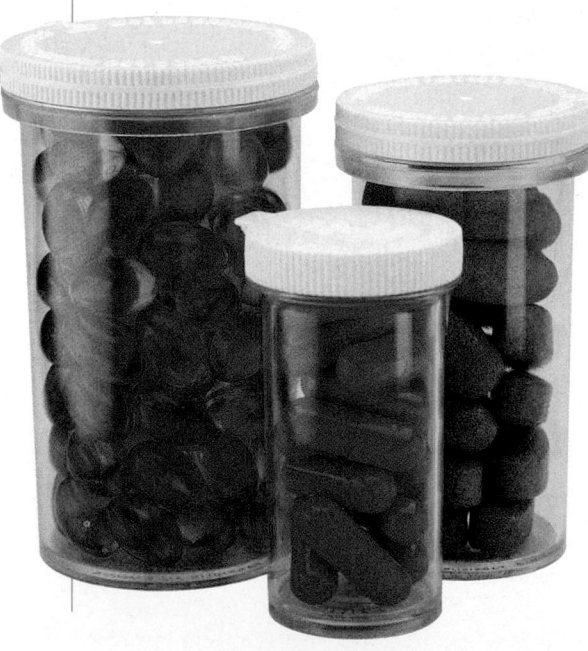

from beta-carotene, a compound that converts to A in the body, which is shown to be safer than straight-up A.

B vitamins (B_6, B_{12}, riboflavin, thiamin, and niacin) (100 percent DV for all except for 50 percent DV for niacin). Bs are in plenty of foods, especially vitamin-spiked cereals, so there's no need for more. (PMS relief claims aren't supported by research.)

Vitamin C 60 mg (100 percent DV). New research suggests the DV of 60 mg is not enough, but it's just fine for your multi. You'll get a lot more through food—one glass of OJ, for example, packs 120 mg of C.

Folic acid 400 mcg (100 percent DV). Between the amount found in this multi and fortified grains such as cereal and breads, you'll get all of the folic acid you need.

Vitamin D 800 IU (200 percent DV). Without D, your body can't absorb calcium. Because it's not in a lot of foods, it's hard to get through your diet, and too much of the other source—sunlight—can cause skin cancer. Several studies have shown that you need at least 600 IU (the DV is 400) combined with calcium to reduce fractures, which is why the 800 IU in One-A-Day Women's makes this multi stand out from the rest. Still consider taking an additional D supplement of 200 IU. You won't OD—the upper limit is 2,000 IU. WH pick: Nature Made Calcium with Vitamin D (200 IU vitamin D, 500 mg calcium).

Vitamin E 30 IU (100 percent DV). There's no evidence you need more than what's found here: Research has failed to prove that extra E protects against cardiovascular disease or cancer.

Vitamin K 25 mcg (31 percent DV). Vitamin K works with vitamin D and calcium to build bones, yet some multis leave K out altogether because it can interfere with blood-thinning drugs like coumadin that are used to treat heart disease. If you're at risk, you should check with your doctor before taking extra K. Women with healthy hearts, on the other hand, should probably add a supplement that contains about 100 mcg. WH pick: Puritan's Pride All Natural Vitamin K (100 mcg). Take it with your vitamin D pill at dinner. The fat in your food will boost absorption.

Calcium 450 mg (45 percent DV). This multi contains more calcium than most, which is another reason we love it. But you should still take 550 mg more at another point in the day—your body can absorb only 500 mg at a time. WH pick: Nature Made Calcium with Vitamin D (200 IU vitamin D, 500 mg calcium). Yes, it's the same as our vitamin D recommendation—just one pill takes care of both.

Magnesium 50 mg (13 percent DV). Most women don't get enough of this mineral that protects against heart disease, diabetes, and colon cancer—and multis, including One-A-Day Women's, don't provide much either. Aim to get to 320 mg a day with the help of another supplement. WH pick: Nature's Bounty Magnesium (250 mg). Take it with a meal—magnesium on an empty stomach can make you queasy.

Iron 18 mg (100 percent DV). Women tend to be low in iron, but the 18 mg here is enough: The body stores iron, and you don't want to hit the toxic level of 45 mg, which can cause diarrhea in the short term and problems like heart disease over time.

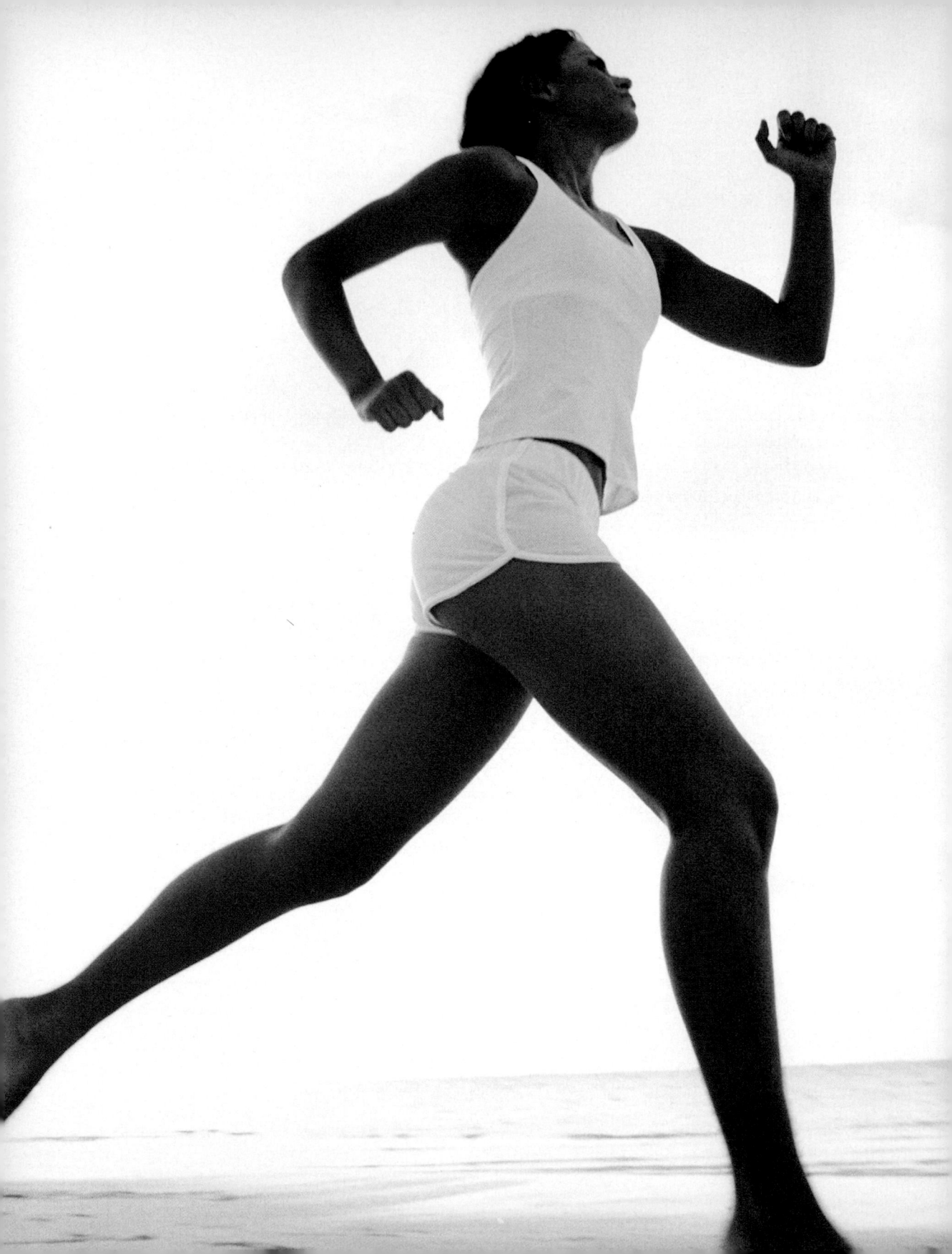

■ PART THREE

scale down, power up

It's time to take things personally! Designing a fat-burning workout plan that shapes your curves and balances your proportions is easier than you think. Here are some expert strategies to slim you down fast.

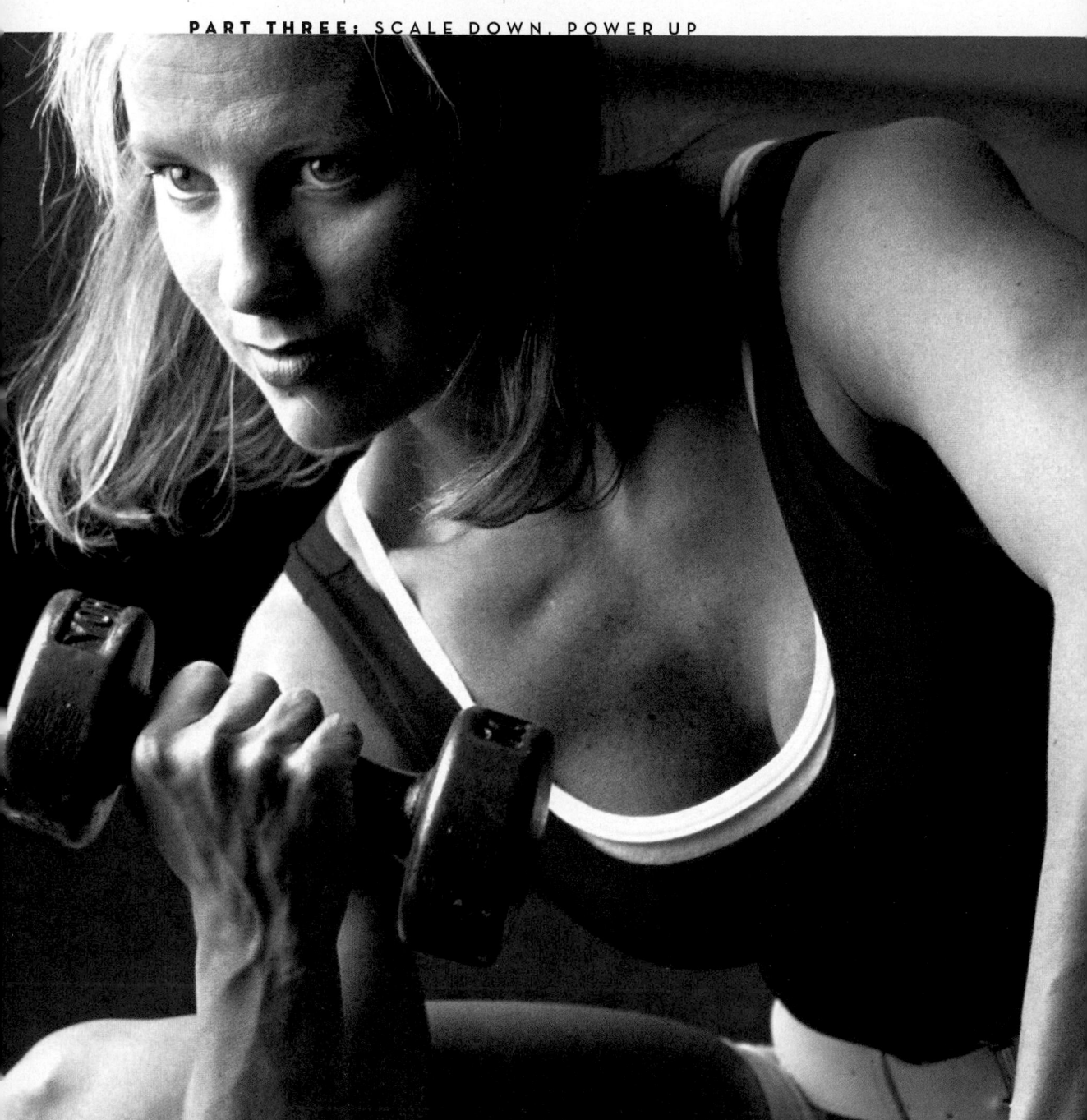

CHAPTER ELEVEN

BURN MORE CALORIES

USE WEIGHTS TO BOOST YOUR METABOLISM.

A GIRL NEEDS A GOAL—but once she has that goal, she needs a plan to carry it out. No matter what your size, this comprehensive exercise plan takes the guesswork out of getting in shape, allowing you to drop pounds and build muscle. An emphasis on weight training means you continue to burn calories after your workout. Follow our foolproof plan designed to sculpt the perfect body —and keep it that way for good.

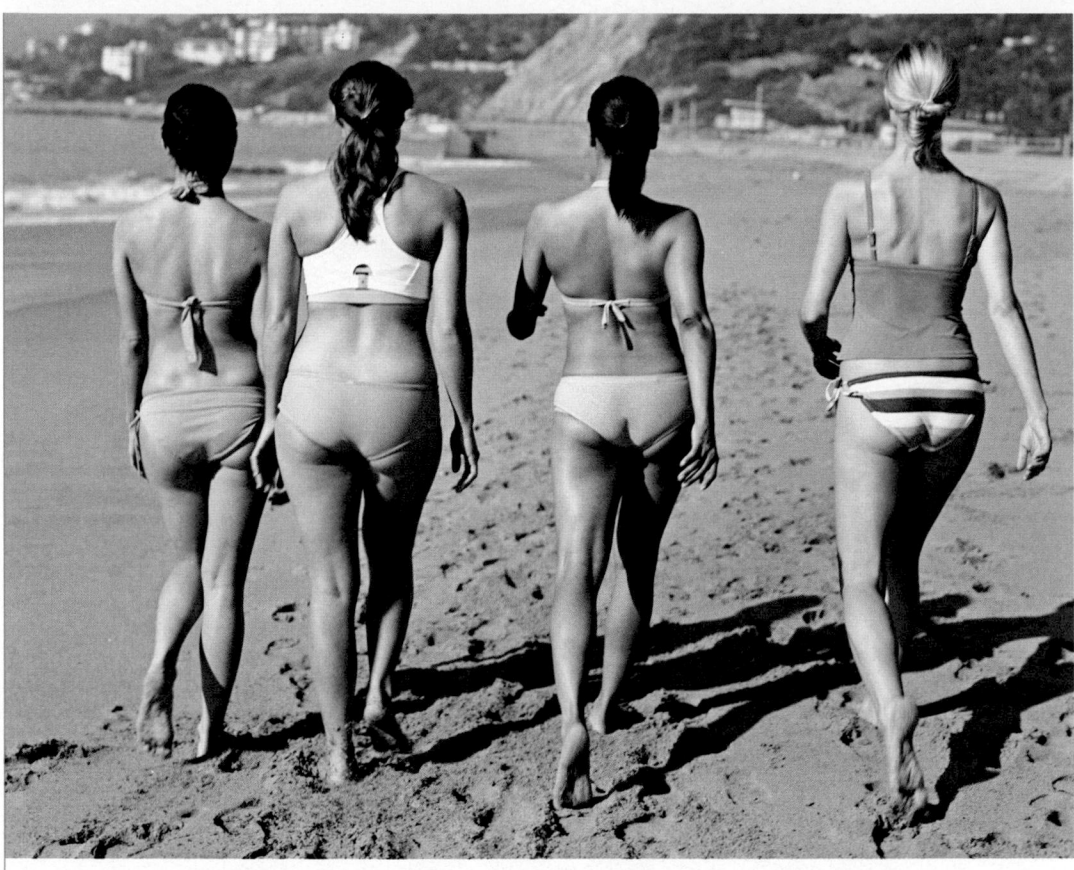

THE PLAN

To burn fat, do two to three sets of 15 repetitions of each exercise, with each rep taking 70 to 80 seconds. Do supersets of each group—that is, A1 followed by A2, back to A1 and A2, before moving on to B exercises, and so on. Rest 2 minutes after you finish the series, then complete the set with a dynamic cardio routine designed to burn maximum calories. As fast as you can, perform dynamic lunges and 24 (12 each leg) jump lunges, alternating them with 24 jump squats (see box on page 120). Rest the same amount of time it took you to complete the first set, then repeat. Time yourself and try to pick up your pace with each set. (If you're just beginning to work out, cut the number of repetitions in half and do only 12 of each.)

To add more muscle tone, increase your weight to one that makes 8 to 12 reps hard (you should not be able to do more than 12 reps) and decrease the length of each set to 40 to 70 seconds—the shorter, more intense sets have been shown to put your body in muscle-building mode. Do 10 to 15 repetitions of each exercise following the same superset guidelines. If you're trying to maintain your weight, cut back the routine to 2 days a week and aim for about 12 repetitions per exercise.

THE MOVES

A1 STEP UP

Place your right foot on the bench and your left foot on the floor. Pushing through with your right foot, lift your body up until you're standing on top of the bench. Do not allow your left leg to touch the bench. Pause, then repeat. Complete all reps for one side before changing legs. Use your body weight, then add dumbbells as you get stronger.

A2 DUMBBELL ROW WITH SINGLE LEG

Stand on your right leg and hold the dumbbell with your left arm. Bend over at the waist, pushing out your hips to keep your back flat. Bend your right leg and lean forward. With your left arm down by your side, fire your glutes and straighten your right leg, pulling your left elbow back and retracting your shoulder blades to row the weight.

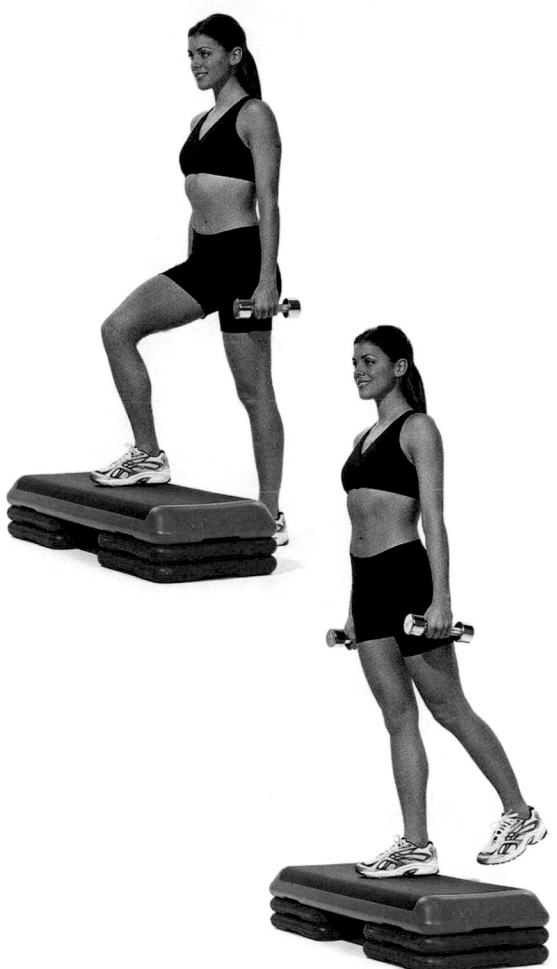

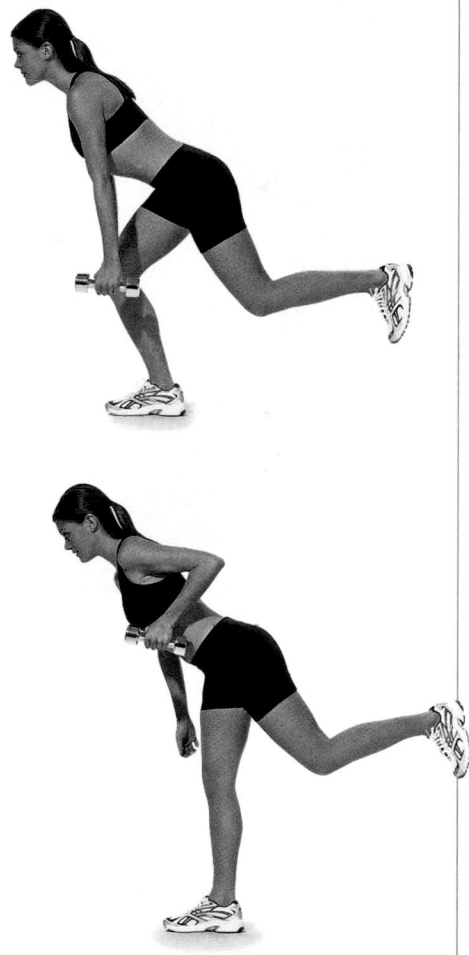

W|H

D1 SHE (SUPINE HIP EXTENSION)

Lie on the floor with your calves on a Swiss ball, arms out to your side. Push down on the ball with your feet, extending up from your hips until your feet, hips, and shoulders form a straight line. Slowly lower your hips to the starting position.

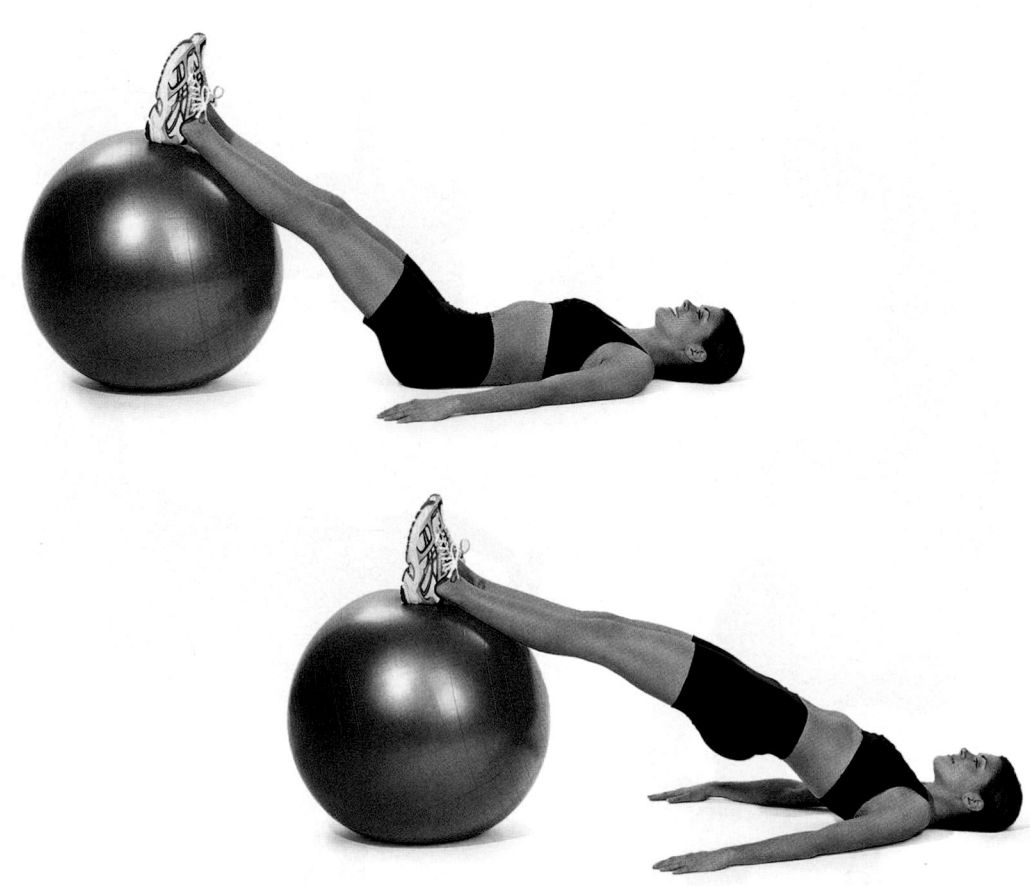

D2 LUNGE WITH OVERHEAD PRESS

Stand with your left foot on a step and your right foot a couple of feet in front of the step. With a dumbbell in your left hand, press your arm overhead as you drop your glutes into a lunge position. Return to start and repeat on the right side.

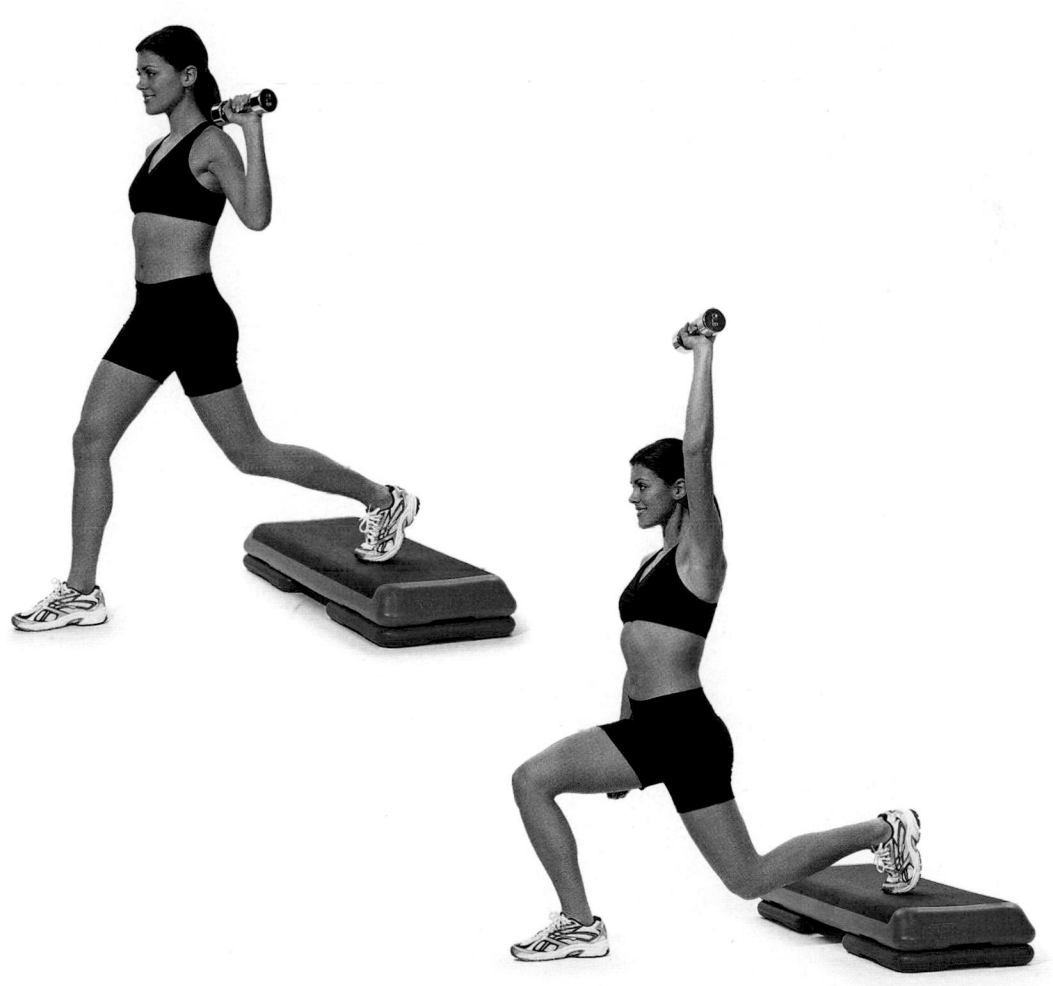

E1 SWISS BALL CRUNCH

Lie face up on a Swiss ball, with your navel at the center of the ball. Place your hands behind your head. From this position curl your torso up, pause, and then reverse into the fully stretched position. As you get stronger, hold a dumbbell directly under your chin.

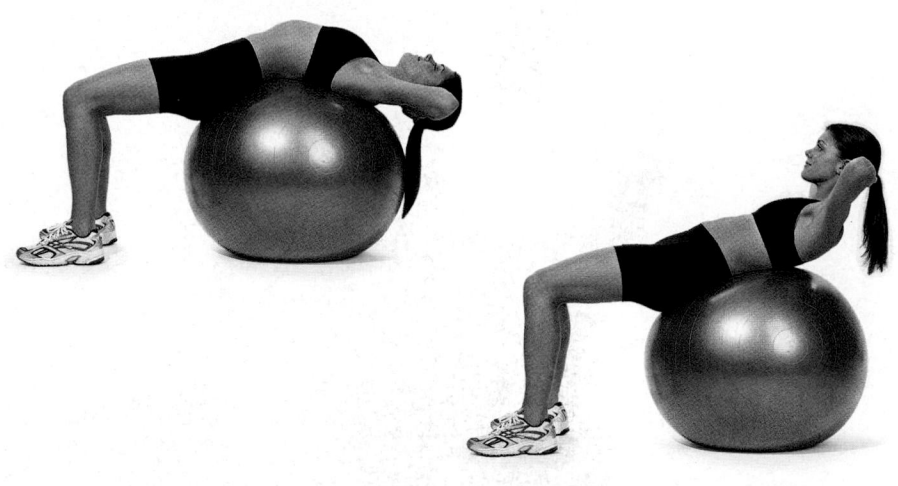

FAT-BURNING CARDIO

THIS ROUTINE PROVIDES A MUCH-NEEDED BREAK FROM THE TREADMILL

SQUATS

Stand with feet shoulder-width apart. Keep your back straight, contract your abs, and lower your hips while pushing your glutes out until you're in a seated position, keeping your knees aligned over your toes. Push up against the floor to return to a standing position.

E2 PRONE KNEE DRIVES

Place your feet on the floor and your hands on a Swiss ball. There should be enough space between the ball and your feet so that your spine is straight and you're in a pushup position. With arms straight, draw your belly button in and raise one knee toward your chest. Return to start. Repeat.

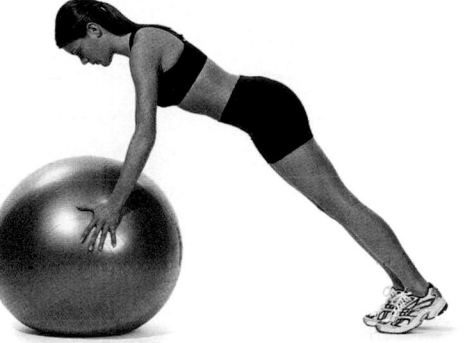 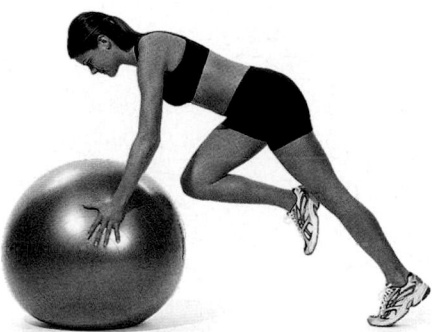

DYNAMIC LUNGES

These are your standard-issue lunges. Start with your legs together, shoulder-width apart, then step forward with your right leg, keeping your back straight, and lower your hips so that your right quad is parallel to the floor and your knee remains in line with your toes. Step back into startling position. Repeat with your left leg.

JUMP LUNGES

Start with a regular lunge, but instead of stepping back to center and stepping out with your left leg, immediately jump to a left-leg lunge once you're lunging with your right. Jump back and forth between legs, always keeping your back straight and your glutes low.

JUMP SQUATS

Finish off the circuit with 24 jump squats. After you reach the seated squat position, use power from your legs to jump up, then land in the seated squat position. Repeat all 24 in rapid succession.

RAISE THE BAR

BARBELL MOVES FOR A
LOOK-AT-ME SPRING BODY

STEPUP

WORKS CORE, GLUTES, HAMSTRINGS, AND QUADS

Grab a 10- to 15-pound barbell with an overhand grip and stand facing a 12-inch-high step. Carefully lift the barbell over your head and rest it across the tops of your shoulder blades, keeping your wrists in line with your elbows. Place your right foot on the step. Squeeze your glutes while you straighten your right leg and lift your left foot until your knee is at hip height. Lower your left foot onto the step. Step down with your left foot, then your right. Return to start and repeat, leading with your left leg.

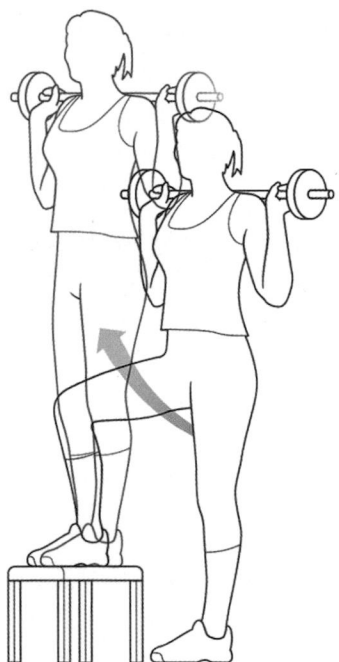

PUSH PRESS

WORKS SHOULDERS

Grab a 10- to 15-pound barbell with an overhand grip and stand with your feet slightly wider than your hips. Raise your hands toward your shoulders until the bar is an inch in front of them and your palms are facing forward. Do a quarter squat, then immediately push back up to standing while extending your arms straight overhead. Return the bar to shoulder level and repeat, starting with the squat.

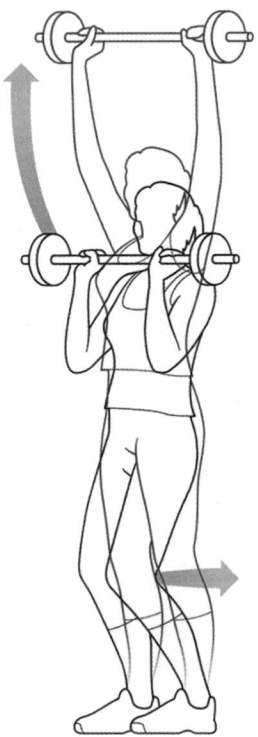

PULLOVER CRUNCH

WORKS ABS AND ARMS

Grab a 5- to 10-pound barbell with an overhand grip and lie on your back with your arms fully extended behind your head. Bend your knees and plant your feet hip-width apart on the floor. Contract your abs as you raise the bar with straight arms until it's directly above your chest. Then do a crunch, lifting only your shoulder blades off the floor. Lower your torso, then your arms.

Counteract your bar habit (be it chocolate covered or beer splattered) with the barbell. When you hoist a weighted bar instead of dumbbells, the poundage is distributed evenly across your body, says Jonathan Sexsmith, C.S.C.S., a personal trainer in New York City. This gives you a stabler base, so you can safely do more reps. To maximize fat burn, Sexsmith suggests this circuit: Warm up by jumping rope for 30 seconds. Then do 12 to 20 reps of each exercise, taking about 10 seconds to set up between moves. Repeat the circuit three times, resting 1 minute between sets.

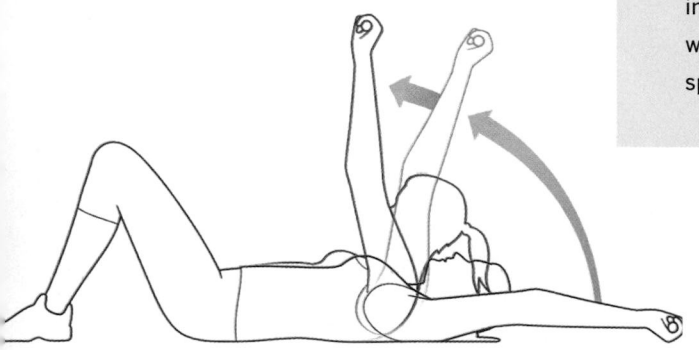

BELL BEHAVED

Use this three-point checklist to make sure your form is spot-on and avoid bar brawls that will land you in the doc's office.

1. **YOUR BACK**

   Form fix: Lift your chest and squeeze your shoulder blades together.

   Because: A rounded back and shoulders can compress your spine.

2. **YOUR HEELS**

   Form fix: As you squat, press your hips back as if you're hovering over a rest-stop toilet seat. Toes should point straight ahead. Focus on pressing down with the center of your feet.

   Because: If your heels rise off the floor as you lower your hips, weight gets shifted to the balls of your feet, straining joints—ankles, knees, hips, and back.

3. **YOUR WRISTS**

   Form fix: Make sure wrists are in line with your forearms and aren't bending forward or back. If you can't maintain this position, the weight is too heavy.

   Because: Flexing your wrist excessively in any direction while it is loaded up with weight can lead to upper-body sprains and strains.

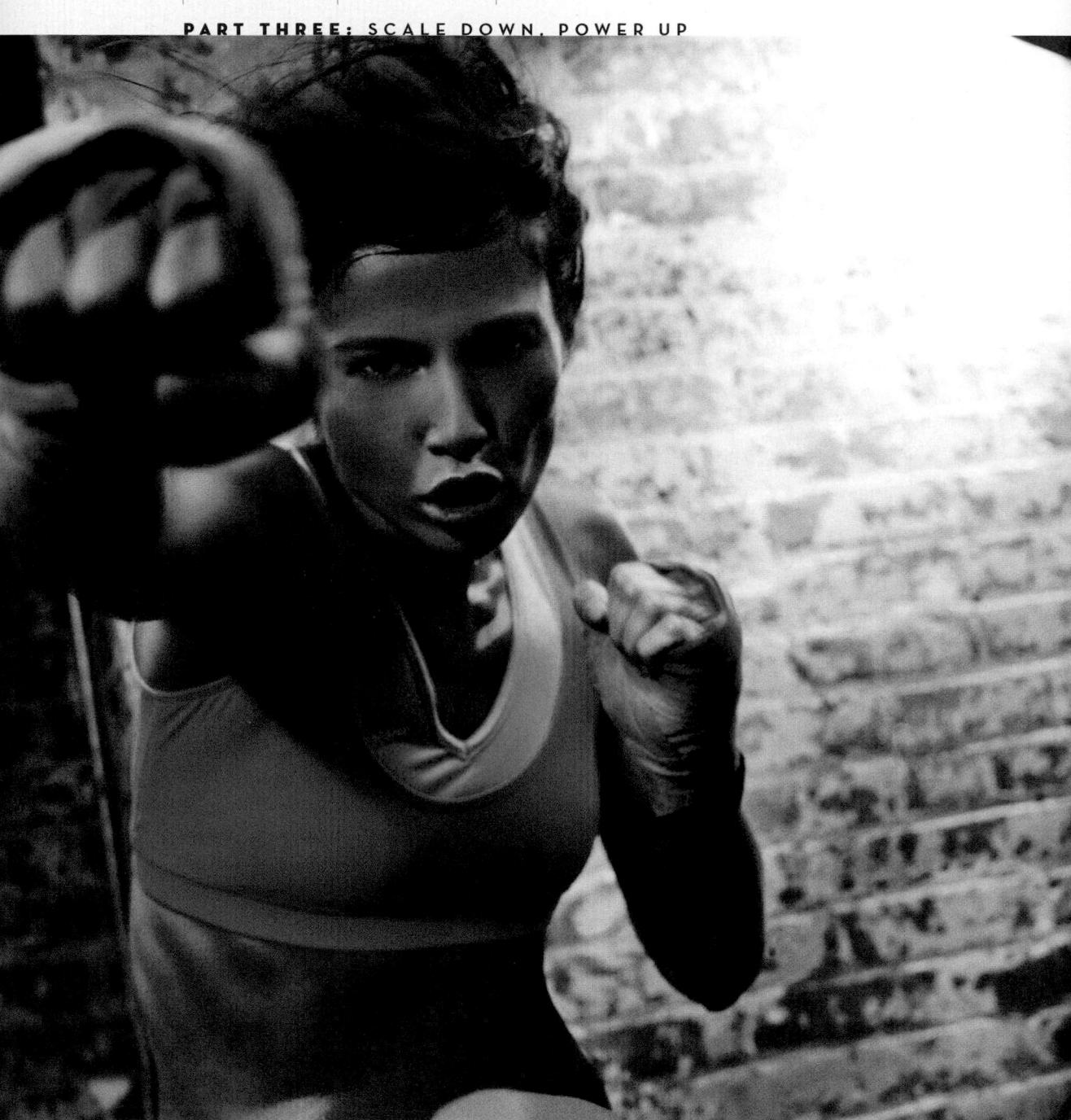

CHAPTER TWELVE

THE FAT-FRYING WORKOUT

SPEED UP YOUR METABOLISM AND TONE UP ALL OVER WITH THESE MOVES

ANY EXERCISE—be it for your arms, abs, or heart—is going to help make you leaner, stronger, and healthier. But only certain exercises can *really* burn fat fast. These moves, designed by Gregory Florez, spokesperson for the American Council on Exercise, torch extra calories because they work several major muscle groups at the same time. And when you combine them into one 30-minute workout, they tap your cardiovascular system, too, keeping your heart rate revved and your metabolism cooking.

Body Burners

Do two to three sets of 15 reps for each exercise. (Increase the reps or the weight when that gets too easy.) To keep your heart rate up, rest for only 45 seconds between sets.

STABILITY BALL BACK EXTENSION

WORKS BACK AND GLUTES

Lie facedown on a large stability ball so it supports your pelvis. Keep the balls of your feet on the floor and rest your hands at your sides. Next, tighten your glutes and gently lift your chest. Hold for 3 seconds, then lower back to start. If this is too easy, clasp your hands behind your head for more of a challenge.

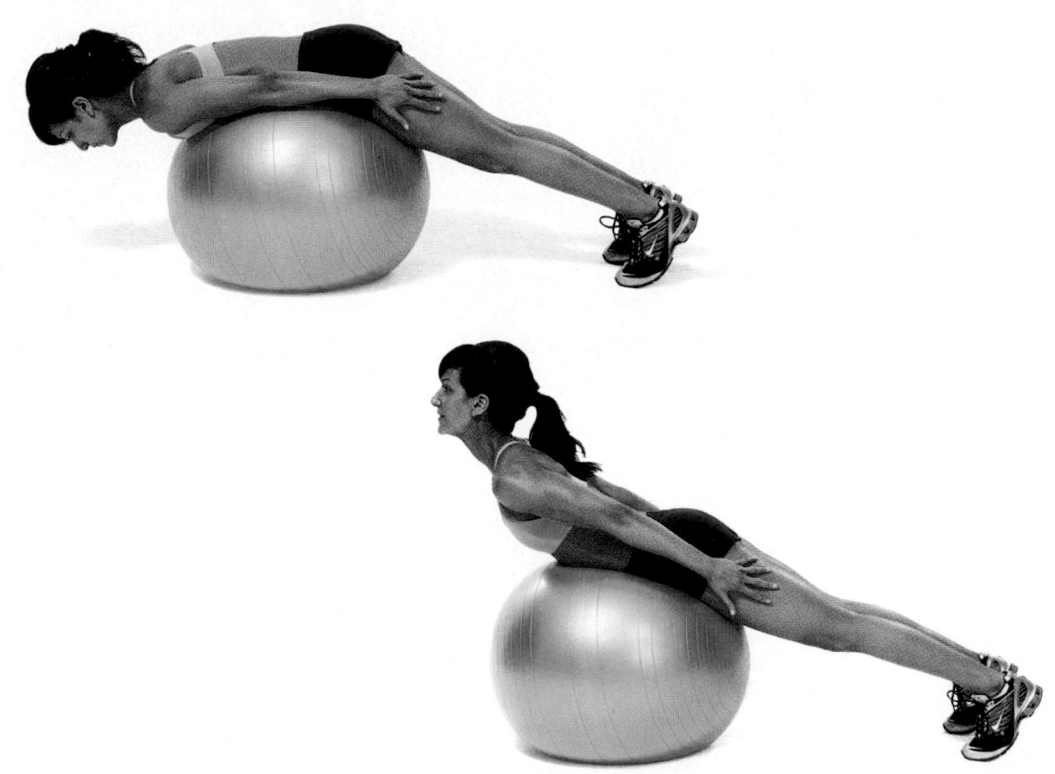

STANDING BODY BAR
SPLIT JUMP

WORKS LEGS AND HEART

Stand with your knees slightly bent, gently holding a
6- to 9-pound body bar at the back of your neck. Drop
your hips and jump slightly so that your right leg lands
about 3 feet in front of your left leg. Repeat with the
left leg. Work up to a total of 30 jumps. Start slowly
and don't sink all the way into a lunge.

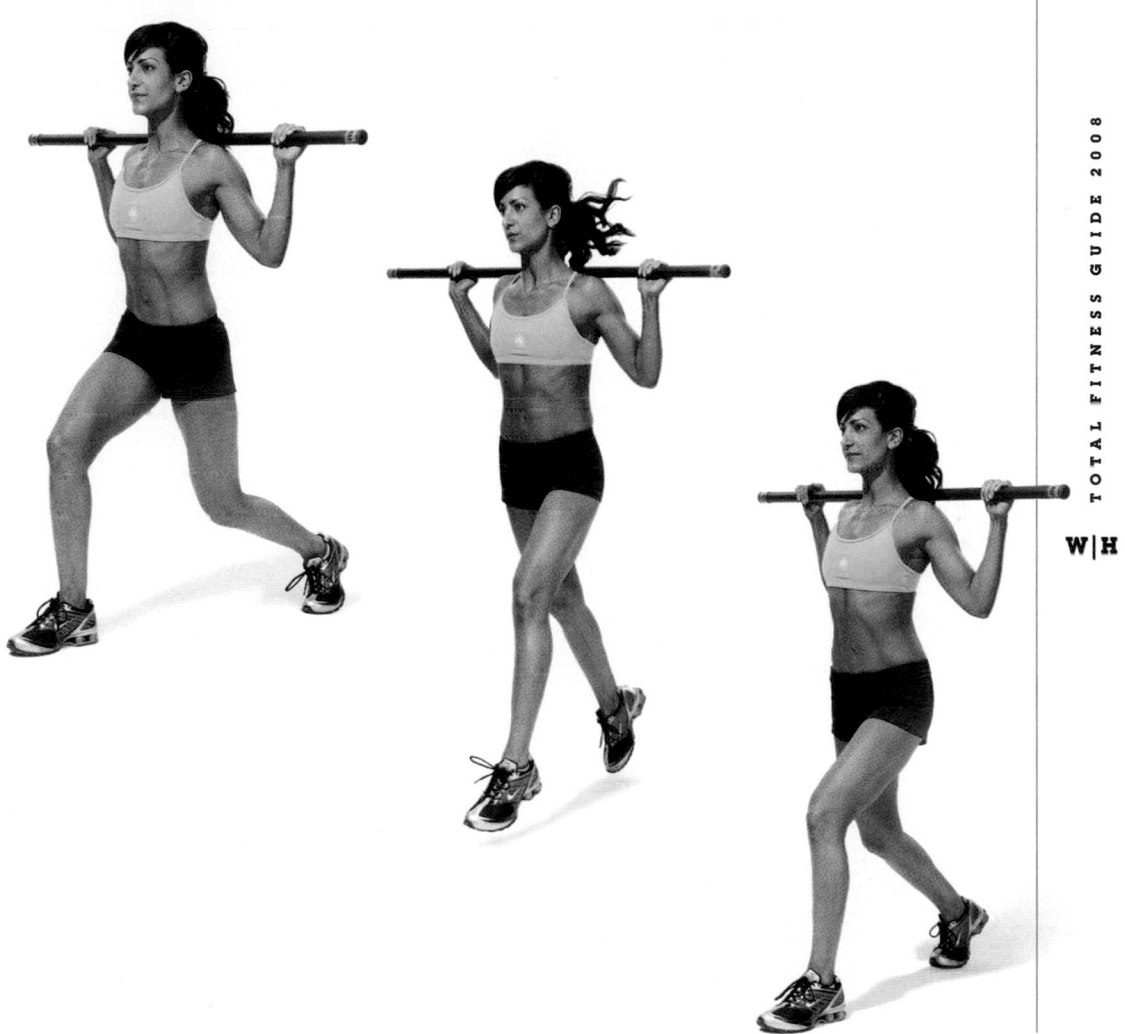

TOTAL FITNESS GUIDE 2008

W|H

WOBBLE BOARD BALANCE AND SIT

WORKS LEGS, CORE, GLUTES, AND LOWER BACK

Stand on a wobble board with your knees slightly bent and try to balance for 5 seconds. Next, lower your hips, keeping your back straight. If you can, lower enough to perform an actual squat and hold for another 5 seconds. Return to start and repeat. If balancing is too hard, try this move on a Bosu or foam pad first; once your body is more stable, return to the wobble board.

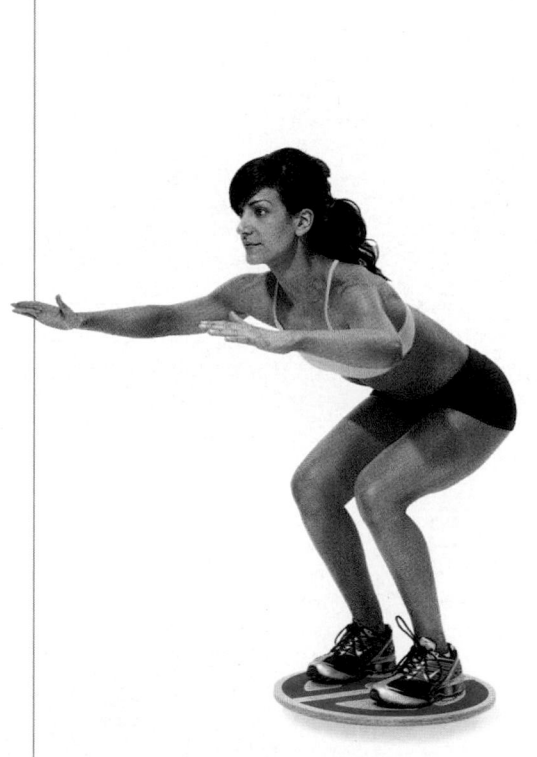
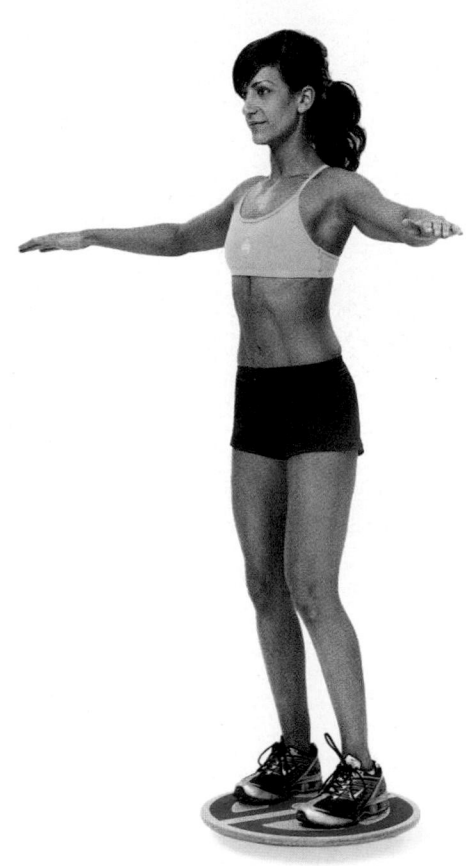

STABILITY BALL CHEST PRESS

WORKS CHEST, SHOULDERS, AND CORE

Grab a pair of 8- to 15-pound dumbbells. Lie on a stability ball (positioning it underneath your mid to upper back) with your feet flat on the floor, knees bent about 90 degrees, and abs pulled tight. Hold the dumbbells by your chest, palms facing forward, and press them straight up toward the ceiling. Lower the weights and repeat, using your abs to keep your body still.

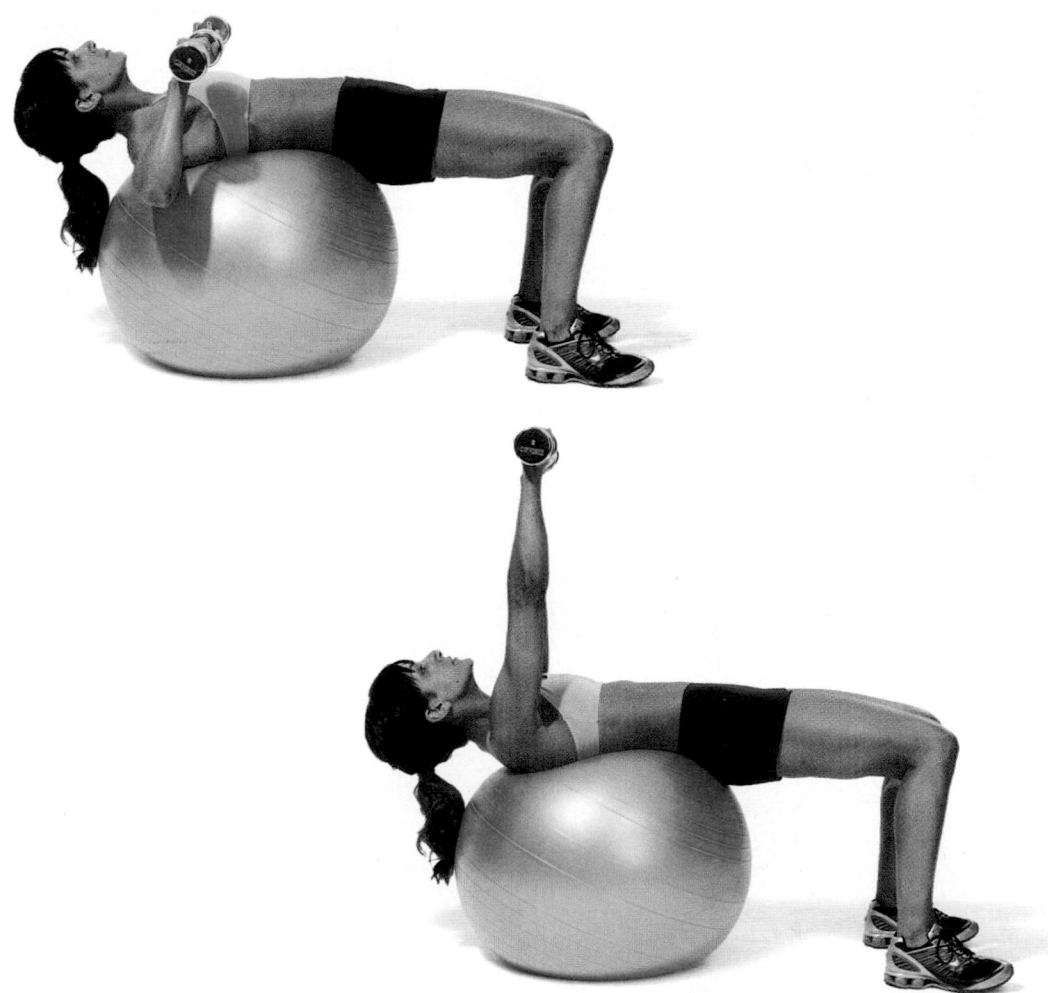

W|H

WEIGHTED BICYCLE CRUNCH

WORKS ABS AND THIGHS

Lie on your back with your knees bent. Hold a 5- or 6-pound medicine ball directly on your chest. Curl your upper body and right leg, and at the top of the crunch rotate your torso so that your left elbow meets your right knee. Extend your left leg at the same time, as if you're pedaling. Return to start and repeat on the other side.

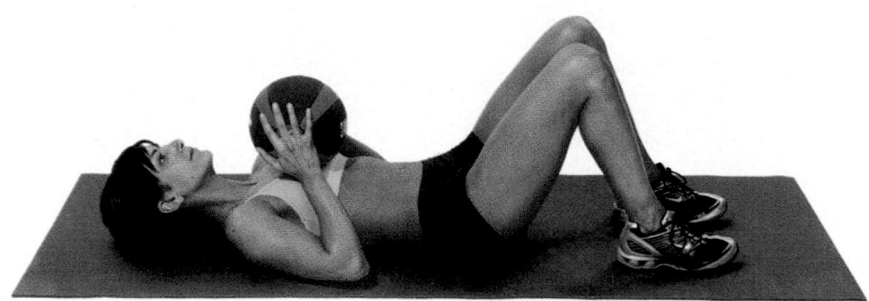

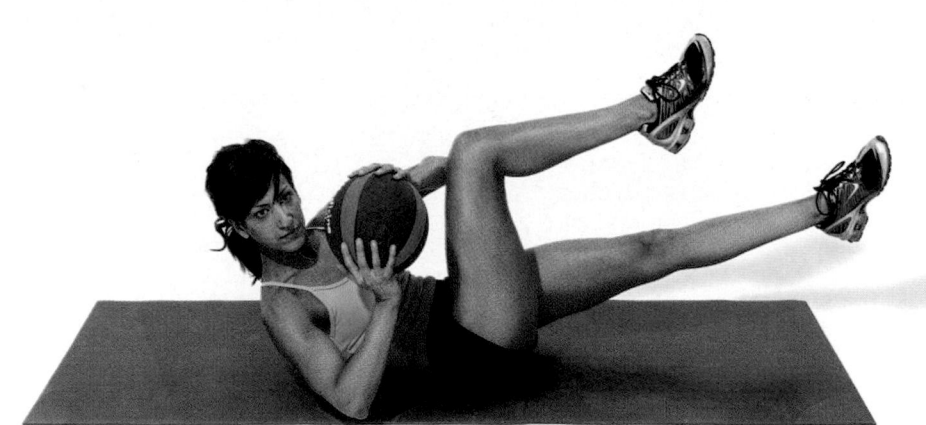

SEATED BALL STABILIZER

WORKS ABS, BACK, AND HIPS

Sit upright on a stability ball with legs hip-width apart and feet flat on the floor. Slowly lower your torso about 6 inches forward, keeping your back straight. Tighten your glutes as you lower and return to start. Then, keeping your abs tight, slowly lift your right leg off the floor. Hold for 3 to 4 seconds and release. That's one rep. Repeat the whole sequence, lifting your left leg next. Alternate until you complete your set.

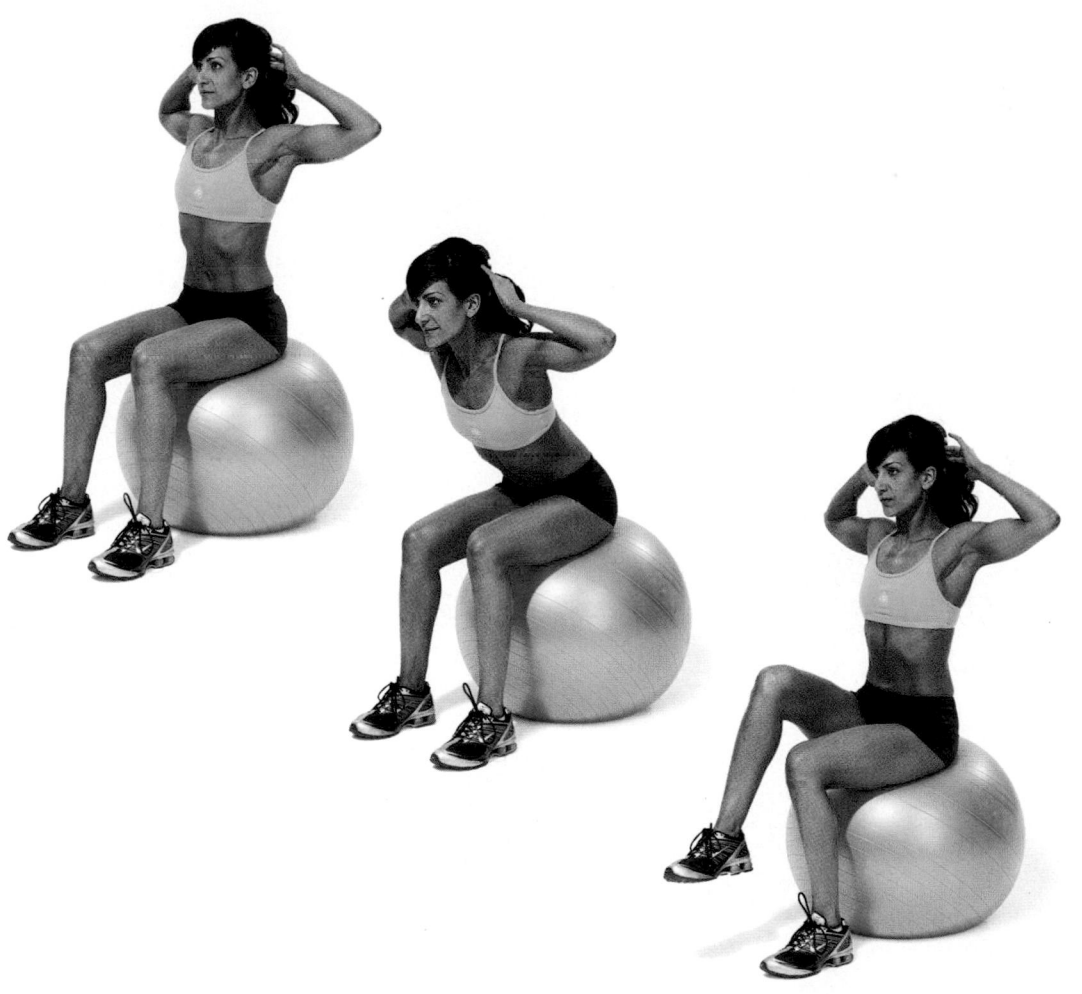

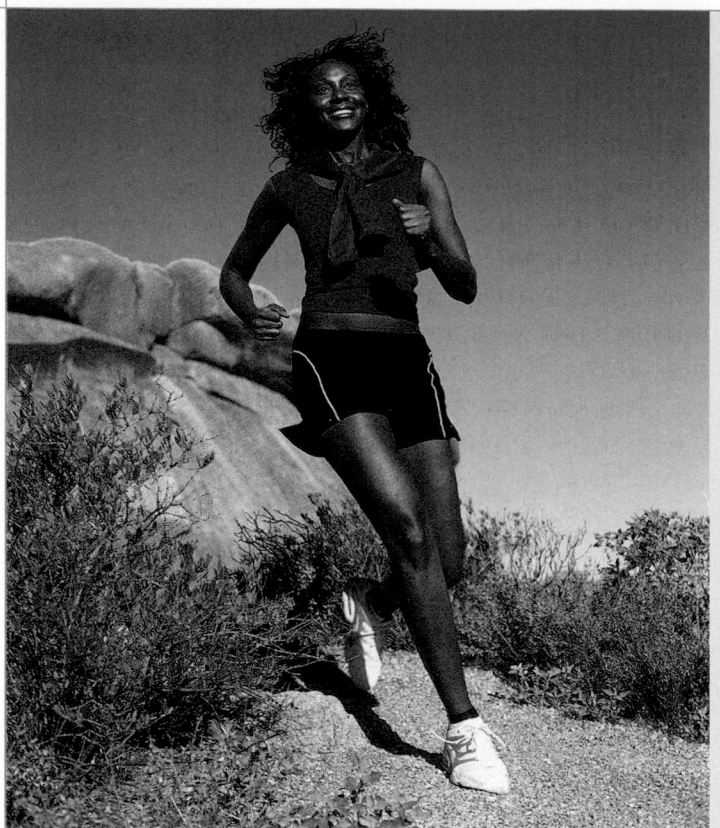

WALK AWAY: HOW TO POWER UP YOUR PACE

Long, low-intensity cardio sessions with more intense intervals are a surefire way to burn fat (it takes at least 30 minutes of continuous aerobic exercise to really dip into your fat stores; the longer you go the better), and walking is the easiest way to do it. Plus, daily walking has less risk of overuse injuries than more intense activities. Use these three items to get the most out of your strides.

PEDOMETER

Studies have shown that pedometers can help motivate because they hold you accountable and keep your goals visible. The New-Lifestyles NL-2000 pedometer ($65, new-lifestyles.com) not only monitors your steps, it also tallies the total number of calories you burn each day. Plus, it can determine your basal metabolic rate based on your input (your age, gender, height, and weight), so you'll know how many calories you burn at rest.

WEIGHTED VEST

It adds a strength-training component to your walk, so you're forced to work harder and burn more calories. We like the Resistance Wear F2PRO weighted vest ($80, resistancewear.com) because it looks like a sports bra instead of a bubbled life preserver. The removable ½-pound weights are nearly invisible. Each vest comes with 4 pounds, but it can hold up to 10.

STURDY SHOES

Tired feet will shorten your workout, so wear ultrasupportive sneakers. The Nike Air Max Imum walking shoes ($80, nike.com) are built with extra cushioning (that's not too squishy) to comfort your feet during long-distance jaunts. A special stabilizing rail system allows your foot to rock easily from heel to toe during every mile.

SIDE STEPUP WITH TRICEPS KICKBACK

WORKS THIGHS, CORE, AND TRICEPS

Stand sideways next to a step, holding 5- to 8-pound dumbbells with arms in a relaxed position and elbows slightly behind your body. Next, step laterally onto the step. At the top of the step, tighten your abs and lean forward slightly. Press the dumbbells behind you and straighten your arms. One stepup and press counts as one rep. Step down and repeat for a complete set before switching sides.

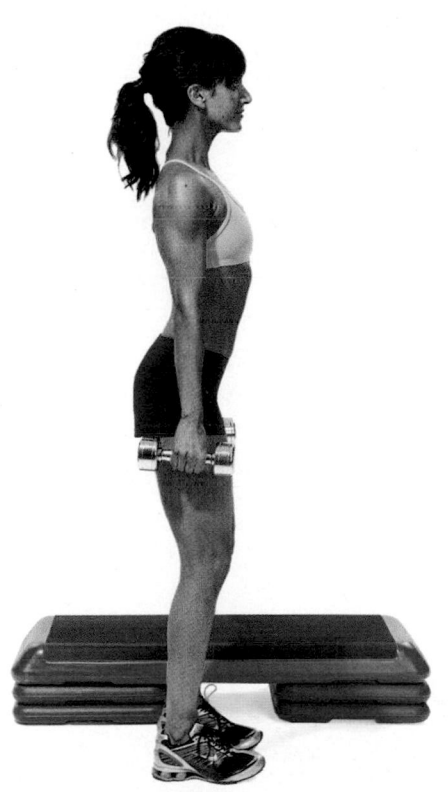

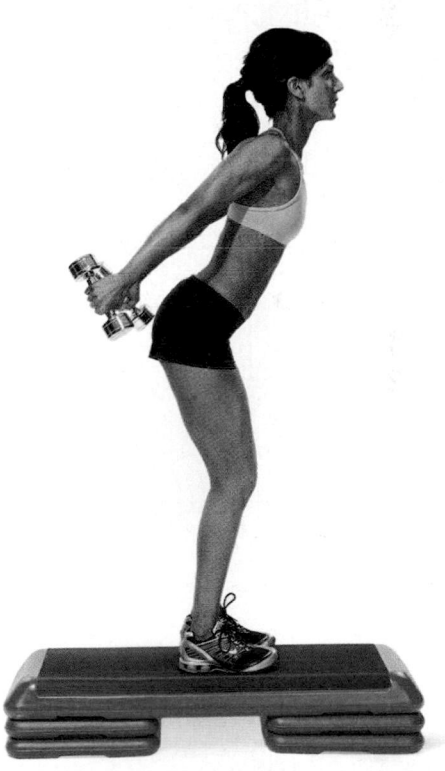

TOTAL FITNESS GUIDE 2008

W|H

TRAVELING LUNGE WITH BICEPS CURL AND SHOULDER PRESS

WORKS LEGS, BICEPS, AND SHOULDERS

Holding a pair of 5- to 10-pound dumbbells, step forward with your left leg into a lunge. Make sure that your left thigh is parallel to the floor, keeping your knee behind your toes. Curl the dumbbells to your chest as you sink down, and as you rise, rotate your wrists so that your palms face forward and press the dumbbells overhead when you are in the standing position. Bring your feet together. Then repeat, stepping your right leg forward. Do one set (two if you're fit).

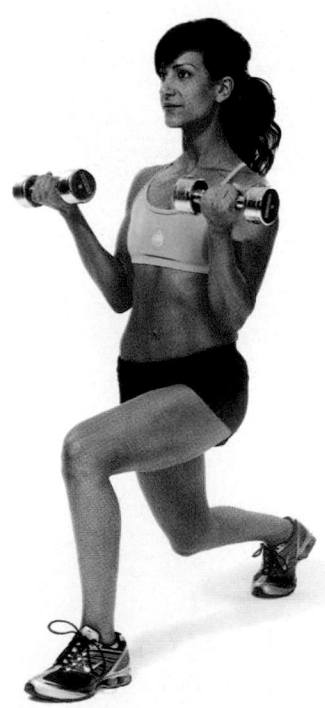
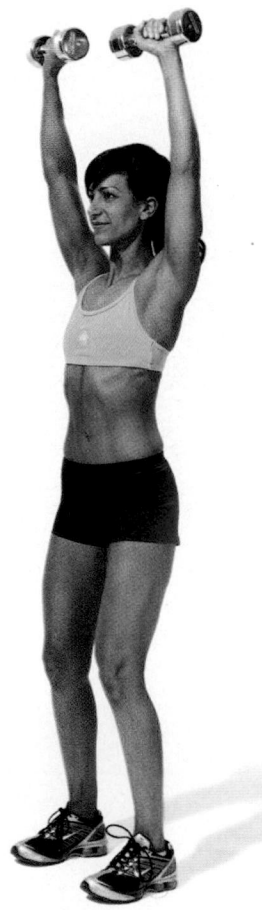

BONUS SECTION

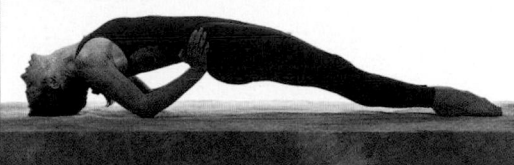

FRY FAT ON THE MAT

TO LOSE WEIGHT, ADD HEART-REVVING YOGA TO YOUR ROUTINE

Maybe you contort into all kinds of wacky positions wriggling into those skinny jeans, but you should save the bending and twisting for your workout. An active sequence of yoga flows—a form called vinyasa—burns more than 450 calories an hour, according to Sara Ivanhoe, host of *20-Minute Yoga Makeover: Weight Loss*. (To bust your belly yoga style, see Chapter 26.)

FLOW 1 CHAIR POSE

TARGET LOWER BODY

1. BACKBEND

Stand with your feet hip-width apart. Lace your fingers behind you (palms facing up). Inhaling, bend from your upper back, lift your chest, and press your shoulders down.

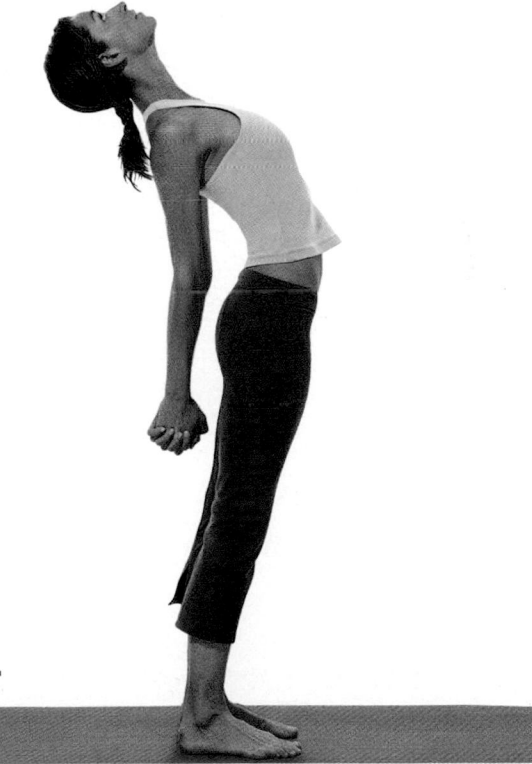

1.

W|H

2. FORWARD BEND

Soften your knees and bend forward as you exhale, letting your torso hang in front of your thighs. Keeping your arms straight and fingers locked together, lift them up and over your head (ultimately reaching toward the floor in front of your feet).

3. CHAIR

Inhale and bend your knees into a squat. Unlock and straighten your fingers, then separate your arms. When your thighs are nearly parallel to the floor, move your arms toward your ears. Keep your weight on your heels. Inhale, stand up, and lower your arms to your sides. Exhale.

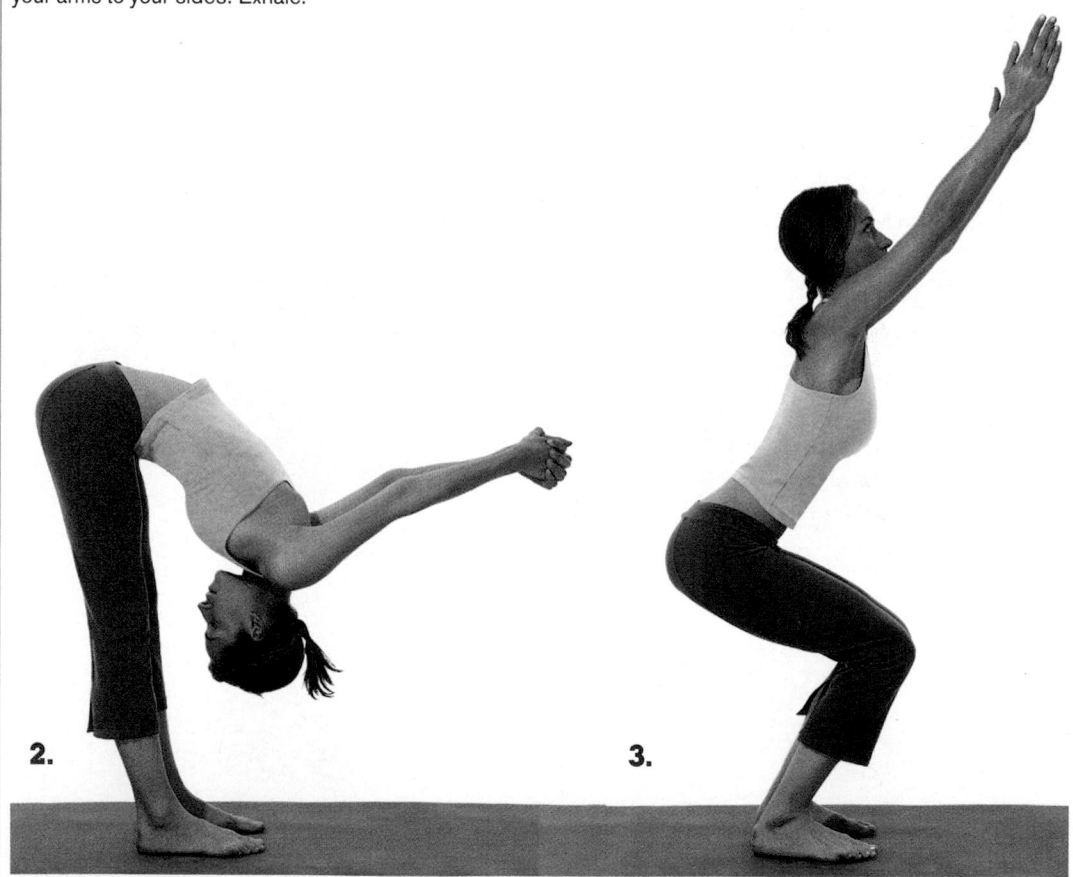

2.

3.

FLOW 2 DOG POSE

TARGET UPPER BODY

1. DOWNWARD-FACING DOG

Get on all fours, lift your hips, and straighten your arms and legs.

2. PLANK

Inhale as you shift forward into the top of a pushup position with your arms straight. Exhale, bend your elbows (keep them pointing back and hugging your body), and lower your body until your chest is on the ground.

3. COBRA

Uncurl your toes so the tops of your feet are touching the ground and press your tailbone down. Hug your elbows in as you inhale, straighten your arms (keep a slight bend), and lift your chest off the ground. Exhale as you gently release your body back to the ground. Inhale, curl your toes under, and press your hips up and back into downward-facing dog. Exhale.

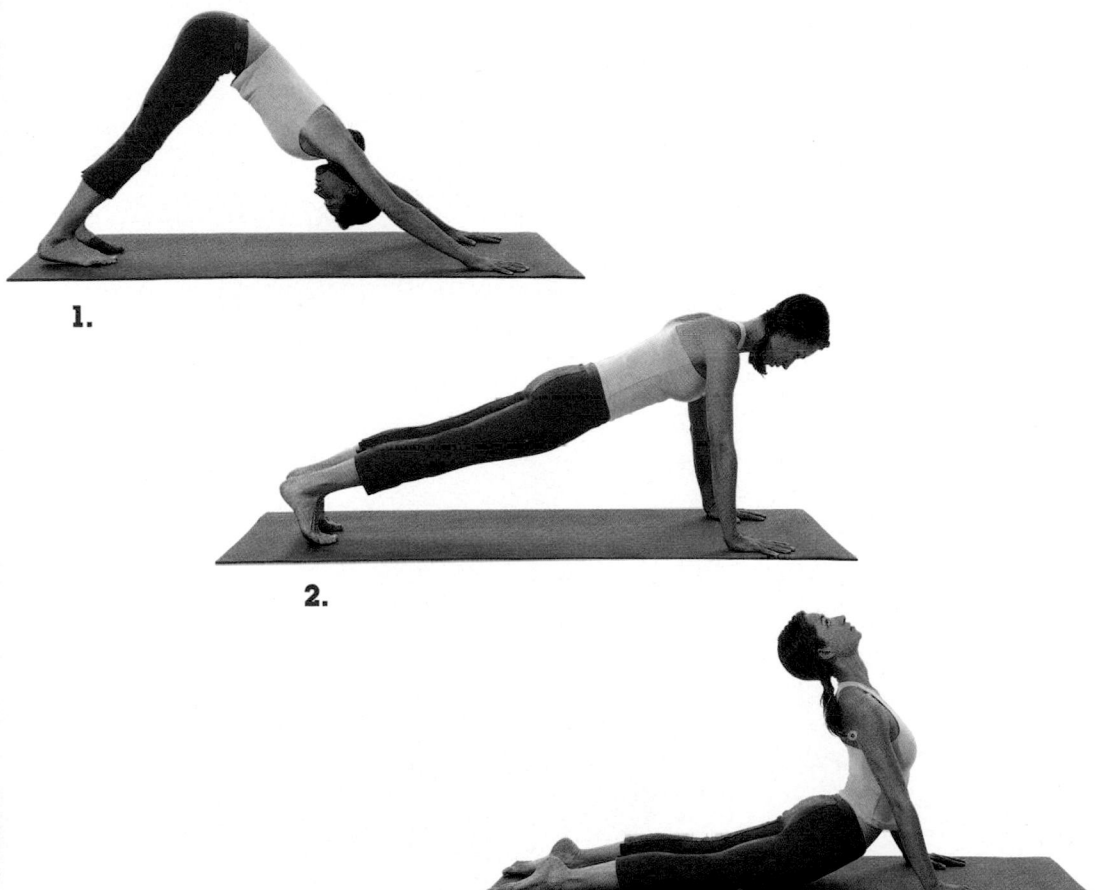

1.

2.

3.

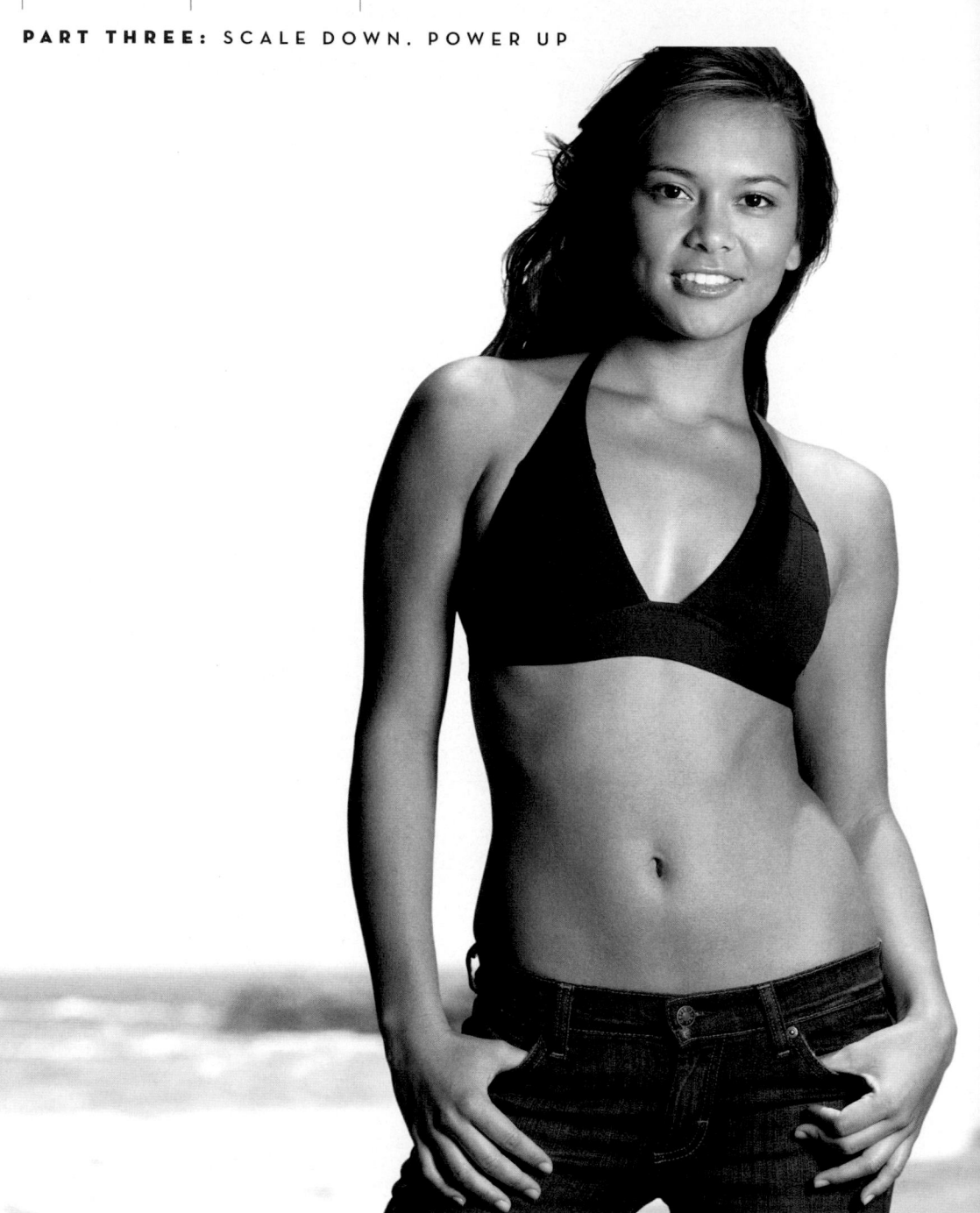

CHAPTER THIRTEEN

MIDDLE
MANAGEMENT

YOU HAVE ABS–UNCOVER THEM TODAY
WITH THESE 10 MIDSECTION MOVES.

TOTAL FITNESS GUIDE 2008

W|H

IT'S SIMPLE: To show off your abs, you have to burn fat. To burn fat, you have to stoke your metabolism by building muscle. Replacing just 1 pound of fat with muscle will force your body to fry up to an additional 50 calories a day. These straightforward moves work major muscle groups—with an emphasis on your midsection—without adding bulk. (To get truly awesome abs in the comfort of your own home, try the moves in Chapter 25.)

DO THIS WORKOUT THREE TIMES A WEEK.
Complete 1 set of each ab exercise (designed
to work key regions of your core: upper abs,
lower abs, obliques, and lower back), then do
the rest of the circuit twice. On other days, do
light cardio like swimming, walking, or cycling.
Make sure you take 1 day completely off. Find a
weight you're comfortable lifting—not too easy,
but not one that tortures your body either. And
get pumped! You'll be in Tiny Town in no time.

EXERCISE	REPETITIONS	REST	SETS
Medicine Ball Blast	12 to 15	None	1
Seated Ab Crunch	12	None	1
Saxon Side Bend	6 to 10 each side	None	1
Back Extension	12 to 15	None	1
Squat	10 to 12	30 sec	2
Pulldown	10	30 sec	2
Leg Curl	10 to 12	30 sec	2
Military Press	10	30 sec	2
Triceps Pushdown	10 to 12	30 sec	2
Biceps Curl	10	30 sec	2

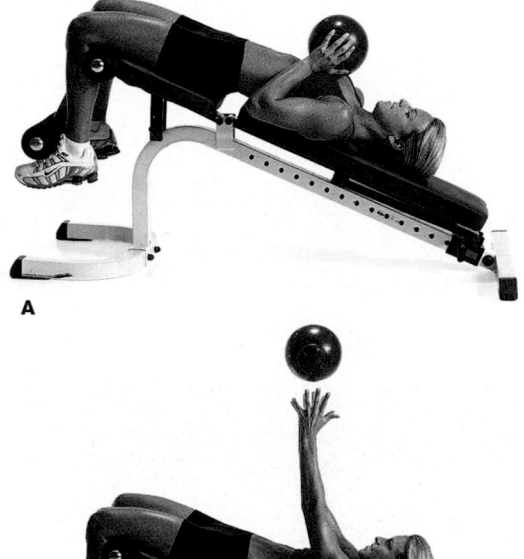

A

B

MEDICINE BALL BLAST

Set an adjustable ab bench at a 45-degree angle.
Lie down on it with your head toward the floor and
hook your feet under the padded support bar. Hold a
medicine ball at your chest as you lower yourself (**A**).
As you come up, chest-pass the ball straight up (**B**).
Catch it at the top of the movement, then lower
yourself and repeat.

SEATED AB CRUNCH

Sit on the edge of a stable chair or bench. Place your hands next to your butt and grip the front of the seat. Lean back slightly and extend your legs down and away, keeping heels 4 to 6 inches off the floor (**A**). Bend your knees and slowly raise your legs toward your chest. At the same time, lean forward with your upper body, allowing your chest to approach your thighs (**B**).

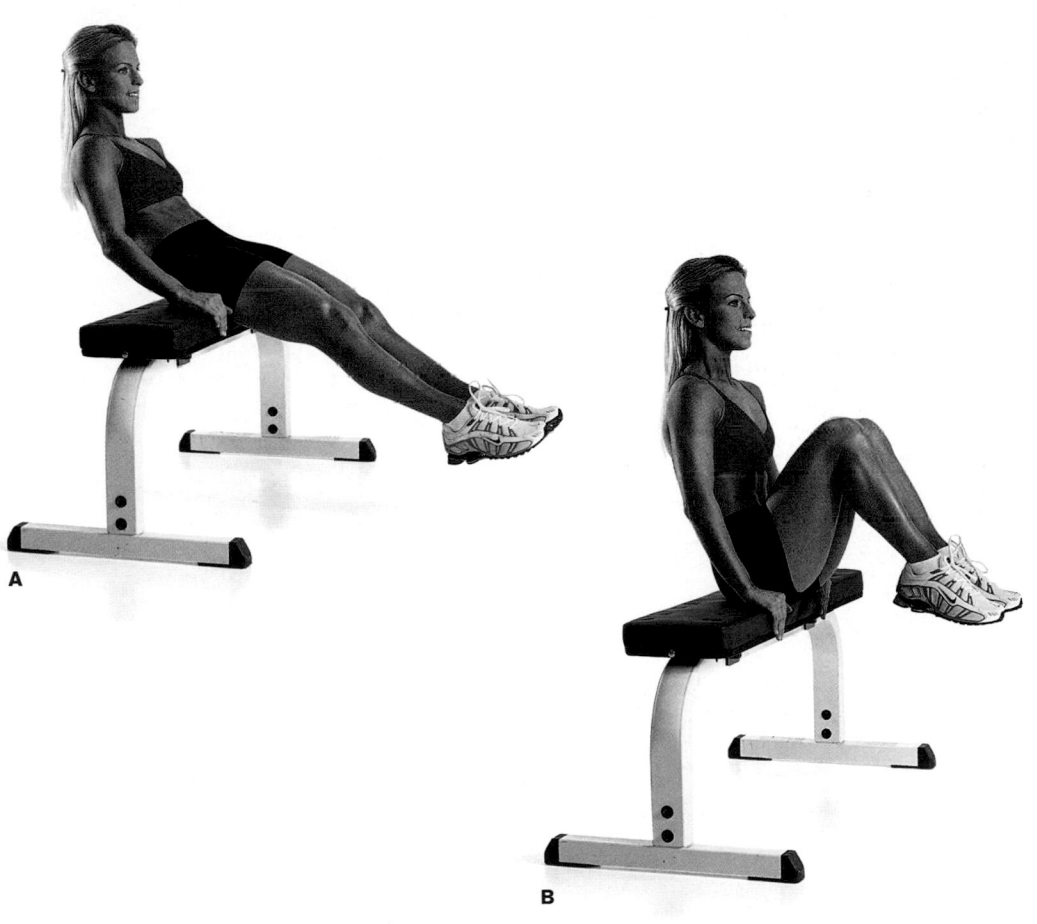

W|H

SAXON SIDE BEND

Hold a pair of lightweight dumbbells over your head, with your elbows slightly bent (**A**). Keep your back straight and slowly bend directly to your right as far as possible without twisting your upper body (**B**). Pause, return to an upright position, then bend to your left as far as possible.

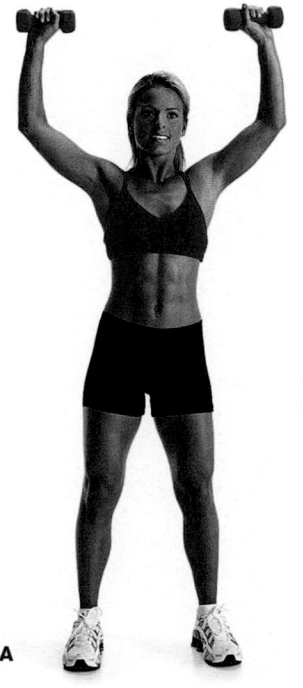

A

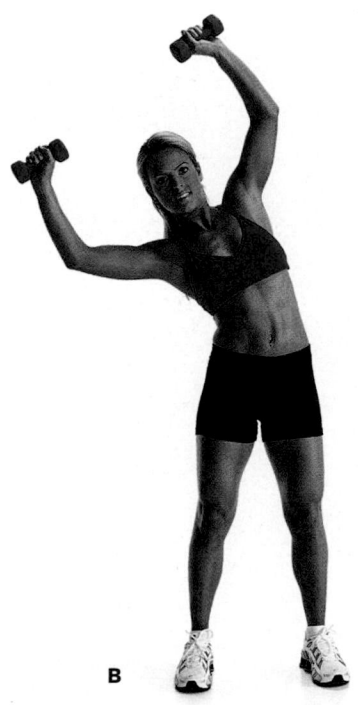

B

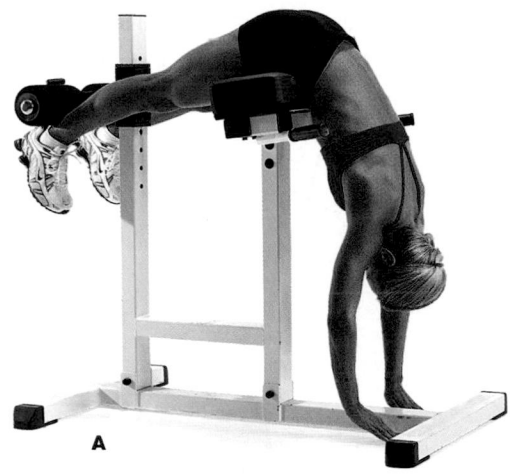

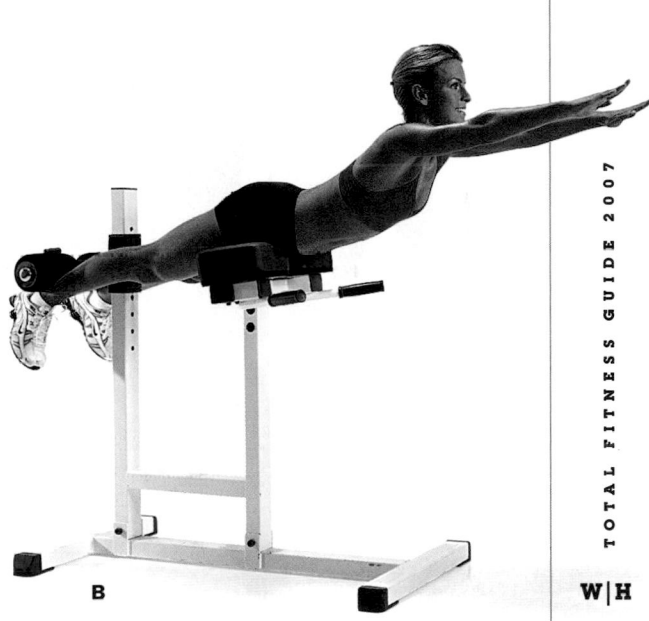

BACK EXTENSION

Position yourself in a back extension station and hook your feet under the leg anchor. Hold your arms straight out in front of you. Your body should form a straight line from your hands to your hips. Lower your torso, allowing your lower back to round, until it's just short of perpendicular to the floor (**A**). Raise your upper body until it's slightly above parallel to the floor (**B**). At this point, you should have a slight arch in your back, and your shoulder blades should be pulled together. Pause for a second, then repeat.

LEG CURL

Lie facedown on a leg curl machine and hook your ankles under the padded bar (**A**). Keeping your stomach and pelvis against the bench, slowly raise your feet toward your butt, curling the weight up (**B**). Come up so that your feet nearly touch your butt and slowly return to start.

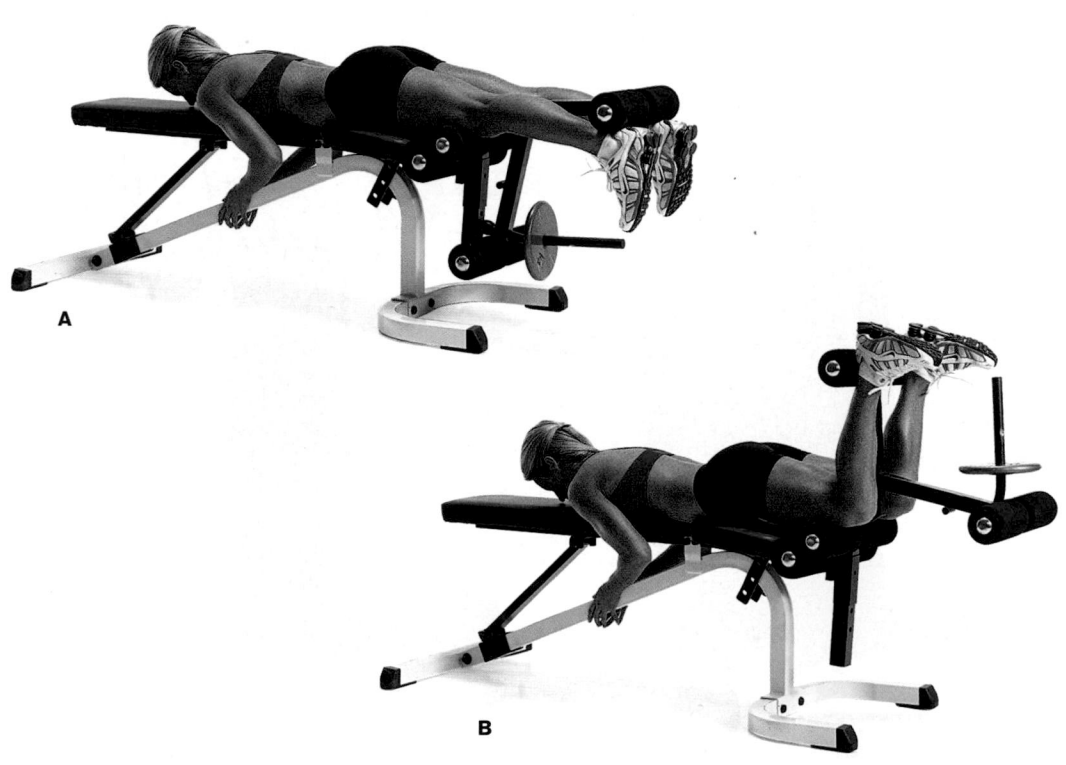

A

B

MILITARY PRESS

Sitting on an exercise bench, hold a barbell at shoulder height with your hands shoulder-width apart (**A**). Press the weight straight overhead so that your arms are almost fully extended (**B**). Hold for a second, then bring it down in front of your shoulders.

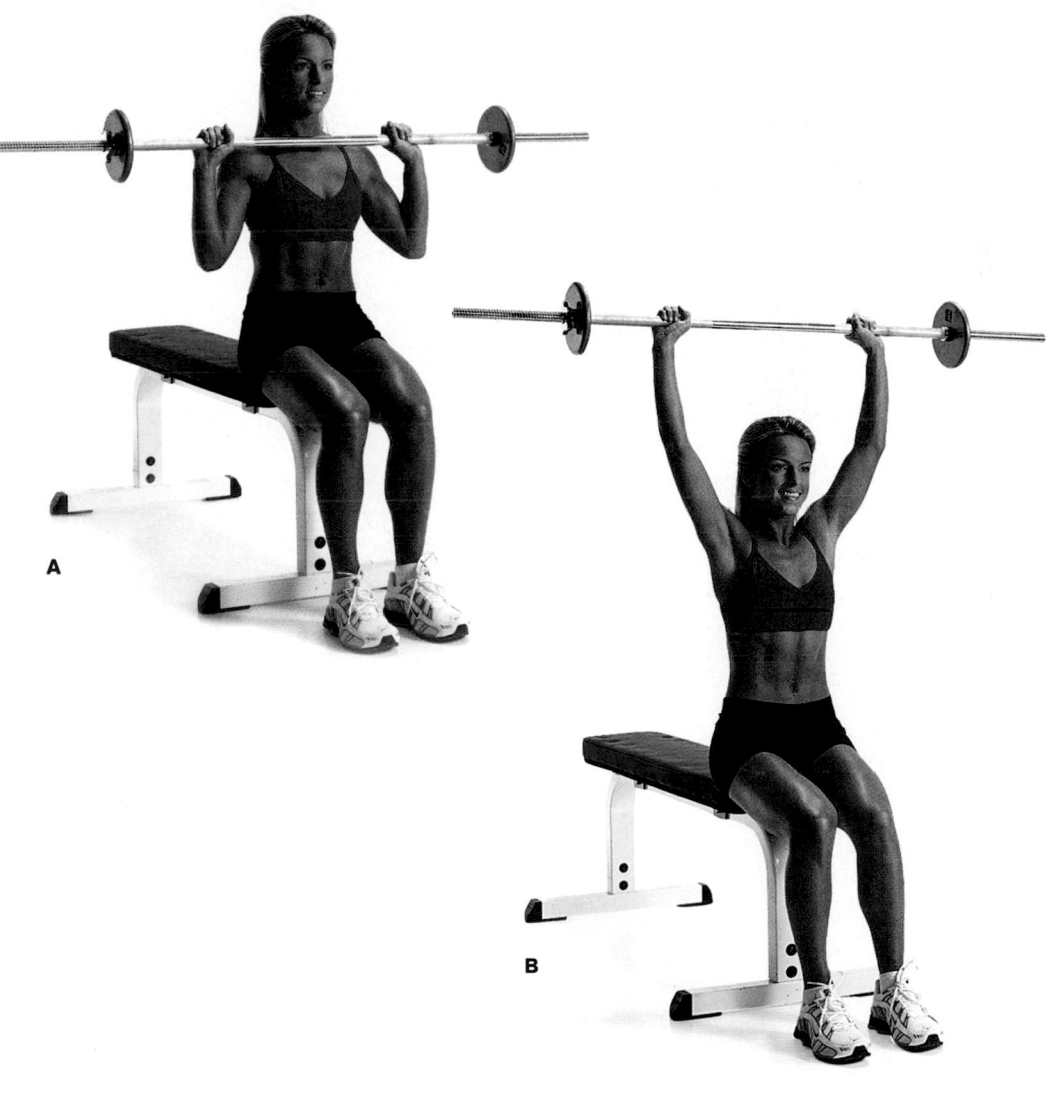

A

B

TOTAL FITNESS GUIDE 2008

W|H

TRICEPS PUSHDOWN

While standing, grip a bar attached to a high pulley cable or lat machine with your hands about 6 inches apart. With your elbows tucked against your sides, bring the bar down until it's directly in front of you (**A**). With your forearms parallel to the floor (the start position), push the bar down until your arms are extended straight down with the bar near your thighs (**B**). Don't lock your elbows. Return to start.

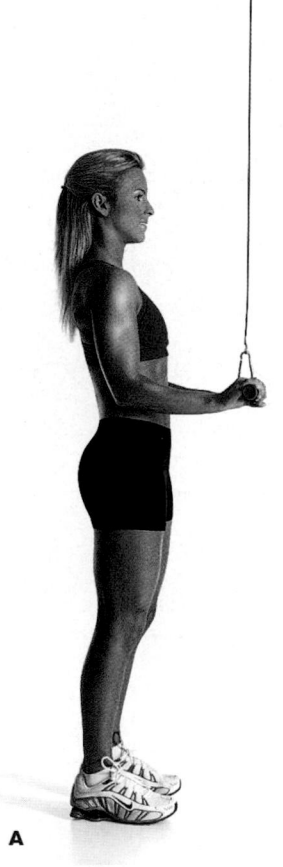

A

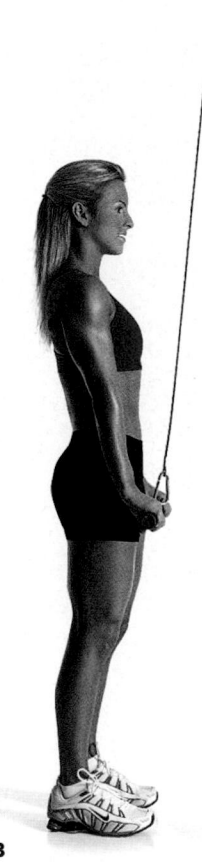

B

BICEPS CURL

Stand while holding a barbell in front of you, palms facing out, with your hands shoulder-width apart and your arms hanging in front of you (**A**). Curl the weight toward your shoulders (**B**). Hold for a second, then return to start.

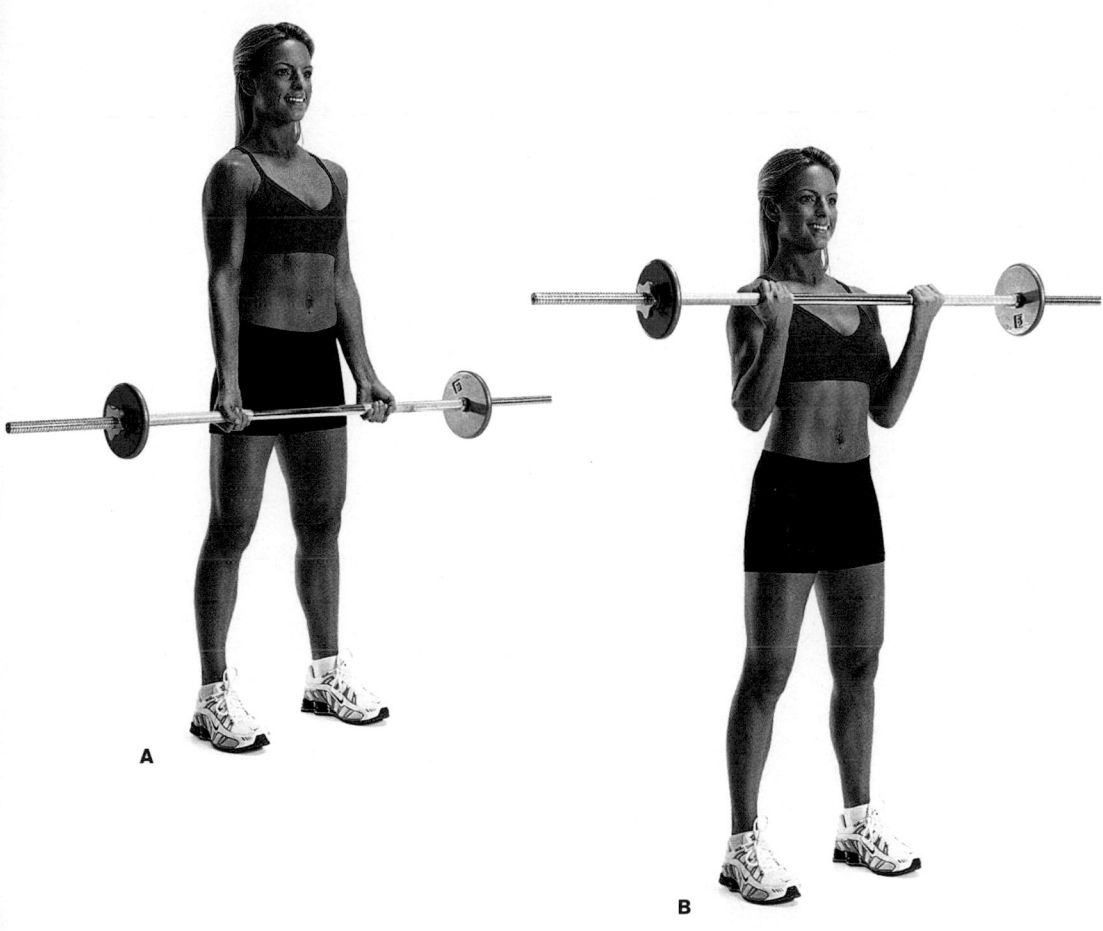

A

B

TOTAL FITNESS GUIDE 2008

W|H

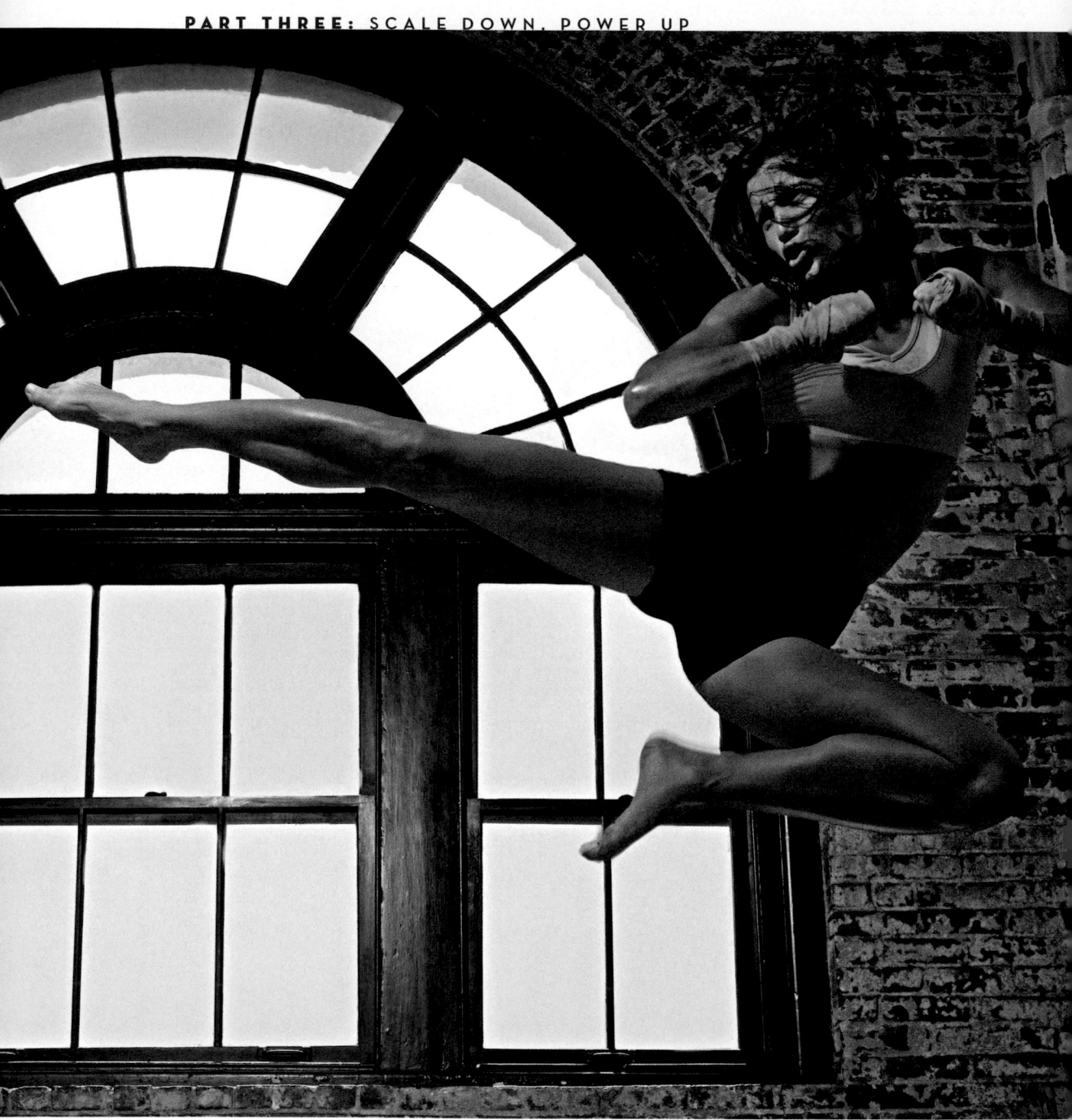

CHAPTER FOURTEEN

SURPRISE YOUR MUSCLES

ADD THESE SMALL BUT POWERFUL CHANGES TO YOUR FAVORITE WORKOUT–AND BURN MORE FAT!

WORKOUTS, LIKE SNOW GLOBES and Snapple lemonade, benefit from a good shaking up. You may love your 5-mile loop around the park, but if you always pass the old oak at minute 12 and the mail carrier at minute 18, your workout routine has officially become, well, routine. Familiarity might be comfortable, but it's not effective—certainly not when it comes to a sweat session. Doing the same thing over and over leaves your muscles unchallenged and your calorie burn pretty much fizzled.

The good news: You don't need to ditch your current workout to see more results. You just need to learn how to rev it up. Follow these tips from some of the top trainers around the country for an ultra-efficient workout that zaps more calories and burns more fat.

Treadmill

Your comfort zone: Flipping channels on the tube, you lope along, either running or walking, at the same ho-hum speed you were at yesterday. And the day before. And the day before that.

BLAST MORE FAT

Don't bounce. You're not in an allergy-drug ad, running through fields of flowers. Keep your movement forward, not up and down, says Los Angeles–based personal trainer Gunnar Peterson. "Anything vertical is wasted energy: It doesn't help you," he says. By focusing on what's ahead, you'll go faster and burn more calories in a shorter period of time.

Squeeze your glutes. "Do it as you push off your toes," says Jan Griscom, a personal trainer at New York City's Chelsea Piers. By focusing on your backside, you'll contract—and tone—the muscle (and make it, not the fat surrounding it, the star of your Sevens). And the more muscle you have, the more calories you'll need to maintain it—and the more fat you'll burn.

Challenge your muscles. At the end of a workout, slow your speed to 2.5 to 3.5 miles per hour. Skip for 30 seconds, walk for 30; walk backward for 30, forward for 30; stand sideways and shuffle with your right foot leading for 30 seconds, walk for 30, and repeat with left foot leading. "You'll call into action other muscles that don't work while going forward," Peterson says. "Which means they'll be surprised"—as will the person on the treadmill next to you—"and add to the calorie burn."

Elliptical trainer

Your comfort zone: Gliding along at a medium pace, your legs are on autopilot. And, if the machine has arms, your upper body is too.

BLAST MORE FAT

Never stop working. To maximize fat burning, don't let the machine's gliding momentum dictate your pace. Your leg muscles should push the pedals around. If there are rails, lightly rest your hands on them—but no white-knuckling, since you may end up supporting your body weight that way.

Use intervals. During every third song on your MP3 player or every commercial break, ramp up the intensity and go as hard as you can. "A steady pace at a sustainable speed burns calories consistently, but intervals blast up the count," Peterson says.

Use your whole body. Every other minute, concentrate on strengthening your arms or core—you'll recruit more muscles and incinerate more fat. For example, if you're on a full-body machine, consciously engage your arms; push and pull with the same intensity as you're using for your legs. If it's a lower-body machine, put your arms in an athletic position—elbows bent, upper arms close to your ribs—to strengthen your core.

Stair stepper

Your comfort zone: You're bent forward at the hips, elbows locked, hands on the rails to ease your load on your beloved hills program, where you've been slogging away at level 7 since Christmas.

BLAST MORE FAT

Stand up straight. Pretend you're squeezing a

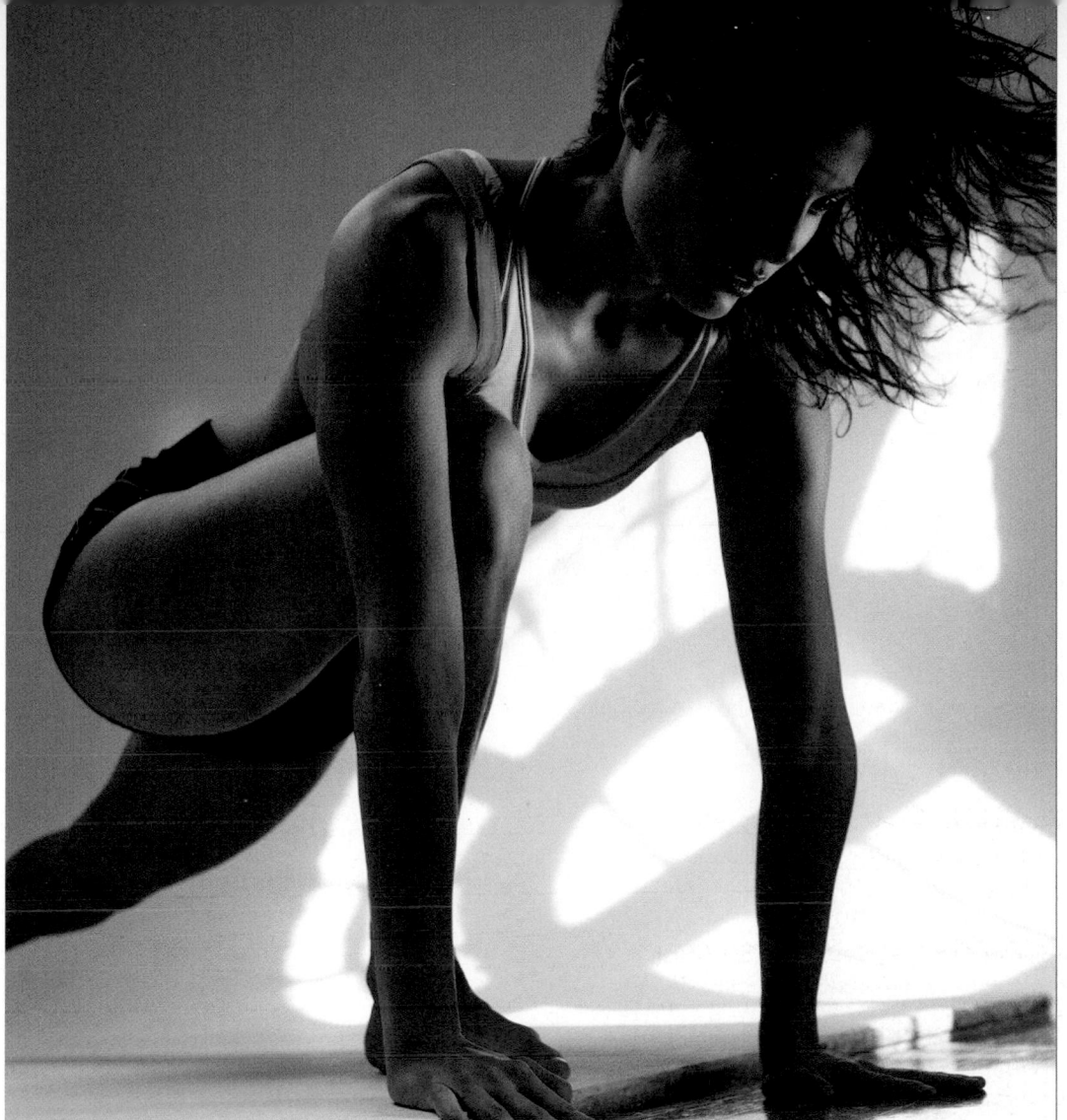

balloon between your shoulder blades, says Brooke Siler, author of *The Ultimate Pilates Body Challenge*. Use the rails for balance only, not support. Picture-perfect posture forces your core and back muscles to contract—great for toning. And engaging more muscles means burning more fat.

Mix up the depth of your stepping. In doing so, you'll surprise your muscles, which leads to an increased calorie burn. If you're a short stepper, add 1 minute of long, slow steps every 5 minutes. "Chal-lenge your leg muscles in a way that they're not used to being challenged," Peterson says. If you usually go long and slow, pick up the pace and shorten the step to about 6 inches to make your muscles react and there-fore adapt—that's where the change comes in.

Tuck your glutes under your hips. And make sure your feet are flat on the pedals. If you originate all movement in your core, not your legs, it will (a) hurt like a bitch and (b) work new muscles hard [see (a)], giving you—you guessed it—a more intense burn.

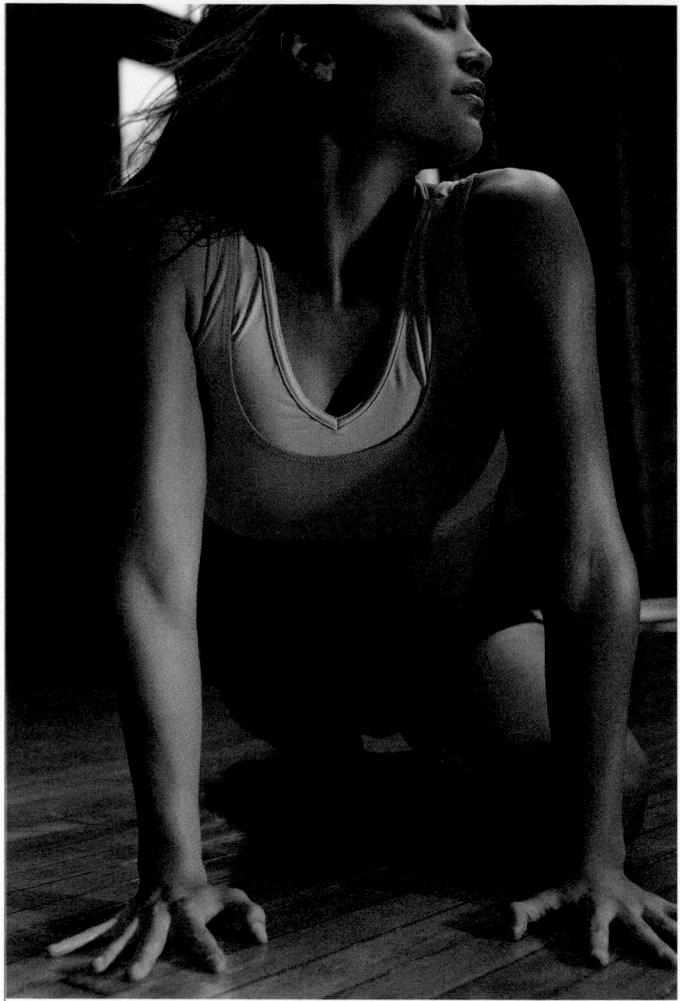

whittle your thighs to swimsuit-worthy slimness. Dixie Douville, R. N., a master spinning instructor with Mad Dogg Athletics in Flanders, New Jersey, advises a pace of 60 to 80 revolutions per minute on hills. Find yours by counting how many times one foot goes around in 15 seconds and multiplying by four.

And keep it there. On flat terrain, aim for 80 to 110 rpm. That way, you'll use your muscles, not the momentum of the weighted front wheel, to power the bike. Go faster and you risk momentum taking over. "If you're going above 110, you need to increase resistance" until you're back in the 80 to 110 range, Douville says. "That makes the workout much harder and the calorie burn more significant than just pedaling faster."

Sit when you climb. This increases your muscular endurance and incinerates more fat. When you stand, you can use your whole leg for leverage and your body weight for momentum; sitting means you have to push more weight around with less help. "Unless you increase the resistance significantly, standing is basically bailing out of a climb," Douville says.

Spinning class

Your comfort zone: Forget sweating—you haven't even started glistening yet. And you're about to start the cooldown. What was that about indoor cycling being such a good workout?

BLAST MORE FAT

Crank it up. God created the resistance knob for a heavenly reason. Use it, especially on hills, to

Running

Your comfort zone: You pass the yellow house 7 minutes into your run, the coffee shop 10 minutes later. Thirteen minutes after that, you're home—where you take off your shoes so you can find them tomorrow to do the exact same route.

BLAST MORE FAT

Run tall. Think about running tall. "Doing that immediately stops you from slouching and forces your arms to go front to back, not side to side," says Greg McMillan, a personal trainer and running coach in Austin, Texas. "Your hips stay tucked under, your butt doesn't stick out, and as a result, your stride is much more effective: You go farther with less energy expended." The result? You can suddenly run longer—and burn more calories.

Mix it up. Run your regular route in the opposite direction so your body doesn't know when to expect the hills. Better yet: Change your speed. "People shuffle when they run at the same pace all the time," McMillan says. "The body gets very efficient and doesn't have to work." If you typically run 30 minutes, try this 3-day routine: Day 1, go slower than your usual pace, but run for 40 minutes. Day 2, speed it up a notch, but run for only 20 minutes. Day 3, throw in some intervals: Run fast for 1 minute, easy for 2, and repeat 6 to 10 times. "Not only does that make the workout go by fast," McMillan says, "but it also burns more calories."

Drill it in. At the end of a workout, slim down your legs, bump up your heart rate, and build speed by doing drills. For 15 seconds, do knee pulls: Pull one knee high until your quads are parallel to the ground, then alternate with the other knee in rapid succession. Jog for 1 minute. Do 15 seconds of butt kicks: Try to hit your glutes with your heel. Jog for 1 minute. Finally, do grapevine (moving sideways, step your left foot over your right foot, then your left foot behind your right foot). Do 15 seconds, leading with one foot, then 15 seconds with the other. Jog for 1 minute, then cool down. As your strength increases, add sets.

Weight training

Your comfort zone: Intimidated by heavy metal, you stick to the light stuff—nothing more than 10 pounds, please—then saunter over to the watercooler for an extended drink.

BLAST MORE FAT

Pop some veins. Forget vanity. The weight you're hoisting should leave you red-faced and weak. "By the last rep, you should feel as though you have to put the weight down," says Brad Jordan, a personal trainer in Dayton, Ohio. "Three sets are plenty." Each day you lift, change it up. On one day, choose a weight you can lift for 8 to 12 reps; the next session, go with a lighter weight and lift 12 to 15 reps; on the last session, increase the load and lift only 6 to 8 reps. It won't make you huge. It will build more muscle, which (all together now) burns more fat.

Minimize downtime. Allow 1 minute between sets for maximum burn. You'll keep your heart rate elevated and your metabolism juiced—both helpful calorie-burning boosts.

Recruit all muscles. To use as many muscles as possible, stand instead of sitting. Or, even better, stand on a Bosu or balance board. Don't let machines be an excuse to rest, Griscom says. For example, on the chest press machine, don't let your back touch the seat (or drop the seat all the way down). Get into a squatting position and do the reps from there.

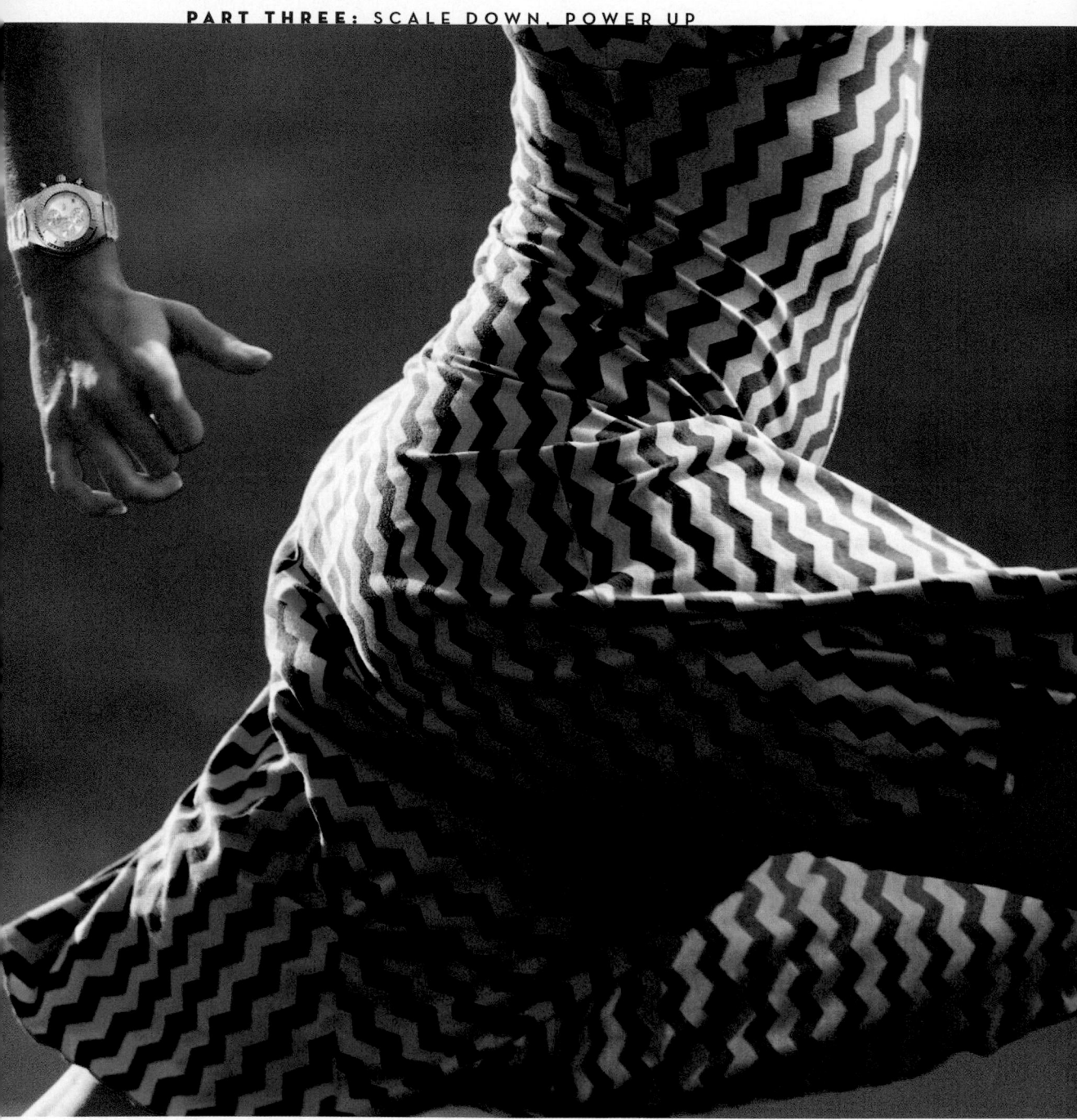

CHAPTER FIFTEEN

LOOK GOOD AT THE LAST MINUTE

WORKOUT SOLUTIONS FOR BIG OCCASIONS.

WE'VE LIVED OUR WHOLE LIVES procrastinating—studying for exams, preparing our taxes, relying on takeout because we haven't had time to hit the store. When it comes to getting in shape for a big night out (a reunion or wedding) or an upcoming getaway (bikini in the Bahamas), you don't want to be doing the kind of cramming that takes place between you and your clothing. With a little planning, you can hone your body in no time—just by focusing on the very parts you plan to show off.

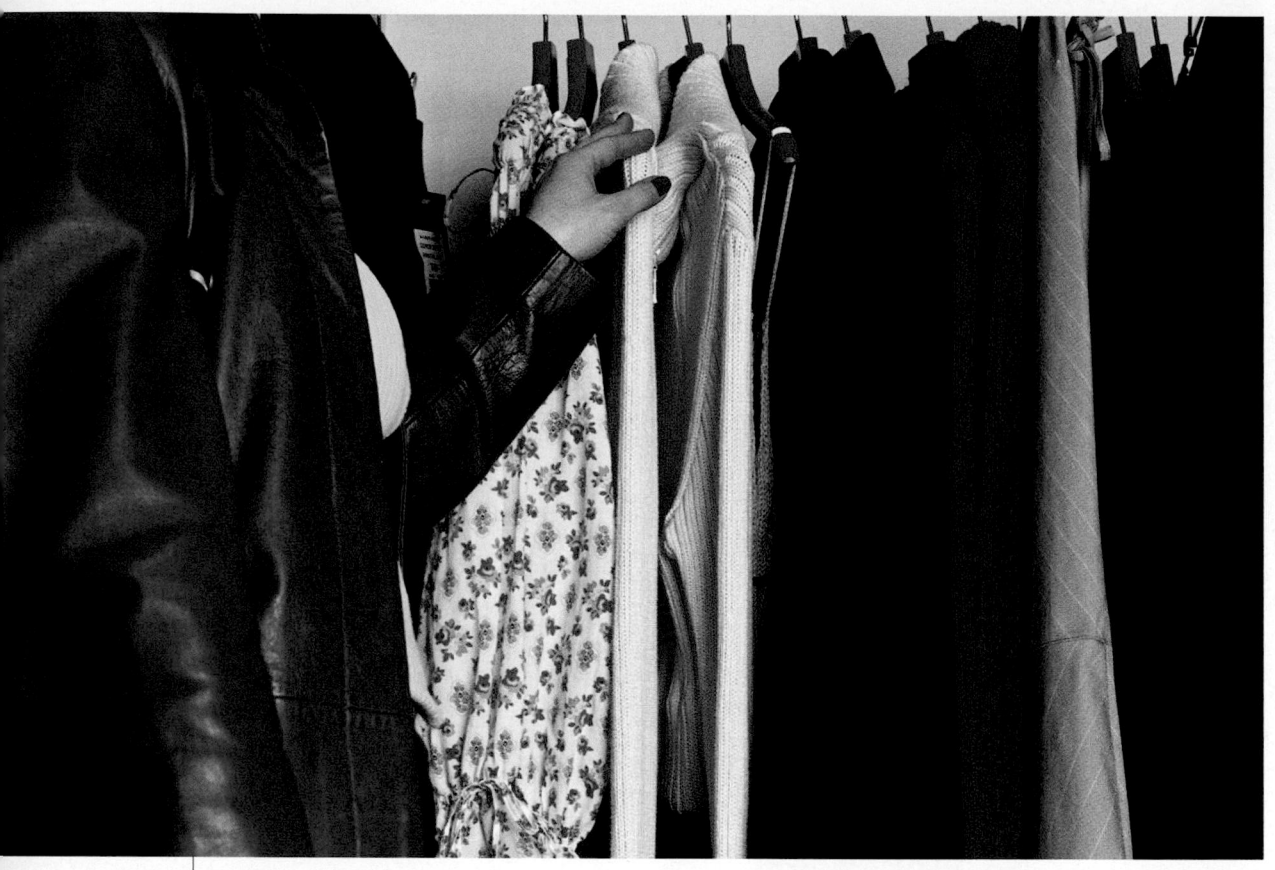

A Strapless or Backless Dress

YOU WANT TO TARGET: BACK, TRICEPS

WHAT YOU NEED: 3- TO 5-POUND WEIGHTS, EXERCISE MAT

BENT OVER ROW

With both weights in your left hand and your right hand resting on your right thigh, bend your right knee and your torso forward, leaving your left leg straightened behind you. Keep your belly tight and pull the weights up toward your chest, and then return to the bottom. Do it with the left arm 8 times, then switch legs and do the same on the right side.

TRICEPS KICKBACKS

Hold one weight in each hand. Rest your right hand and weight on your right thigh, and bend your knee. Straighten your left leg behind you. With weight in hand, make your upper left arm even with your body. Without moving your upper arm, drop the weight toward the ground with your lower arm. Extend the lower arm so it's even with your upper arm. Repeat 8 times, then switch sides.

YOU WANT TO TARGET: BICEPS

HAMMER CURLS

With shoulders squared and belly tightened, hold the
weights in each hand at your sides, fists facing the
floor. Keeping elbows at your sides, use the biceps
to bring the forearms up to your shoulders for 2 slow
counts (so that the ends of the dumbbells just touch
the shoulders), and then bring them back down for
2 counts. Do 12 reps.

ANGLED BICEPS CURLS

With feet shoulder-width apart and one weight in
each hand, bring your elbows against your sides and
face palms out to the sides. Slowly raise the weights
up toward your shoulders for 2 counts and then back
down for 2 counts. Do 8 reps.

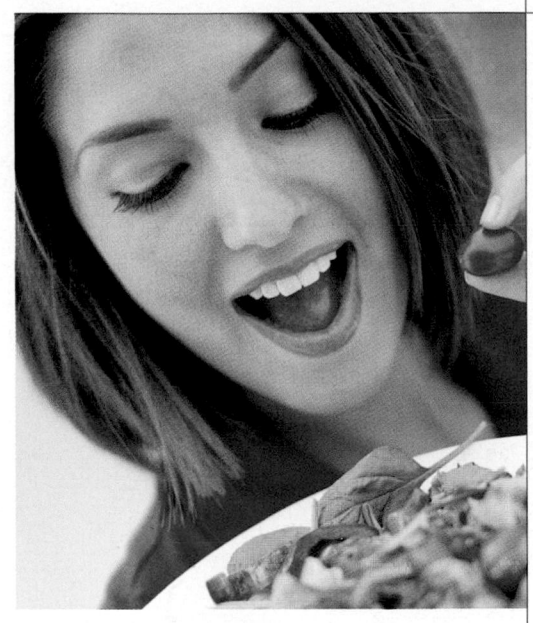

YOU WANT TO TARGET: CHEST, SHOULDERS

CHEST PRESS

Lying on a bench, the floor, or stability ball, hold one
weight in each hand. Push the weights up by
straightening your arms. Lower the weights and
repeat. Do this 8 times.

SHOULDER PRESS

Begin with one weight in each hand, feet hip-width
apart, holding arms straight above the head, weights
touching ends (arms should make a triangle above
head). Pull the weights down toward the floor (biceps
should arrive horizontally above the floor). When
elbows align with shoulders, stop and raise arms
again to repeat. Do 8 reps.

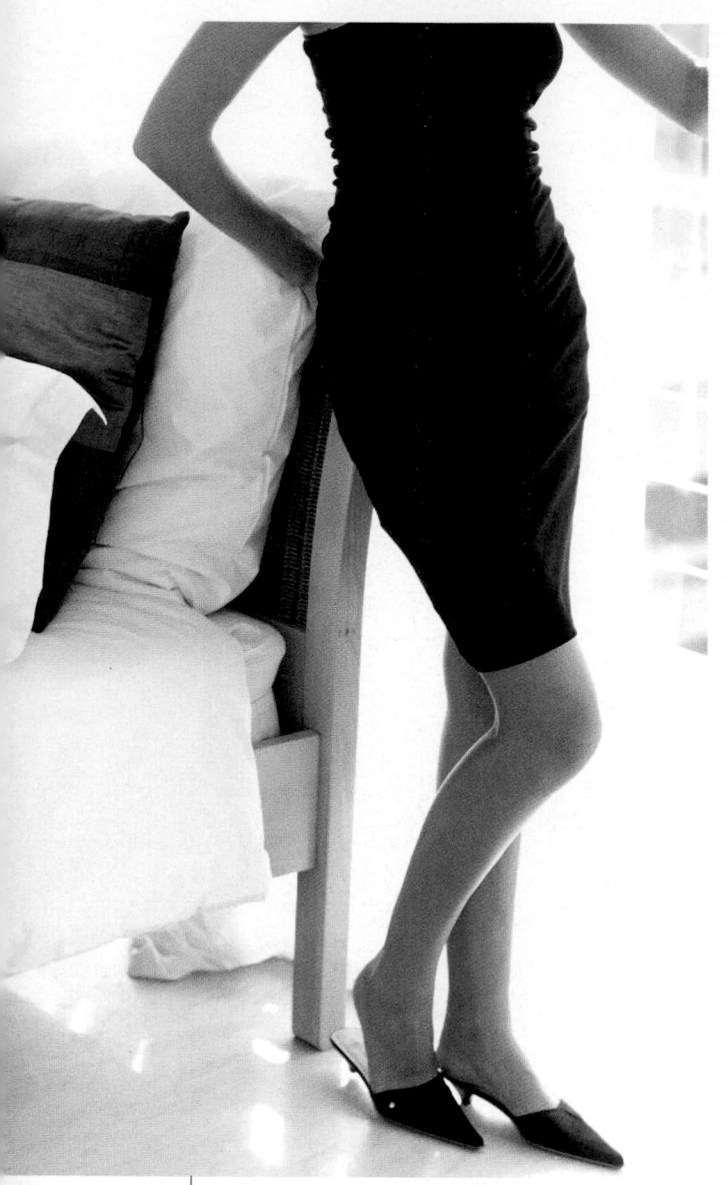

A Little Black Dress

YOU WANT TO TARGET: QUADS, INNER & OUTER THIGHS, CALVES, GLUTES

ALTERNATING SQUATS

Begin with your knees slightly bent and feet one foot-length apart, with your hands on your hips or out in front of you like in a classic kickboxing stance. Extend the right leg to the right side, and squat by bending your knees and sitting back into the heels, with your thighs parallel to the floor. After you squat, bring the feet back together, keeping your knees bent. Repeat 8 times, alternating legs each time.

ALTERNATING LUNGES

Begin with your knees slightly bent and feet next to each other. Step back onto your toes and bend your right knee (keeping it suspended just above the floor) while lunging the left leg forward. (Make sure your left knee bends only over the ankle, not beyond the toes.) Bring feet back to their original position and repeat using the other leg. Do this 8 times, alternating legs.

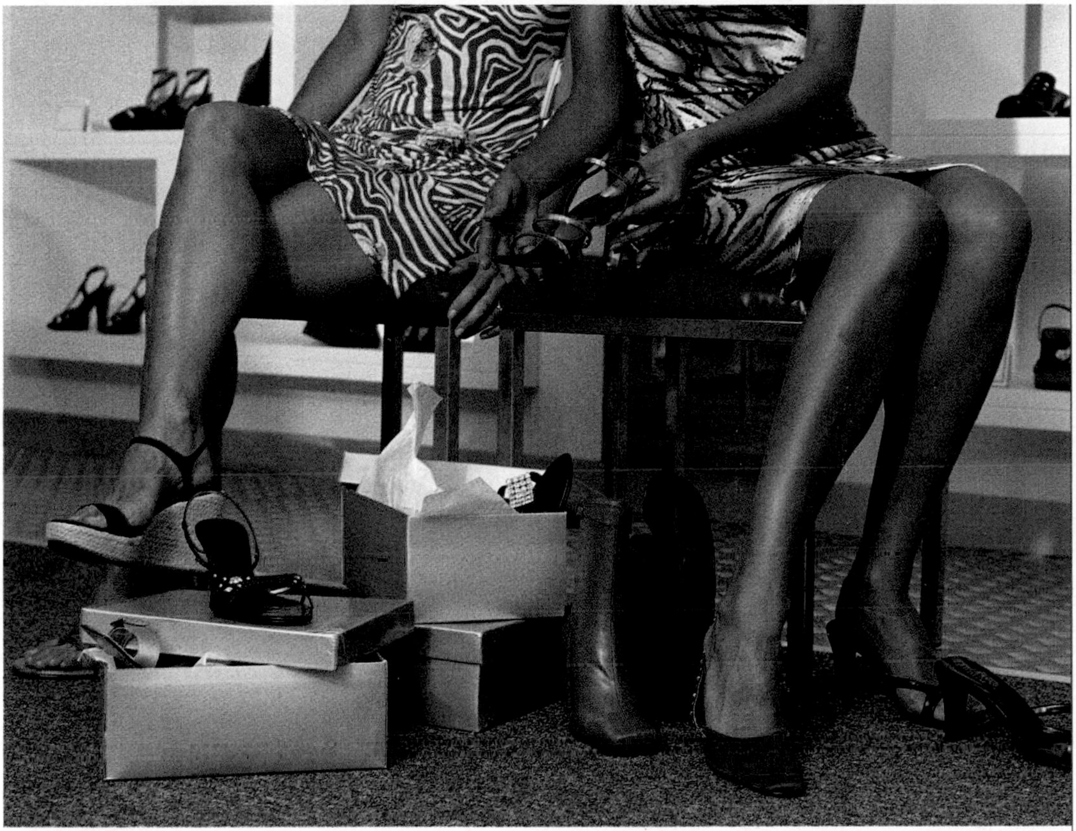

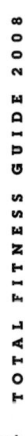

IF YOU PLAN TO WEAR . . .

Heels

YOU WANT TO TARGET: CALVES

CALF RAISE

Begin with your legs shoulder-width apart and knees slightly bent. Lift your heels off of the ground, straightening your legs up toward the ceiling and tightening the calves. Do this 8 times.

LEG LIFT

Beginning with feet together, put your right foot behind you and balance your weight on your toes, bending the left leg into a lunge. Then, lift the same leg up behind you, as if you were kicking the ceiling with the bottom of your sneaker. Do this 8 times, switch legs, and repeat.

W|H

BODY MAKEOVER IN A PINCH
SOLUTIONS FOR MAIN PROBLEM AREAS

Being crunched for time doesn't mean you get to skip crunches, but luckily you can quickly tighten up common problem areas. Use this last-ditch effort to ditch the one-piece and get bikini-ready with these four uplifting moves.

FLOOR DIP (works triceps)

Sit on the floor with your knees bent and hands at your sides, directly underneath your shoulders. Hoist your hips off the floor, like a crab. Next, bend your elbows and lower yourself toward the floor (without touching it), then straighten your arms.
Do two sets of 20 dips.

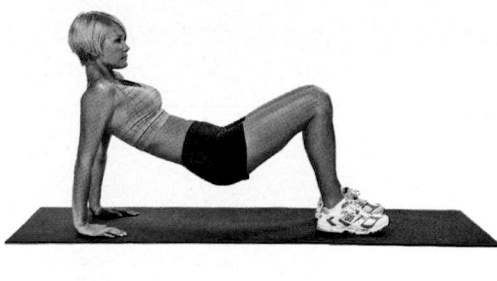

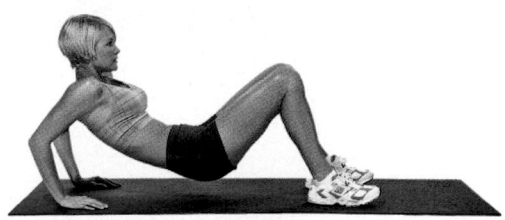

ONE-ARM WALL PUSH (works chest)

Stand at arm's distance from a wall and put your right palm flat against it. Bend your right arm as much as you can, making sure your elbow goes directly behind you and not out to the side. Return to start and repeat 15 times before switching sides. Do two sets.

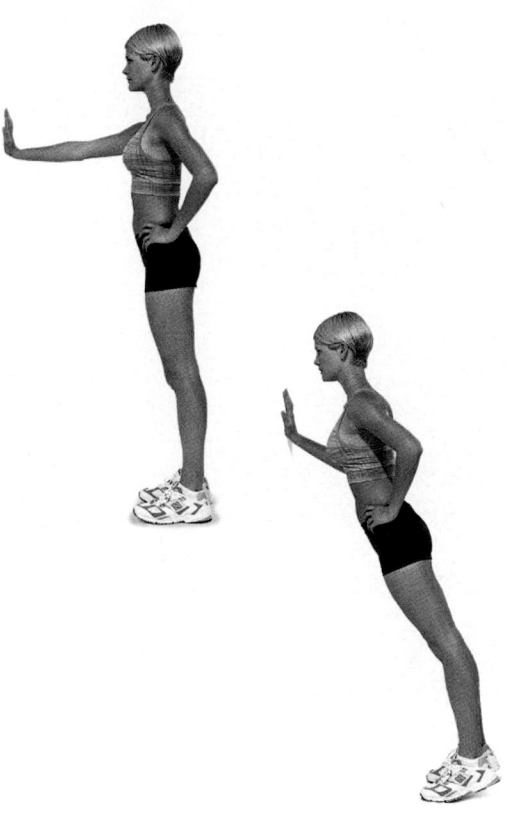

KNEE-DROP CRUNCH (works abs)

Lie on your back with your hands behind your head and knees bent above your hips. Keeping your shoulders flat against the floor, drop your knees to the right in one controlled movement. Do one crunch in that position. Lift your knees back to start, do one crunch there, then drop them to the left and crunch again. Do two sets of 30 crunches.

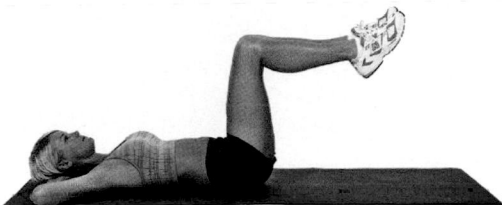

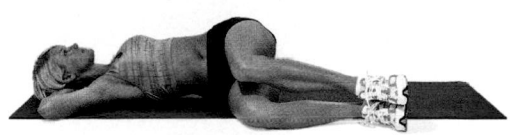

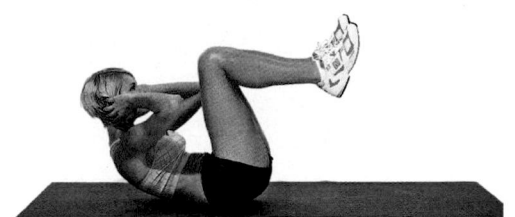

HEELS-UP PLIÉ (works glutes)

FIRM UP THAT BUTT WHILE BRUSHING YOUR TEETH!

Stand with your heels close together and press up onto the balls of your feet. (If you know ballet, this is a relevé.) Next, bend your knees about 45 degrees, pause for a few seconds, and return to start.

Keep your back straight with your tailbone pointed toward the floor. Do two sets of 15.

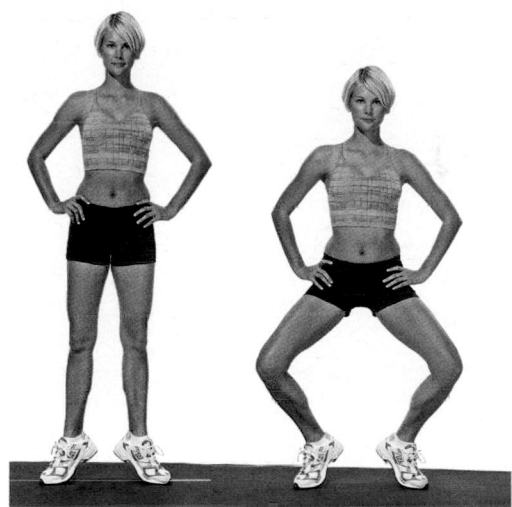

Excerpted from *Women's Health: The Wedding Workout*, distributed by Gaiam. The DVD is also available at womenshealthdvds.com.

TOTAL FITNESS GUIDE 2008

W|H

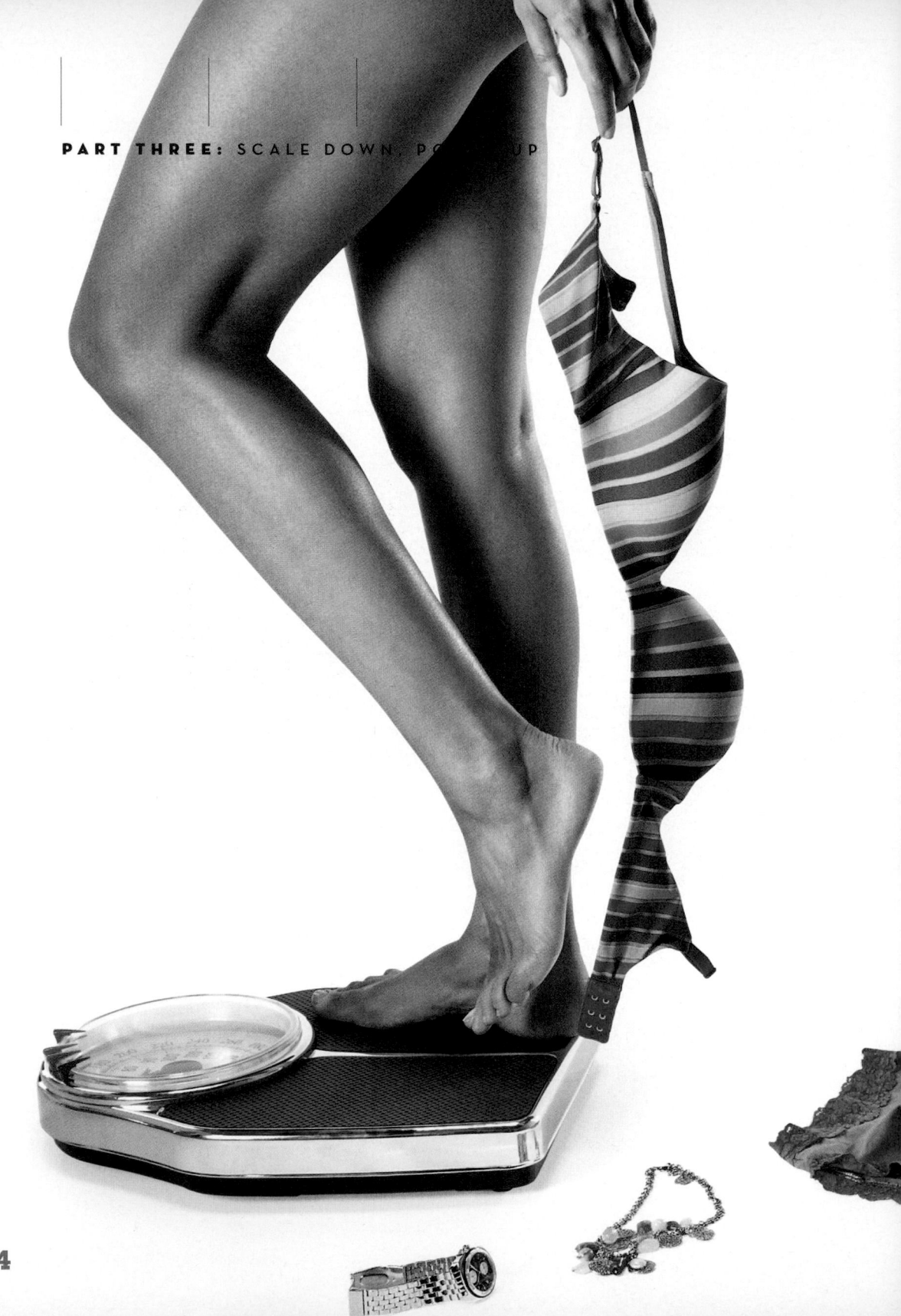

CHAPTER SIXTEEN

BREAK THROUGH THE PLATEAUS

WHEN YOUR WEIGHT LOSS FLATLINES, BUDGE THAT STUBBORN SCALE WITH THESE EXPERT TIPS.

TOTAL FITNESS GUIDE 2008

W|H

BY ALLISON WINN SCOTCH

YOU'VE BEEN EATING FEWER CALORIES, your trainer is your new BFF, and your body has gotten teenier. But now it seems like you couldn't lose a pound unless you cut your arm off. You've hit the dreaded plateau—a frustratingly common dieting phenomenon. "At a certain point in weight loss, usually after losing about 10 percent of your weight, you may have to tweak your diet and exercise to jump-start your body again," says Susan Mitchell, Ph.D., R.D., coauthor of *Fat Is Not Your Fate*. Here's why you might stall and what you can do to rev back up.

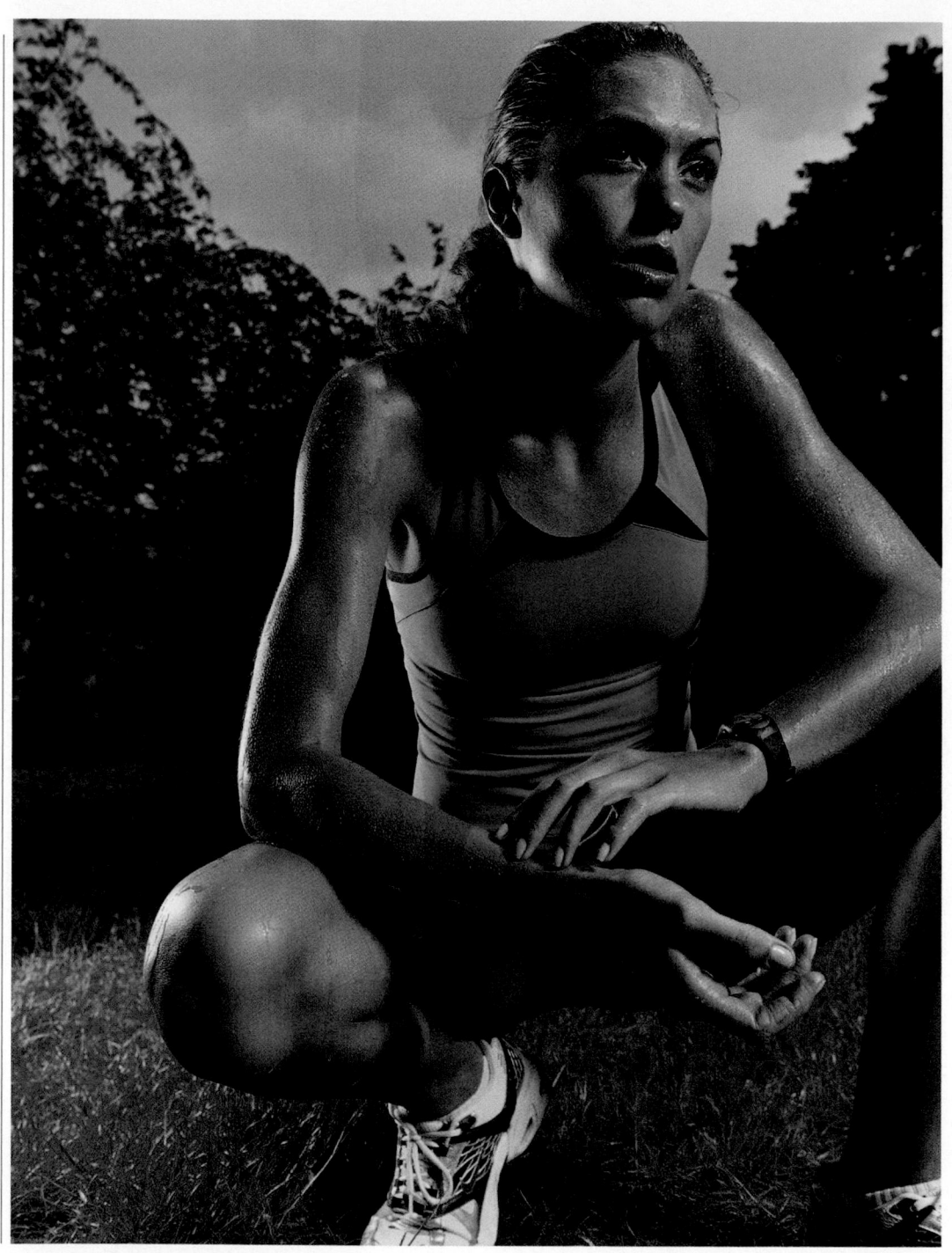

YOU'RE EATING FOR 164 (POUNDS, NOT PEOPLE).

Flatline Yeah, losing mass means you look better in your low-riders, but it also means there's less of you to burn calories. It's a cruel truth: Your basal metabolic rate (BMR)—the number of calories your body needs just to exist—gets lower as you get littler. Keep eating for your old weight and you're going to hit a wall.

Finish line As the number on the scale goes down, so too must your food intake. Figure out your BMR by dividing your current weight by 2.2 pounds, then multiplying this number by 0.9, and then by 24. (Or calculate it at bmicalculator.net/bmrcalculator.) Now multiply your BMR by 1.2 and voilà: You've got the average number of calories your body burns per day when you factor in normal activities. (Add another 300 to 500 on days you do an hour of moderate to intense exercise.) Once you have your final number, shave off 500 to find out how many calories you need to eat to lose a pound a week, or 300 to lose 2 pounds a month. Just don't ever go below 1,200 a day or you'll run into the problem below.

YOU'RE EATING FOR 95.

Flatline Here's the flip side: There's such a thing as eating too little to lose weight. "The body needs a certain number of calories per day to meet minimum metabolic needs, such as cardiovascular function and respiration," Mitchell says. When you're running on empty, your brain sends signals to various organs (like your thyroid), telling them to slow down your metabolism to conserve energy.

Finish line Strategy? Simple: "Increase your calories," Mitchell says. "Many women are afraid to do this because they think they'll gain weight, when actually the body will function more efficiently and

they'll start losing again." If you're stuck (and starving), try adding 100 calories a day for 2 weeks.

YOU COULD WORK OUT IN YOUR SLEEP.

Flatline Been repeating the same moves since you made your New Year's resolutions? You need a kick in your (shrinking) behind. "When your body is used to an exercise, it stops making physiological changes," says Cassandra Forsythe, a nutrition and exercise scientist at the University of Connecticut. Translation: Your bod has become so efficient at doing your current routine that it's burning fewer calories. Want proof? A recent study in the *International Journal of Obesity* found that runners who didn't increase their mileage gained weight over time.

Finish line Mix it up. "To grow more muscle and keep your metabolic rate high, you have to damage the muscles a little by challenging your body with a different workout," Forsythe says. If you're a treadmill rat, get on the elliptical or bike. If you're hell-bent on the treadmill, up the intensity (by adjusting the speed or incline) every other minute, or work up to a longer run by adding a half mile every couple of weeks. In the weight room, forget those 15 reps you usually do with a 5-pounder: "Decrease the number of reps and increase the weight, using one you can lift only five to eight times," Forsythe says.

YOU'VE BECOME AN EXERCISE FANATIC.

Flatline So you've amped up your workout. Great! Now you have to give your body time to recover. If you don't schedule any downtime, the pounds won't budge. "When you're sore after a

UPS AND DOWNS

Feel like your weight seesaws more than your 4-year-old niece on a sunny day at the playground? Relax. Even if you're doing everything perfectly, there are lots of reasons why the number on the scale could be up by a pound or two. According to Melina Jampolis, M.D., author of *The No-Time-to-Lose Diet*, these are some of the usual suspects.

YOU WERE THIRSTY! Downing 16 ounces of any fluid can cause an immediate "gain" of 1 pound.

YOU'RE BACKED UP. Constipation can tilt the scale by as much as 2 pounds if it's been more than a couple of days since your bowels did their thing.

YOU'RE GOING ON VACATION. To Thailand. The changes in air pressure can make you retain water on flights longer than 4 hours, which can show up as an extra 1 to 3 pounds on the scale.

YOU ATE CHICKEN KUNG PAO. Have a salty dinner and you could wake up 2 to 3 pounds heavier—your body retains water to dilute all that sodium.

AUNT FLO'S ON HER WAY. Hormone fluctuations in the 3 days leading up to your period can make you retain up to 5 pounds of water.

workout, it's because you've torn the muscle fiber," explains Angela Corcoran, head of education and corporate development at the American Academy of Personal Training in New York City. "When you rest, the muscle fiber has a chance to heal and comes back more effectively. This drives up metabolism, so you burn more calories at rest."

Finish line Take a day off! Corcoran says she's seen clients lose weight after logging a few days of rest. But this doesn't mean you get a week to lie around watching *Lost* reruns (nice try): 24 to 48 hours is all your body needs to recover and recharge. Forsythe suggests working out 2 consecutive days followed by a day of rest, taking no more than 3 days off in a row.

YOUR BODY BALKS.

Flatline Like it or not, you have a "set point," Forsythe says—a genetically determined weight where you're most comfortable. To stick to this number and regulate its fat stores, your body uses a gazillion physiological mechanisms, like interactions between hormones and molecules that affect hunger levels. So if you're trying to drop 20 pounds below your set point, you're getting in the ring with Mama Nature: When you don't eat enough to maintain your set point, your body thinks you're starving and "responds by lowering its metabolic rate, which reduces the number of calories you burn," Forsythe says.

Finish line The best way to conquer your set point is to speed up your metabolism with regular exercise—at least 30 minutes of cardio, 5 days a week. It also helps to increase the amount of good fats (such as monounsaturated) and lean protein (think fish and poultry) in your diet—these foods can accelerate your metabolism.

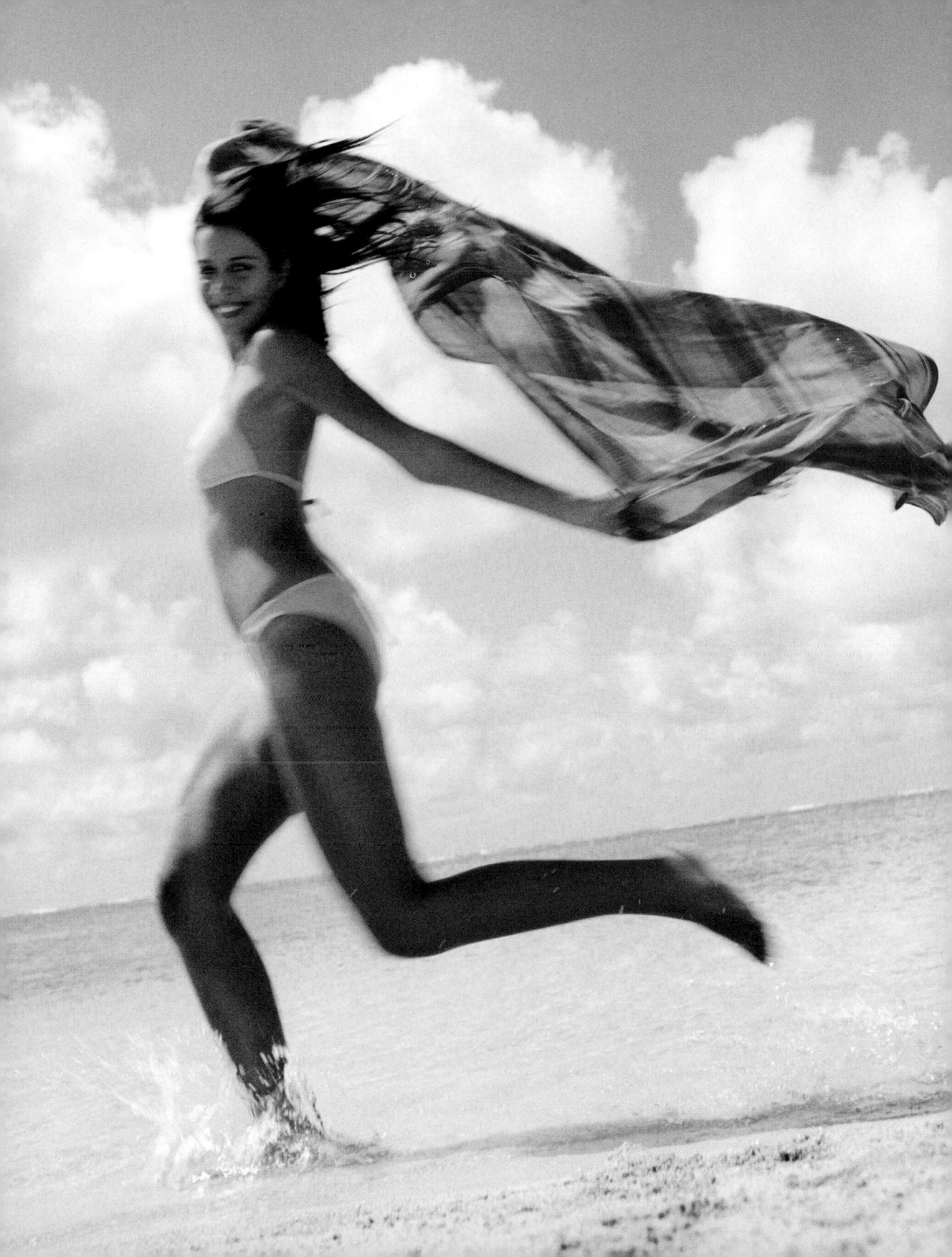

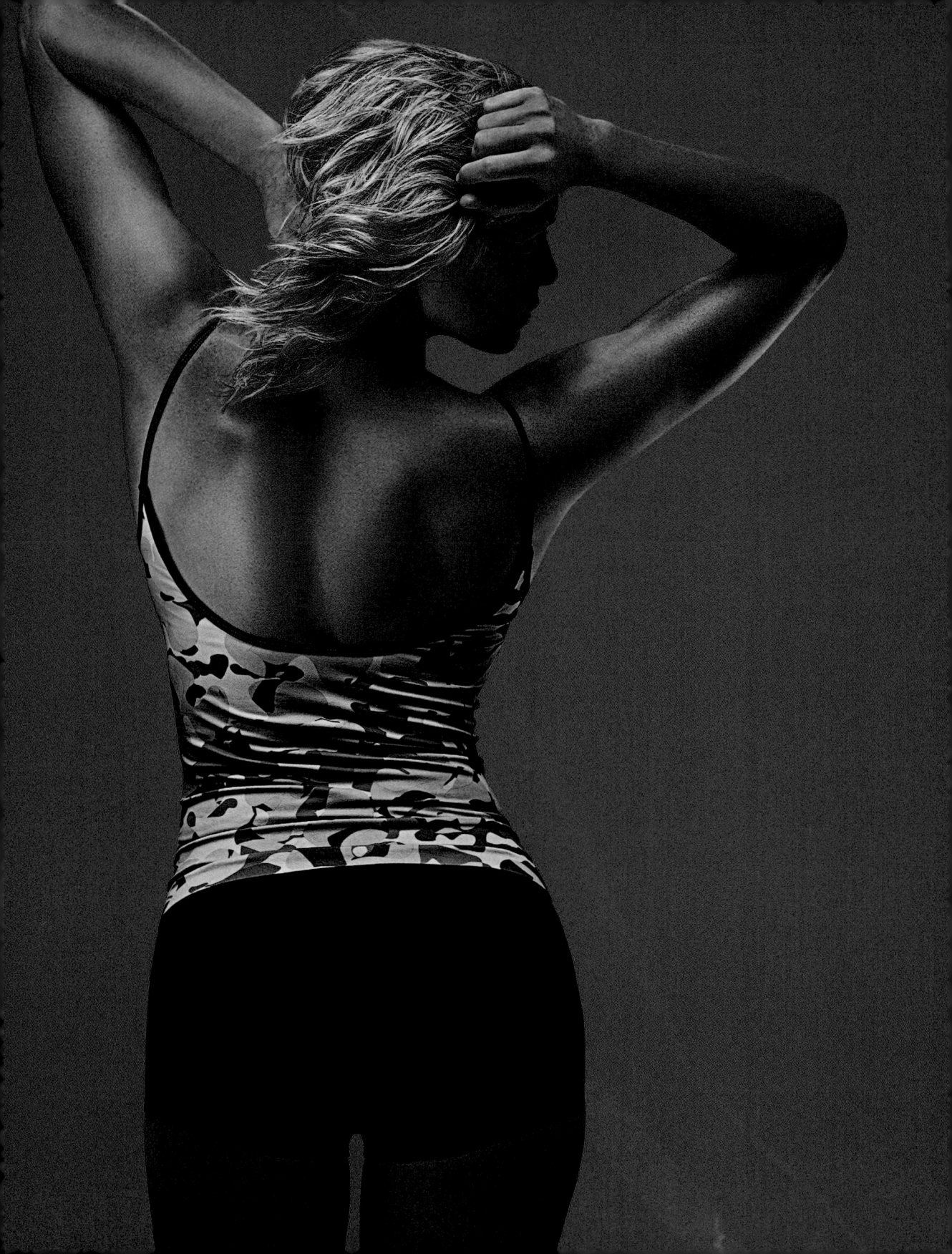

■ PART FOUR

tone and strengthen from head to toe

Want to run longer, ride faster, or power through a killer Pilates class? Or are you simply hoping to carry a few more grocery bags in one hand? Look no further. Your prescriptions for power start here.

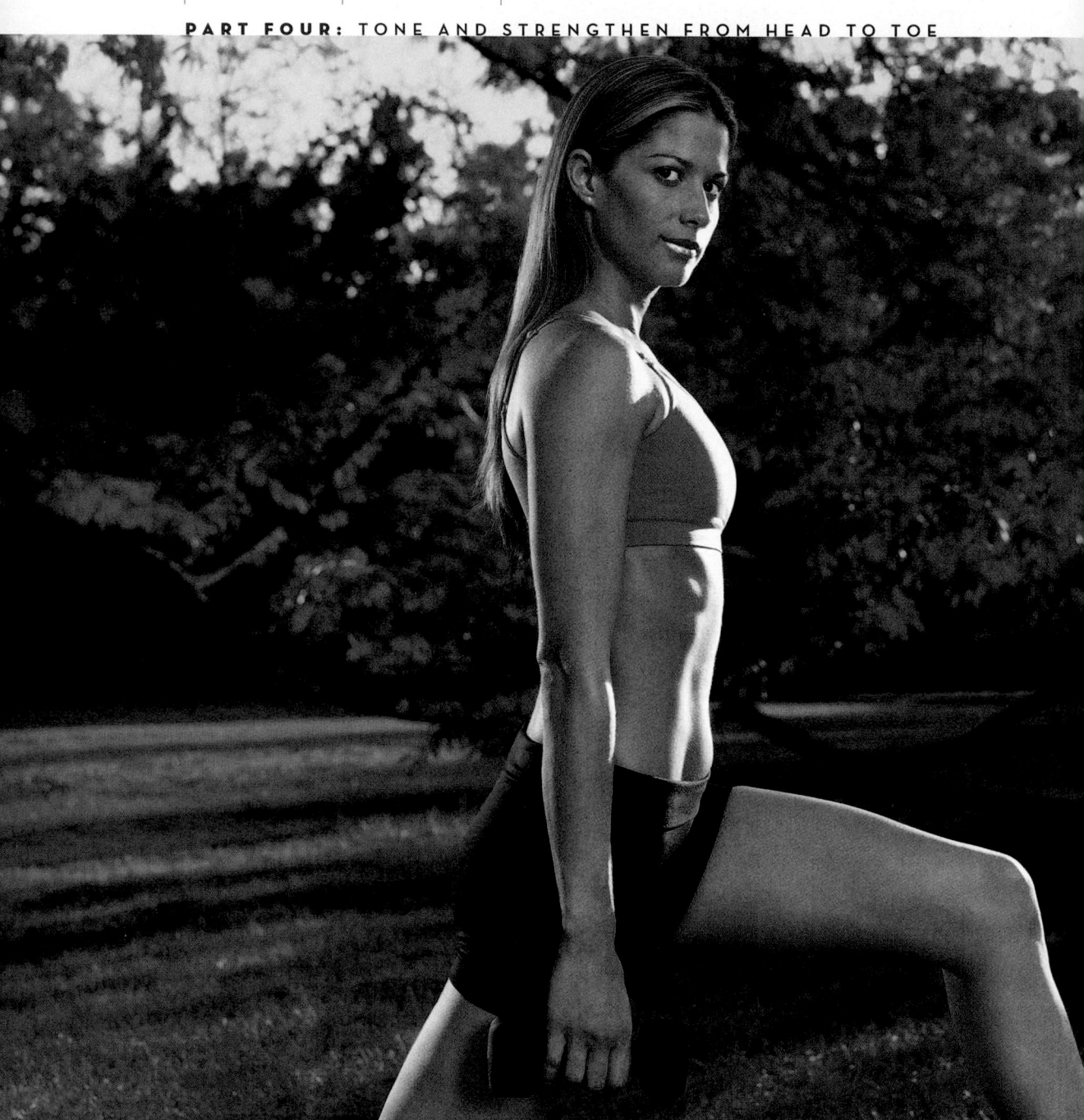

CHAPTER SEVENTEEN

TONE FOR YOUR TYPE

MAXIMIZE YOUR ASSETS WITH MOVES THAT MAKE EVERY BODY FRUITALICIOUS!

FACT: YOUR BODY SHAPE and ability to burn fat and build muscle were predetermined the minute your parents did you-know-what. Well, that's terrific news (and alarming imagery). But here's another fact: It doesn't mean you're stuck with Mom's wobbly arms or Dad's flat patooty. You can improve on these genetic "gifts" with targeted exercises that even out your proportions while optimizing calorie burn and muscle mass.

We asked two top trainers—Geralyn Coopersmith, C.S.C.S., author of *Fit + Female: The Perfect Fitness and Nutrition Game Plan for Your Unique Body Type*, and Mike Mejia, C.S.C.S., author of several books including *Men's Health Better Body Blueprint*—to help us devise a quickie way for you to figure out exactly what you've got and how to take advantage of it.

First, identify your silhouette as either an apple or a pear, those fruitalicious terms physiologists use to describe body shapes. Simply measure your waist-to-hip ratio by dividing the circumference of the narrowest part of your waist by that of your hips at their widest point. If the ratio is 0.8 or more, you're an apple. Less than 0.8 makes you a pear.

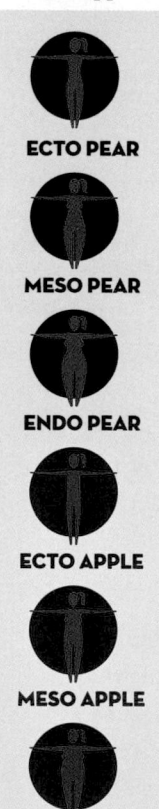

ECTO PEAR

MESO PEAR

ENDO PEAR

ECTO APPLE

MESO APPLE

ENDO APPLE

Next, determine whether your metabolism sizzles, simmers, or does something in between—in lab-speak, whether you're an ectomorph, endomorph, or mesomorph. Just scan the characteristics listed beneath each body type on the following pages. If you identify with at least two of them, bingo, that's your body type. If you don't fit one of the categories neatly, pick the illustration at left that looks the most like your bod.

Now, follow the specific instructions for cardio and strength building—and max out your assets in just 8 weeks.

YOU'RE AN

ECTO PEAR

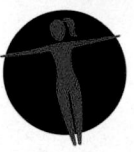

If you...

1. Can enjoy the whole buffet–twice–without gaining an ounce.

2. Aren't totally void of hips and have some junk you know where.

3. Get frustrated because no matter how much you lift, you can't seem to carve muscles in your arms and shoulders.

YOUR ASSET The potential to build killer curves.

MAX IT OUT Do just enough cardio to keep your heart healthy (30 minutes at least three times a week). Really long aerobic sessions, say, 60-plus minutes, could burn needed muscle. The moves on the following pages target several muscles at once to maximize tone, focusing on glutes, the biggest muscle group and the easiest to sculpt. Use heavy weights (load up until you can perform only eight reps, the last almost impossible) to activate mucho muscle mass. Complete three sets of each move before doing the next, resting up to a minute between sets. Do the workout three times a week before cardio or on opposite days.

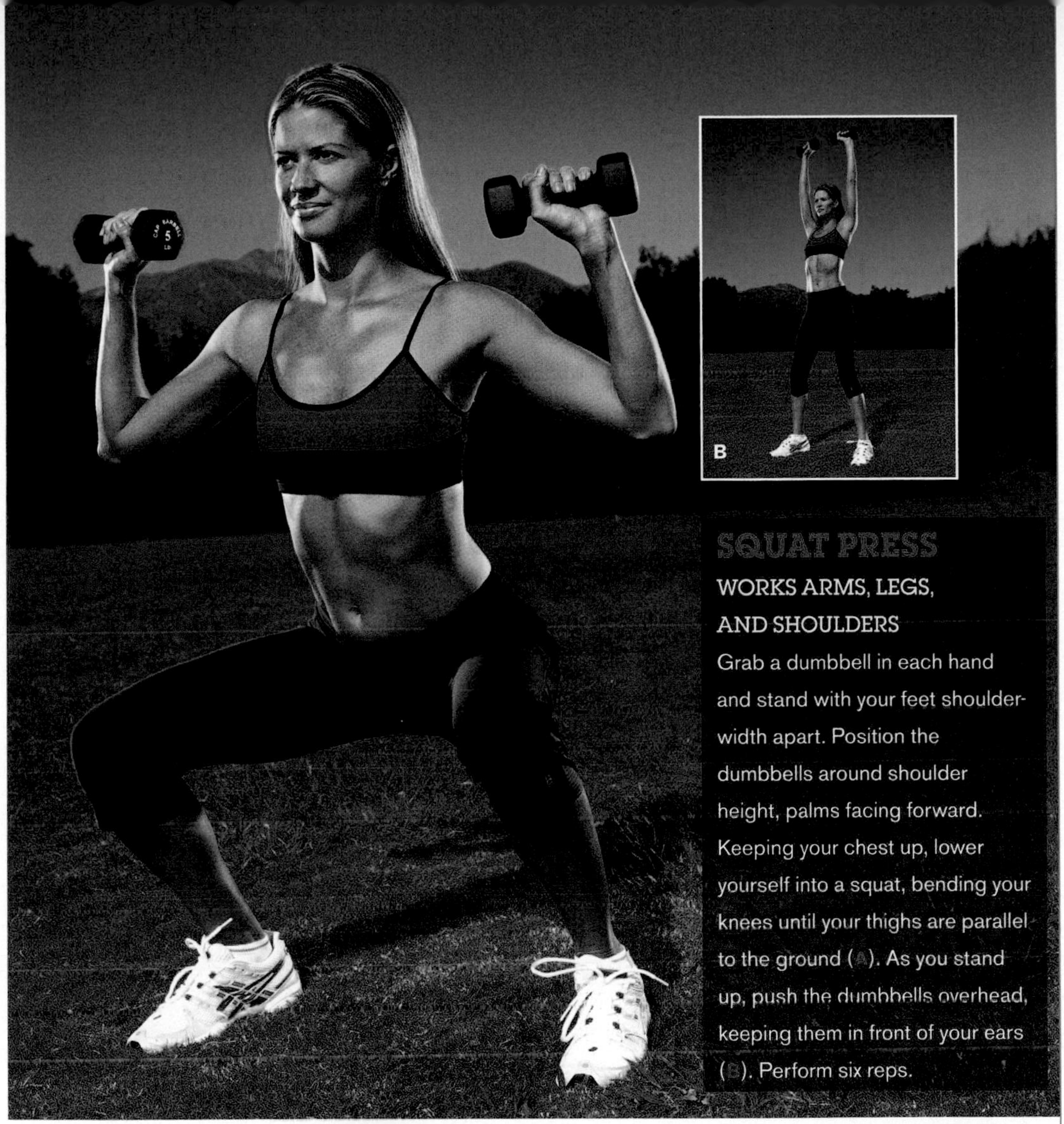

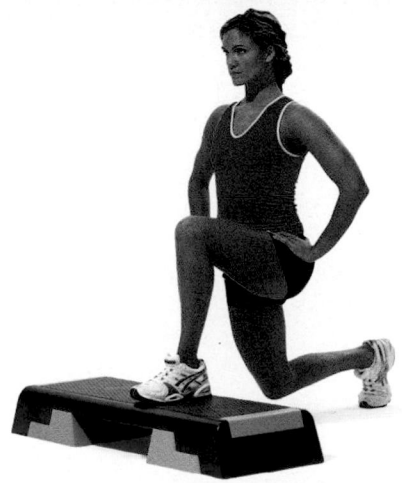

SQUAT PRESS

WORKS ARMS, LEGS, AND SHOULDERS

Grab a dumbbell in each hand and stand with your feet shoulder-width apart. Position the dumbbells around shoulder height, palms facing forward. Keeping your chest up, lower yourself into a squat, bending your knees until your thighs are parallel to the ground (A). As you stand up, push the dumbbells overhead, keeping them in front of your ears (B). Perform six reps.

W|H

ELEVATED REVERSE LUNGE

WORKS GLUTES, HAMSTRINGS, AND THIGHS

Stand on a 6- to 12-inch step with your feet hip-width apart. Take a giant step back with your right foot and drop your right knee until it's a few inches from the floor (shown). Squeeze your glutes to push your body up. Return your right foot to the step. Repeat, stepping back with your left foot to complete one rep. Do four.

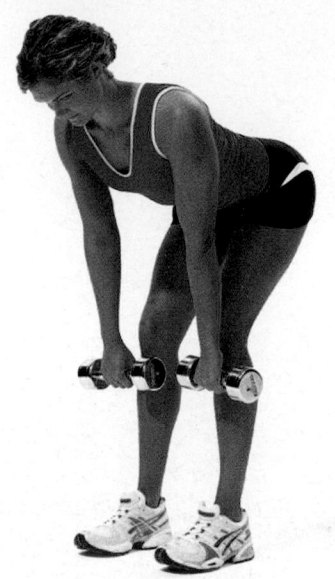

STEP WALKOVER

WORKS ARMS, CHEST, CORE, AND SHOULDERS

Get into pushup position with your palms on a 6- to 12-inch step. Keeping your legs, spine, and neck aligned, shift your weight onto your right arm and place your left palm on the floor. Next, push up with your left hand and place your right palm on the floor. Now, step up with your right hand (shown), then with your left. That's one rep. Repeat, stepping down to the opposite side, and continue alternating for 16 reps.

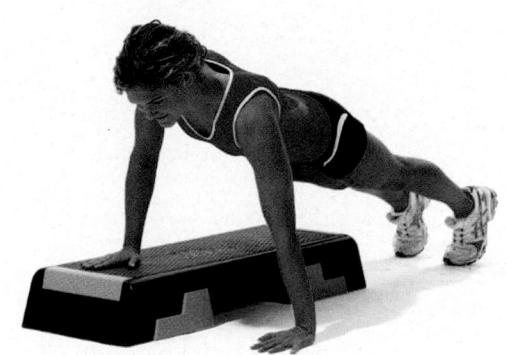

ROMANIAN DEADLIFT

WORKS BACK, GLUTES, AND HAMSTRINGS

Grab a pair of dumbbells with an overhand grip and stand with your knees slightly bent and aligned over your middle toes, arms at your sides. Keeping your arms straight and knees in place, slowly bend at your waist and lower the weights as far as possible without rounding your back (shown). Squeeze your glutes to pull yourself up. Do three sets of eight reps. Up for a bigger challenge? Try them on one leg.

YOU'RE A

MESO PEAR

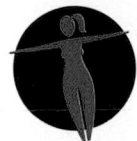

If you ...

1. Have strong athletic thighs.

2. Are slender up top with a defined waist.

3. Have a well-tuned metabolism—in other words, you gain muscle but no jiggle.

YOUR ASSET The toned body of an athlete no matter how little you exercise.

MAX IT OUT Keep your body fat in check with 40 to 60 minutes of cardio at a moderate pace (you can talk but only in one-sentence spurts) twice a week. Build your smaller upper half for a more balanced look. These lower-body exercises elongate muscles, and lots of reps firm them up without adding bulk. The extra quarter rep on the upper-body exercises makes them more intense—you lift more weight for fewer reps to build power and curves. Complete all sets of each move before doing the next, resting up to a minute between sets. Do the workout three times a week before cardio or on opposite days.

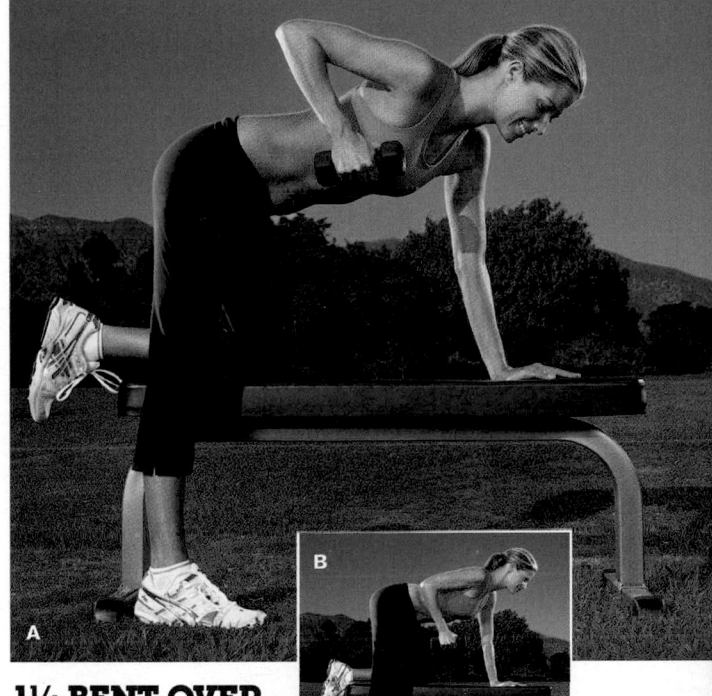

1¼ BENT-OVER ROW

WORKS BACK AND BICEPS

Grab a 3- to 5-pound dumbbell in your right hand. Place your left palm on an exercise bench so it's in line with your shoulder and place your left shin on the bench so your knee is in line with your hip—your torso should be parallel to the floor. Lower the dumbbell until it's hanging straight down. Pull it up to your torso (**A**), then lower it a quarter of the way (about 6 inches) (**B**). Raise it back up, then lower it until your arm is completely straight to finish the rep. Do three sets of six reps.

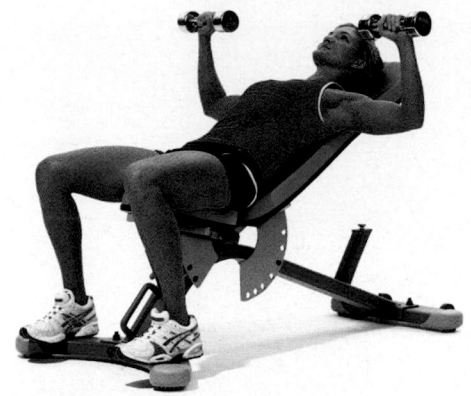

1¼ INCLINE
DUMBBELL PRESS

WORKS ARMS, CHEST, AND SHOULDERS

Grab a pair of 8- to 10-pound dumbbells and lie faceup on an incline bench set at 45 degrees, with hands at your chest, palms facing away from you, and feet flat on the floor. Push the dumbbells up a quarter of the way (shown) and return to start. Next, push them straight up until your arms are fully extended. Lower them to complete the rep. Do three sets of six reps.

STEPUP LUNGE

STRETCHES HAMSTRINGS AND HIP FLEXORS AND STRENGTHENS GLUTES AND THIGHS

Grab 3- to 5-pound dumbbells and stand about 3 feet from a step or bench that's just below knee height. Step forward, placing your left foot flat on top of the step, and sink into a deep lunge (shown). Press up, bringing your right foot flat onto the step to complete the rep. Repeat, stepping back with your right foot. Do two sets of 16 reps.

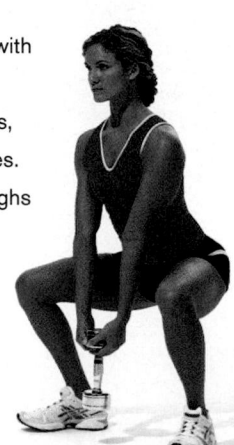

PLIÉ SQUAT

STRETCHES AND STRENGTHENS GLUTES AND THIGHS

Grab a 5- to 8-pound dumbbell with both hands, stand with your feet slightly wider than your shoulders, and turn your toes out 45 degrees. Lower your tailbone until your thighs are parallel to the floor (shown). Press back up to start. Do three sets of 16 reps. Too hard? Ditch the weight and place your hands on your hips instead.

YOU'RE AN
ENDO PEAR

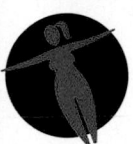

If you . . .

1. Are naturally curvy.

2. Easily pack weight onto your lower half.

3. Have a hard time toning your upper body, which is small in proportion to your bottom half.

YOUR ASSET An hourglass figure the boxy among us covet.

MAX IT OUT Don't even think about extreme dieting or nonstop exercise; you'll just eat up the muscle you need to tighten those curves. Keep body fat in check with regular cardio (40 to 60 minutes at a moderate pace—you can talk but only in one-sentence spurts—three to five times a week). These exercises work your arms, back, chest, and shoulders to counterbalance your lower half. Use light or no weight and do lots of reps to burn fat all over without bulking up below—the circuit is perfect for creating lean tone. For upper-body work, add weight to build more muscle and balance your proportions. Complete all sets of each move before doing the next, resting up to a minute between sets. Do the workout three times a week before cardio or on opposite days.

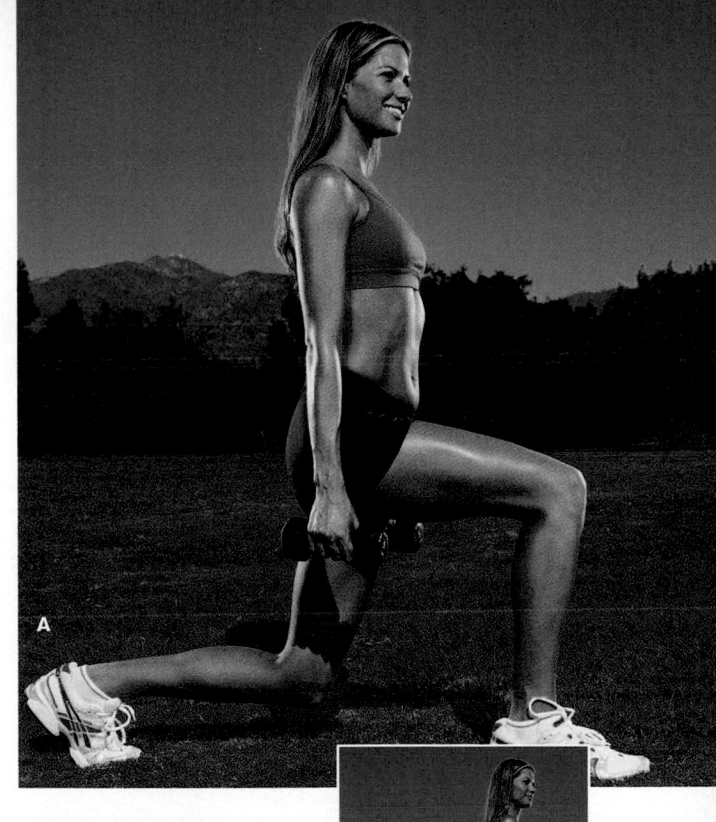

TWO-MOVE CIRCUIT: SQUAT TO LUNGE LEG CURL

WORKS GLUTES, HAMSTRINGS, AND THIGHS

Stand with your feet shoulder-width apart, arms at your sides, and lower your butt until your thighs are parallel to the ground. Push back up to start. Next, take a giant step forward with your right foot and lower your body until your right thigh is parallel to the ground (**A**). Push up with your right leg while curling your left heel toward your glutes (**B**). That's one rep. Repeat, stepping forward with your left foot. Continue alternating the lunge/leg curl sequence for 20 reps. Do three sets of the entire circuit. For a challenge, add 3- to 8-pound dumbbells.

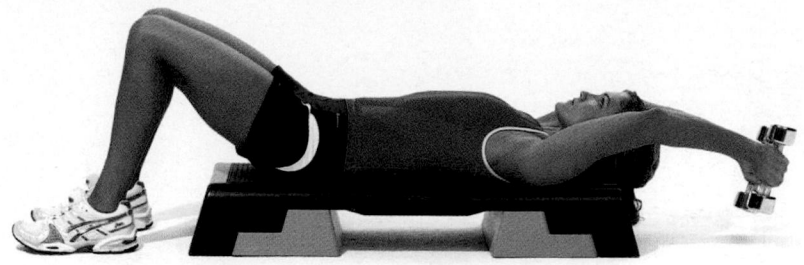

LYING LAT PULLOVER

WORKS SHOULDERS AND UPPER BACK

Grab a pair of 3- to 8-pound dumbbells and lie faceup on a 6- to 12-inch aerobic step, knees bent and feet flat on the floor. Your arms should be parallel to your body with elbows slightly bent. Raise the dumbbells toward the ceiling and lower them behind your head (as far as possible without touching the floor) in one fluid motion (shown). Squeeze your shoulder blades together, then pull the weights back over your head and lower them until your arms are parallel to your body again. Do three sets of 15 reps.

LATERAL BAND RAISE

WORKS ARMS AND SHOULDERS

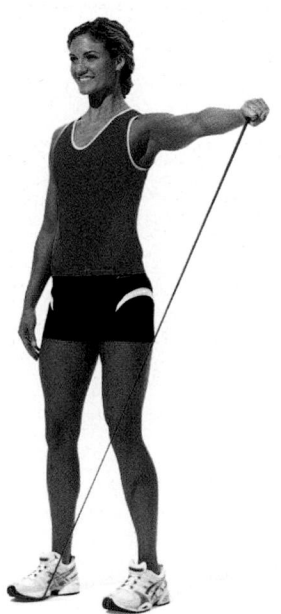

Grab an exercise band and stand with your feet shoulder-width apart. Hold one end of the band in your left hand, at your side with elbow slightly bent, and step on the other end of the band with your right foot. Raise your left arm straight up to the side until it's in line with your left shoulder (shown), then lower it slowly. Do 10 reps to complete one set. Repeat, raising your right arm. Perform three sets on each side.

YOU'RE AN
ECTO
APPLE

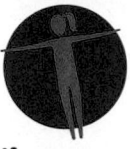

If you . . .

1. Have a metabolism that doesn't just cook, it scorches.

2. Have a hard time gaining muscle or fat.

3. Have poor posture.

YOUR ASSET A runway body—you could slip into Gisele's jeans, no problem.

MAX IT OUT Burning too many calories will make adding muscle tone difficult, so hit the track, bike, or your favorite cardio machine for no more than 30 minutes, three times a week. Hoisting weights will give you a healthier look and even a curve here and there. Upper- and middle-back work will un-hunch your shoulders to make you appear less I'll-blow-away-if-you-sneeze-ish. Complete three sets of each move before doing the next, resting up to a minute between sets. Do the workout three times a week before cardio or on opposite days.

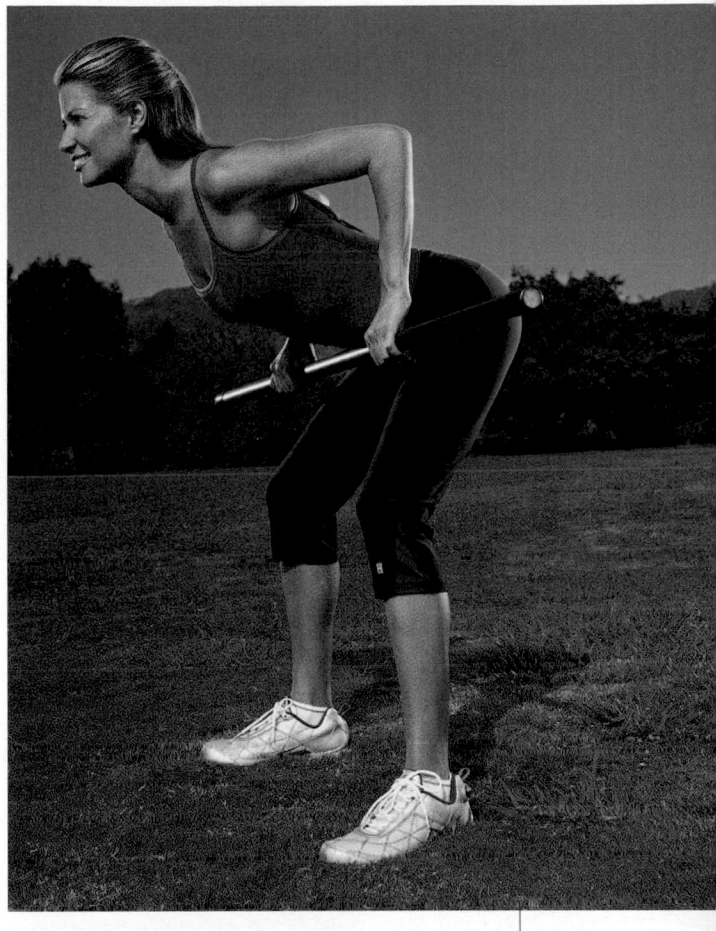

STANDING BAR ROW
WORKS ARMS AND UPPER BACK

Grab a 9- to 12-pound barbell and stand with your feet shoulder-width apart, holding the bar in front of your ribs with hands shoulder-width apart. Bend your knees slightly and lean forward 45 degrees from your hips, keeping your back straight. Lower the bar straight down until your arms are fully extended. Squeeze your shoulder blades together and pull the bar back up to your ribs, keeping your elbows close to your body (shown). Lower the bar. Continue rowing for three sets of 10 reps.

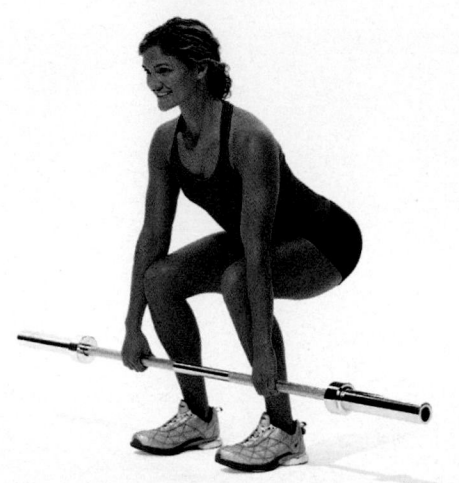

STEPUP LEG LIFT
WORKS HAMSTRINGS AND GLUTES

Stand facing a step or bench that's just below knee height with your feet shoulder-width apart, arms straight at your sides. Place your right foot on the step and step up, extending your left leg behind you (shown). Place your left foot on the step, then step back down (right foot followed by left). Repeat, stepping up with your left foot. Do three sets of 10 reps on each side.

CONVENTIONAL DEADLIFT
WORKS GLUTES AND THIGHS

Stand holding a 9- to 12-pound barbell with your arms straight and shoulder-width apart, palms facing your body. Position your feet shoulder-width apart and lower your butt until your thighs are parallel to the floor. Allow the bar to lower, keeping it close to your body (shown). Return to standing. Do three sets of six reps.

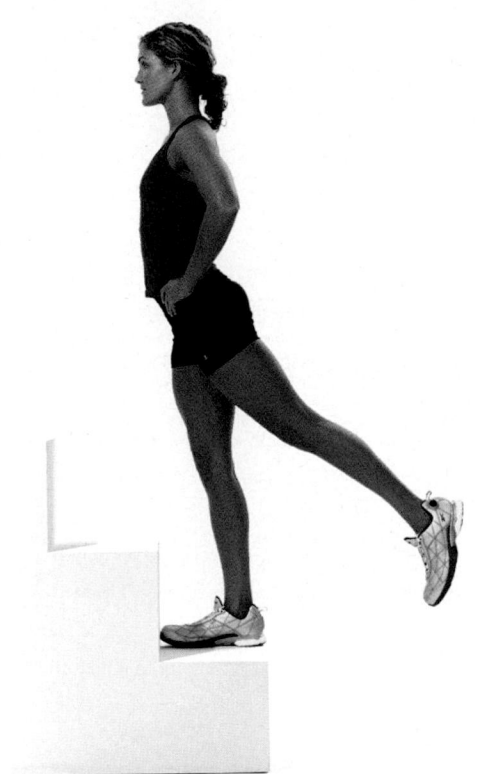

REVERSE DUMBBELL FLY

WORKS SHOULDERS AND UPPER BACK

Grab a pair of 2- to 5-pound dumbbells and stand with your feet shoulder-width apart, knees slightly bent. Position your hands, palms facing each other, in front of your thighs with elbows slightly bent. Lean forward 45 degrees from your hips. Keeping elbows bent, squeeze your shoulder blades together and raise your elbows to shoulder height (shown). Lower the weights. Do three sets of 10 reps.

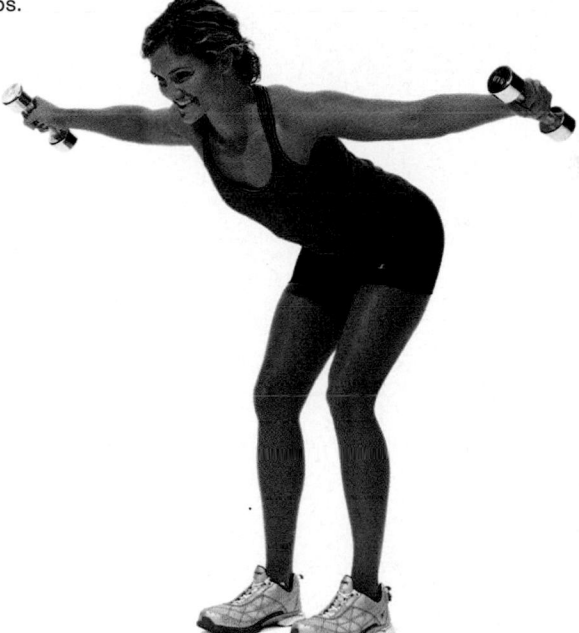

YOU'RE A
MESO APPLE

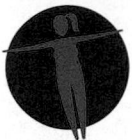

If you . . .

1. Are muscular and can hold your own on any playing field.

2. Have a dancer's slim but strong legs.

3. Are like the best desserts: soft in the middle.

YOUR ASSET A super-fit, powerful look, but washboard abs are unlikely–you tend to store your fat there.

MAX IT OUT Preserve muscle by hitting the track, bike, or your favorite cardio machine for no more than 30 minutes, three times a week. Build strength with exercises that call on your core while working other body parts. Bonus legwork with extra weight and fewer reps will add tone and give you a perkier bum. Sculpt your arms and shoulders without adding bulk by using low weight and doing lots of reps. Complete three sets of each move before doing the next, resting up to a minute between sets. Do the workout three times a week before cardio or on opposite days.

PLANK ROW
WORKS ARMS, CORE, SHOULDERS, AND UPPER BACK

Grab a pair of 5-pound dumbbells and get into plank position. Rest your hands on the dumbbells, palms facing each other. Push the left dumbbell into the floor, and pull your right elbow up until it passes your torso (shown). Lower and repeat with your left arm. That's one rep. Do three sets of seven. Make it easier by dropping your knees to the floor for extra support.

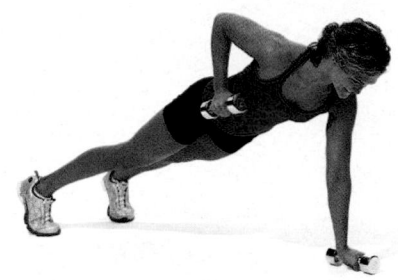

OVERHEAD SQUAT
WORKS CORE, GLUTES, AND THIGHS

Hold a body bar (heavy enough that you're just eking out the last rep) above your head with your feet shoulder-width apart. Lower your tailbone until your thighs are parallel to the floor, keeping your knees behind your toes (shown). Keep the bar in line with your hips and heels as you squat, and use your core to stabilize your body throughout the movement. Do three sets of eight reps. Too hard? Work up to it using a broomstick instead.

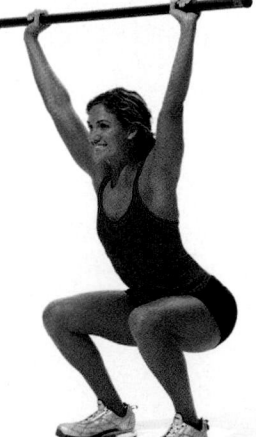

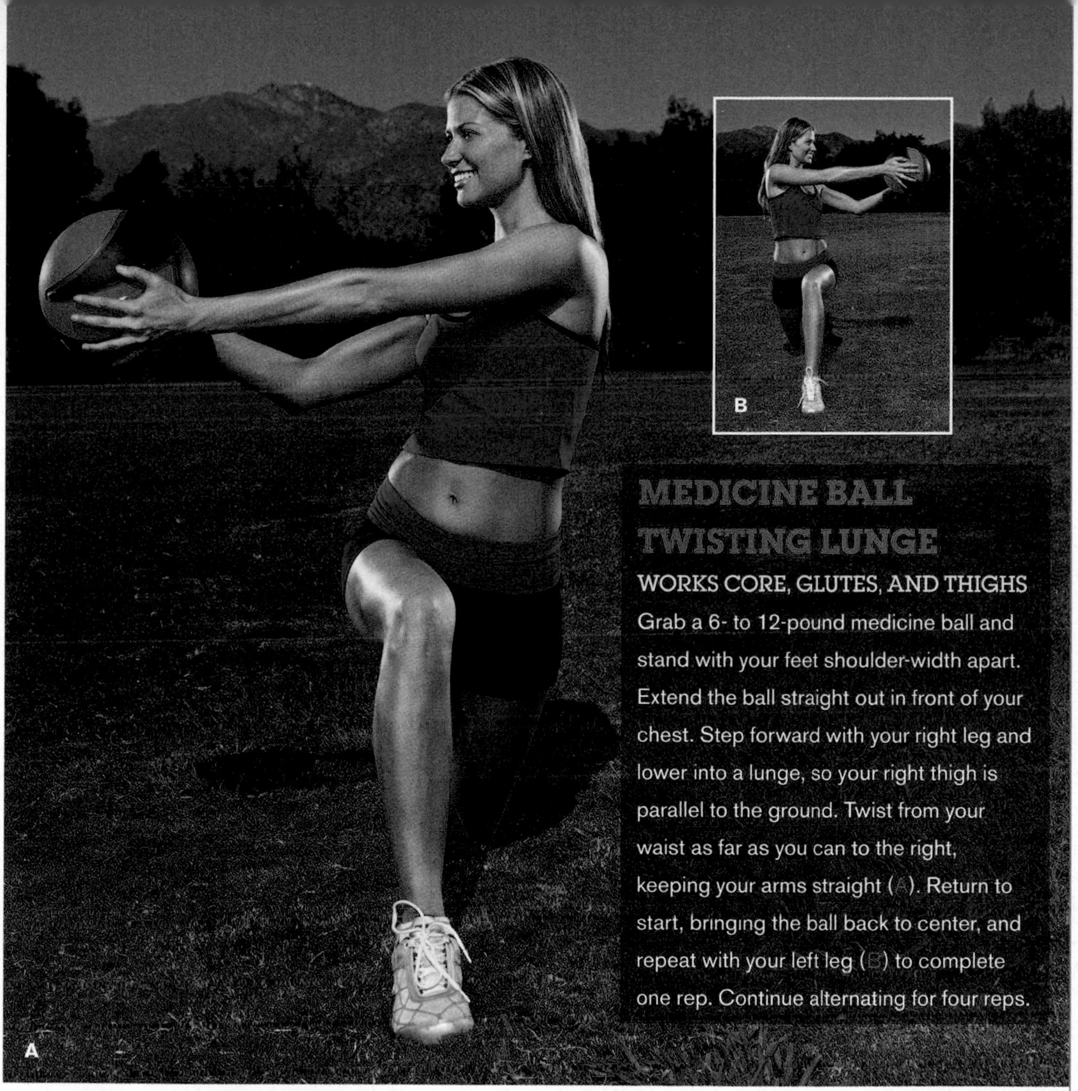

MEDICINE BALL TWISTING LUNGE

WORKS CORE, GLUTES, AND THIGHS

Grab a 6- to 12-pound medicine ball and stand with your feet shoulder-width apart. Extend the ball straight out in front of your chest. Step forward with your right leg and lower into a lunge, so your right thigh is parallel to the ground. Twist from your waist as far as you can to the right, keeping your arms straight (A). Return to start, bringing the ball back to center, and repeat with your left leg (B) to complete one rep. Continue alternating for four reps.

W|H

STABILITY BALL DUMBBELL PRESS

WORKS ARMS, CHEST, AND CORE

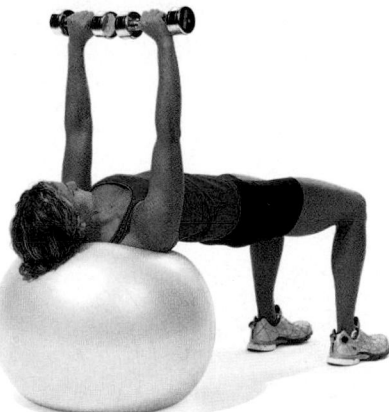

Grab a pair of 5-pound dumbbells and place your shoulders on a stability ball, feet flat on the floor and knees bent 90 degrees. With palms facing forward, raise the dumbbells to chest level. Press the weights up over your chest (shown), then lower them to start. Squeeze your glutes and thighs throughout the movement to stabilize your body. Do three sets of 12 reps.

YOU'RE AN
ENDO APPLE

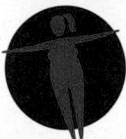

If you . . .

1. Sport sexy, well-defined legs. Your butt? Pretty flat.

2. Have soft arms. Your chest? Definitely not flat.

3. Are constantly pinching the inner tube above your waistband.

YOUR ASSETS Curves to spare.

MAX THEM OUT Melt your middle by doing 40 to 60 minutes of cardio at a moderate pace (you can talk but only in one-sentence spurts) three to five times a week. Toning your arms and maintaining definition in your lower body will balance your proportions. Use low weight (enough to do 20 reps) and high reps (12 to 20) to tighten your upper body. Build your bottom half with heavier weights (enough to do 10 reps). Do three sets of these exercises as a circuit, moving from one to the next without stopping. Rest a minute between each circuit. Do the workout three times a week before cardio or on opposite days.

REVERSE PUSHUP
WORKS ARMS, CHEST, SHOULDERS, AND UPPER BACK

Set the bar on a Smith machine to 3 to 4 feet from the floor. Lie on your back with your chest directly below the bar. Reach up and grab it with a shoulder-width, underhand grip so you're hanging from the bar and your body forms a straight diagonal line from your heels to your shoulders. Keeping your core tight, pull yourself up until your chest meets the bar (shown). Lower and repeat for 10 to 12 reps. If you don't have access to a Smith machine, do regular pushups instead.

CURTSY LUNGE
WORKS GLUTES AND THIGHS

Stand with your feet hip-width apart, hands on your hips. Take a big step back with your left leg, crossing it behind your right. Bend your knees and lower your hips until your right thigh is nearly parallel to the floor (shown). Keep your torso upright and your hips and shoulders as square as possible. Return to start. Perform 10 reps and repeat, stepping back with your right leg. Add dumbbells once you master the movement with perfect form.

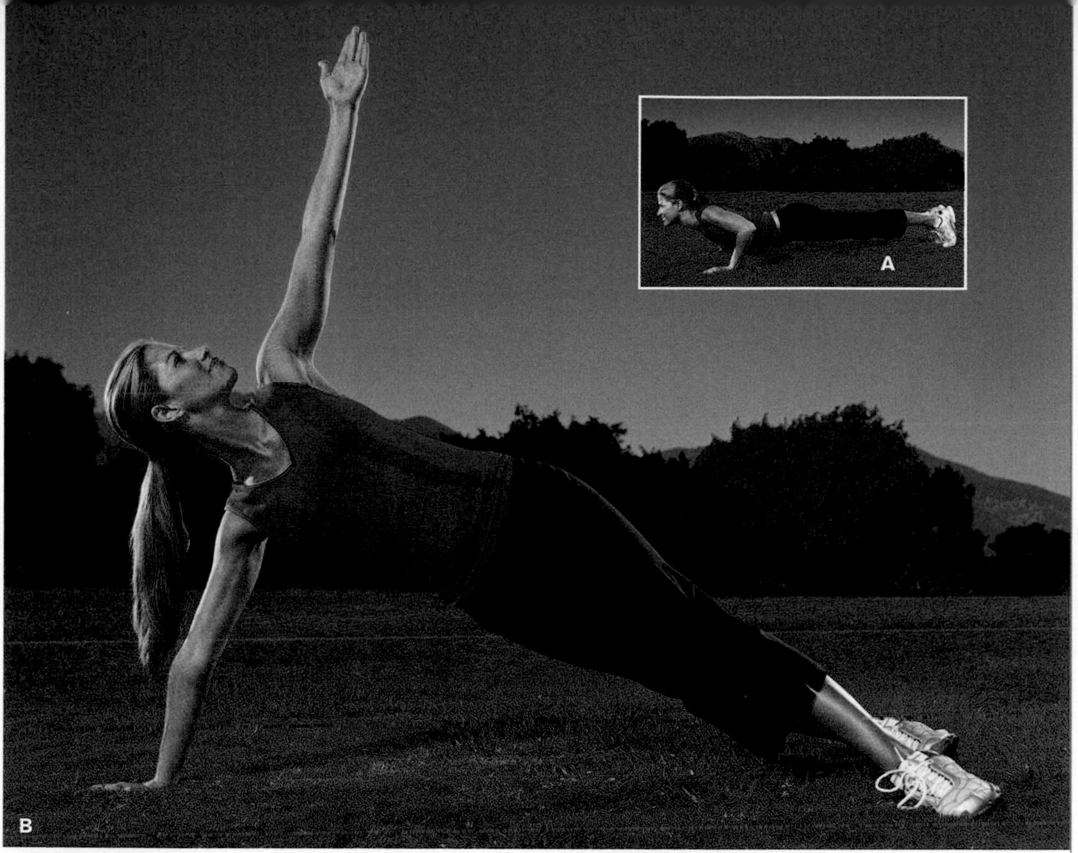

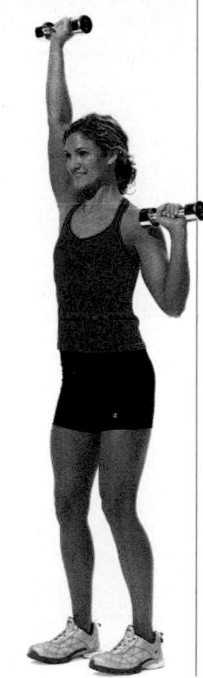

T PUSHUP

WORKS ABS, ARMS, BACK, AND SHOULDERS

Start in a low plank position with your elbows bent so your body is 2 inches off the ground (A). Push up and, as you reach the top, lift your left hand and roll onto the outside of your feet, keeping your body aligned. Straighten your left arm so your fingertips point upward (B). Hold for 1 second before returning to start. Repeat on the other side. That's one rep. Do five. For an additional core and balance challenge, stack your feet as you raise your arm.

STANDING ONE-ARM PRESS

WORKS ARMS AND SHOULDERS

Grab a pair of dumbbells and stand with your feet shoulder-width apart, knees slightly bent. Raise the dumbbells in front of your shoulders, palms facing forward. Press the right dumbbell overhead, keeping your arm in front of your ear (shown). Slowly lower, then raise the left dumbbell. Continue alternating for 14 reps.

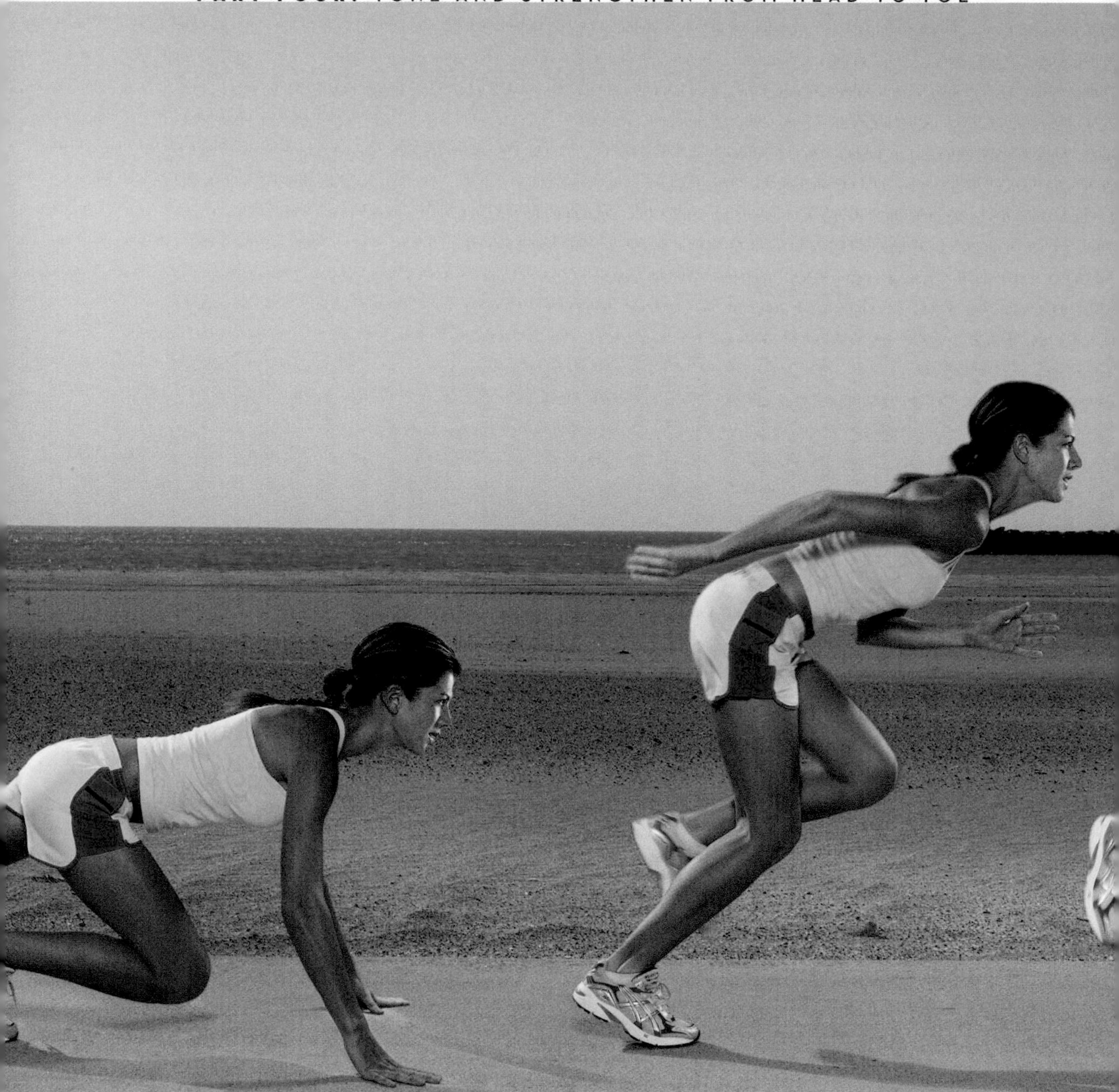

CHAPTER EIGHTEEN

GRAY MATTERS

TRAIN YOUR BRAIN TO MAKE YOU STRONGER AND FASTER WITH THIS (VERY SMART) ONCE-A-WEEK WORKOUT.

YOU'RE IN THE MIDDLE of a power struggle. And, no, it's not the "Why must ESPN be on 24/7?" argument you're always having with your NFL-obsessed significant other. We're talking about physical power—specifically, strength plus explosive speed. The type you'd use, say, to tackle your guy for the remote.

Unlike the never-ending ESPN debate, this power struggle is easy to ignore. Why? For one thing, who wants to look like a lumberjack? For another, you're comfortable with slow, steady weight-training moves that increase muscular endurance and tone. But those don't build power, which you need for dozens of every-day activities like chasing after a wayward toddler, hauling the newspaper bin down the stairs, or heaving your jam-packed gym bag off the shelf. (What's in that thing anyway?)

Luckily, this kind of power doesn't call for wine-barrel quads or Rocky Balboa–style workouts. The changes come from training a different muscle: your brain. Yep, your gray matter. The key is to train it to send signals more efficiently to your muscles via the nerve pathways that connect them, says Cassandra Forsythe, a Ph.D. candidate in exercise science at the University of Connecticut. This means that when your brain tells your legs to jump, they'll do it faster and with more force. And just adding a handful of power-specific moves to your weekly strength regimen will teach that cranium of yours all it needs to know.

That's awesome, but here's even better news: You only need to power train 1 day a week for 4 weeks. Power training is so intense (for your brain and your muscles) that its effects last up to 2 months. By week 4, you'll have the coordination and body (fringe benefit!) to rock that little black dress.

Oh, and you might want to take it outside. All the lunging, running, and medicine-ball-chucking you'll do requires space. Besides, you could use a bit of fresh air.

SUPERCHARGE IT
FOUR WAYS TO AMP UP YOUR POWER MOVES

1 Brace your abs as if Mike Tyson might sucker punch you at any moment. This stability will help your arms and legs produce more force.

2 Soften your set. During jumping drills, make sure you're landing on the right surface. Grass, sand, and rubber mats are best because they absorb most of the force when you hit the ground, reducing the impact on your ankles, knees, hips, and lower back. Bouncing around on harder surfaces, like concrete and asphalt, will pound your delicate joints into submission. Not good.

3 Avoid crash landings. Land as lightly as possible between repeated jumps. As soon as the balls of your feet touch down, bend your knees slightly and let your hips drop (as though squatting) to absorb the shock as you lower your heels.

4 Lighten your load. Hoisting a weight that's too heavy can actually teach your muscles to contract slower— obviously, not what you're going for. Opt for one that lets you complete the explosive part of the exercise (usually when you're moving upward) in less than a second. If it takes any longer, you're lifting too much weight.

MORE POWER TO YOU

FOLLOW THIS PLAN TO GET YOUR MUSCLES FIRING FASTER

DO IT: PERFORM TWO SETS OF 8 TO 10 REPS FOR EACH EXERCISE 1 DAY A WEEK.

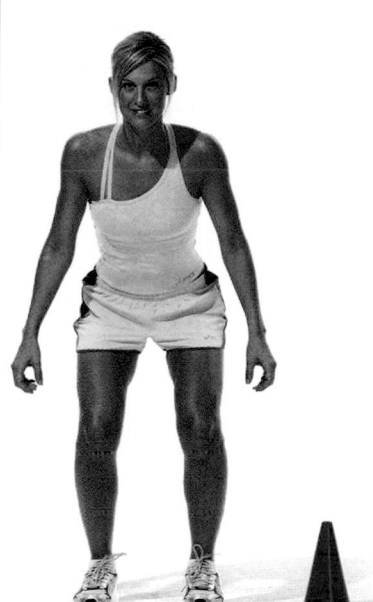

A

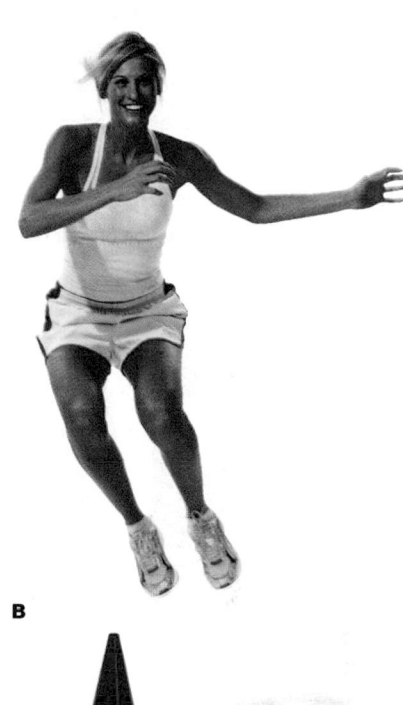

B

LATERAL BOUND

WORKS CORE, HIPS, AND THIGHS

Stand 12 inches to the right of an agility cone (if you can't find one, use an upright dumbbell) with feet hip-width apart (**A**). Push off with both legs and jump sideways over the cone (**B**). Land on the other side as softly as possible, then quickly explode back over. That's one rep.

TRAINING TIP: Swing your arms In the direction you're jumping to help get your body up and over the cone faster.

PUSHUP SPRINT

WORKS CHEST, CORE, LEGS, SHOULDERS, AND TRICEPS

Assume a pushup position, with hands slightly wider than your shoulders and your chest, hips, and legs touching the ground. In one explosive action, push up until you're in the top of a pushup (**A**), then immediately break into a sprint (**B**). After running 10 to 15 yards, stop and repeat in the other direction. Continue alternating.

TRAINING TIP: When you're about three strides away from the end of your sprint, start putting on the brakes so you can quickly switch directions.

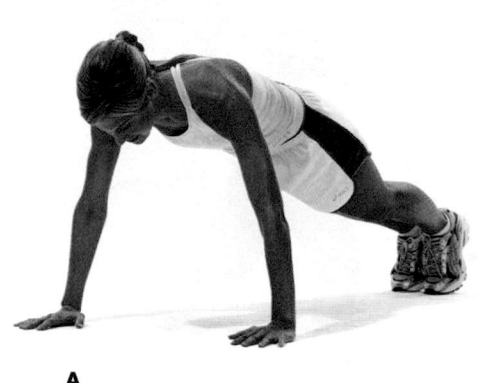

A

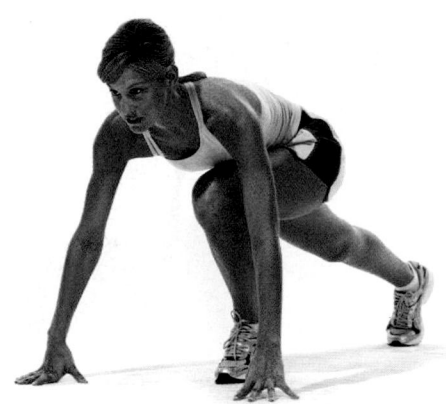

B

REVERSE OVERHEAD THROW

WORKS CORE, HIPS, SHOULDERS, THIGHS, AND UPPER BACK

Grab a 2- to 4-pound medicine ball. Stand with your feet slightly wider than your shoulders and hold the ball straight out in front of you at shoulder height. Perform a squat, keeping your knees behind your toes, and lower your arms until the ball nearly touches the ground (**A**). Quickly reverse directions, jump up, and simultaneously throw the ball up and back so it flies over your head (**B**). Land, retrieve the ball, and repeat.

TRAINING TIP: Use the momentum from your legs to propel the ball.

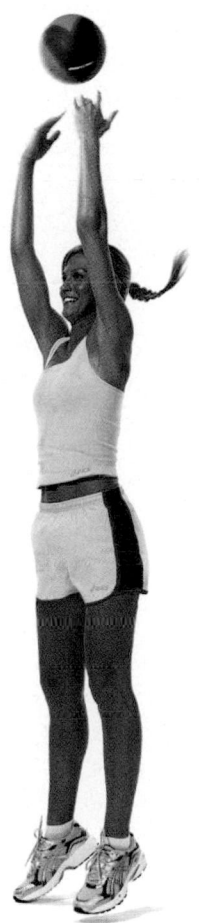

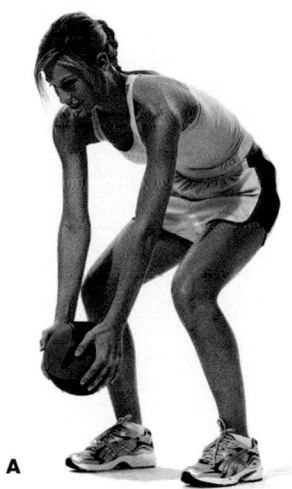

A

B

INSIDER TRAINING

Speedy strength requires stellar balance and core stability–aka coordination and no muffin top. To prime your body for the power workout, do this indoor routine for 4 weeks prior to moving outdoors. These moves will get you ready to jump, throw, and dash without injury.

DO IT:

PERFORM TWO SETS OF 8 TO 10 REPS FOR EACH EXERCISE 1 DAY A WEEK.

DUMBBELL PUSH PRESS

WORKS CORE, SHOULDERS, AND TRICEPS

Grab a pair of 8- to 10-pound dumbbells and stand with your feet shoulder-width apart, knees slightly bent. Position the dumbbells about 12 inches above your shoulders, palms facing each other. Quickly lower your hips into a quarter squat (**A**). Immediately straighten your legs and use that momentum to press the weights straight up with explosive force (**B**). Pause, lower, and repeat.

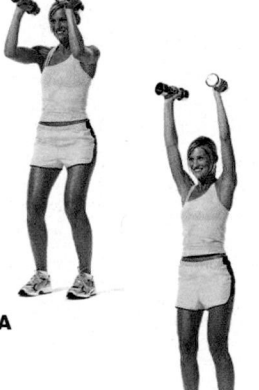

A

B

UNILATERAL SQUAT AND CABLE ROW

WORKS CORE, GLUTES, THIGHS, AND UPPER BACK

Stand facing a low cable pulley machine (set the weight to be challenging without hindering good form), feet hip-width apart and knees slightly bent. Bend at your hips and grab the pulley (like you're shaking hands) with your left hand. As you stand back up, lift your left foot (**A**). Next, lower your hips until your left thigh is parallel to the floor, then immediately push your right heel into the floor to stand up while performing a row with your left arm until your elbow passes your torso (**B**). Pause, lower, and repeat, alternating sides.

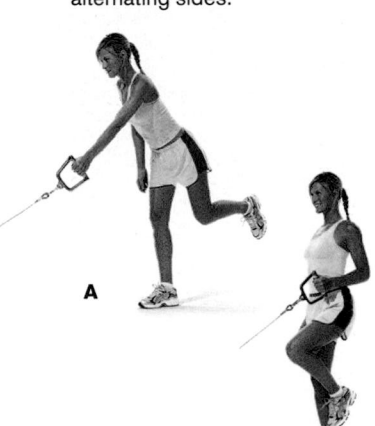

A

B

CABLE ROTATION
WORKS CORE AND ENTIRE UPPER BODY

Stand to the left of a cable pulley machine so the weight stack is on your right. With legs hip-width apart and knees slightly bent, reach across your body with your left arm and grab the pulley. Place your right hand on top of your left hand (**A**). Keeping your arms fairly straight, pull the handle out and away from you in a wide, sweeping motion. In the finish position, the cable should be pressed against your right shoulder (**B**). Pause there for 1 second, then slowly return the weight to start. Complete four to five reps, then face the other direction and repeat, reaching across with your left arm.

STABILITY BALL CHEST PRESS WITH HIP EXTENSION
WORKS CHEST, CORE, HIPS, SHOULDERS, AND TRICEPS

Grab a pair of 8- to 10-pound dumbbells and lie with your shoulders and upper back on a stability ball. Hold the dumbbells right above your chest, palms facing away from you. Position your legs hip-width apart with knees bent 90 degrees and feet flat on the floor, then slowly let your hips sink until your lower back comes as close to the ball as possible (**A**). In one explosive movement, drive your heels into the floor and raise your hips as you press the weights straight up over your chest (**B**). Hold for 1 second, then lower your hips and the weights. Repeat.

STEP-OUT LUNGE
WORKS CORE, HIPS, AND THIGHS

Grab a 2- to 4-pound medicine ball with both hands and hold it against your chest. Position your feet shoulder-width apart with knees slightly bent (**A**). Take a giant step out to the side with your left foot, keeping your toes pointing forward, and sink into a squat until your left leg is parallel to the floor (**B**). Be sure to keep your right leg straight throughout the move. Pause for 1 second, then explosively push back up to start and repeat on the other side. That's one rep.

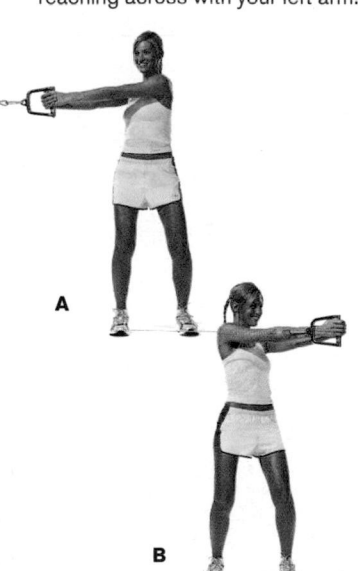

A

B

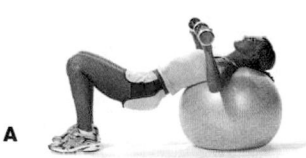

A

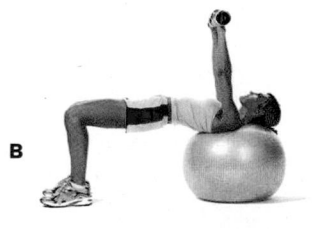

B

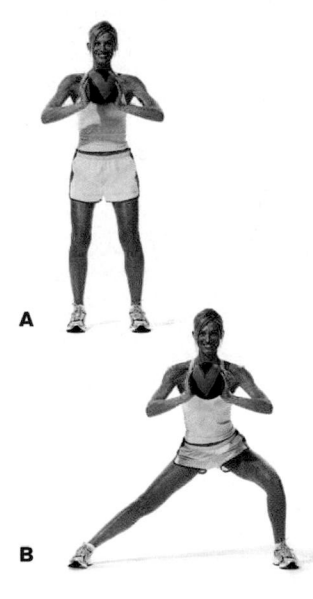

A

B

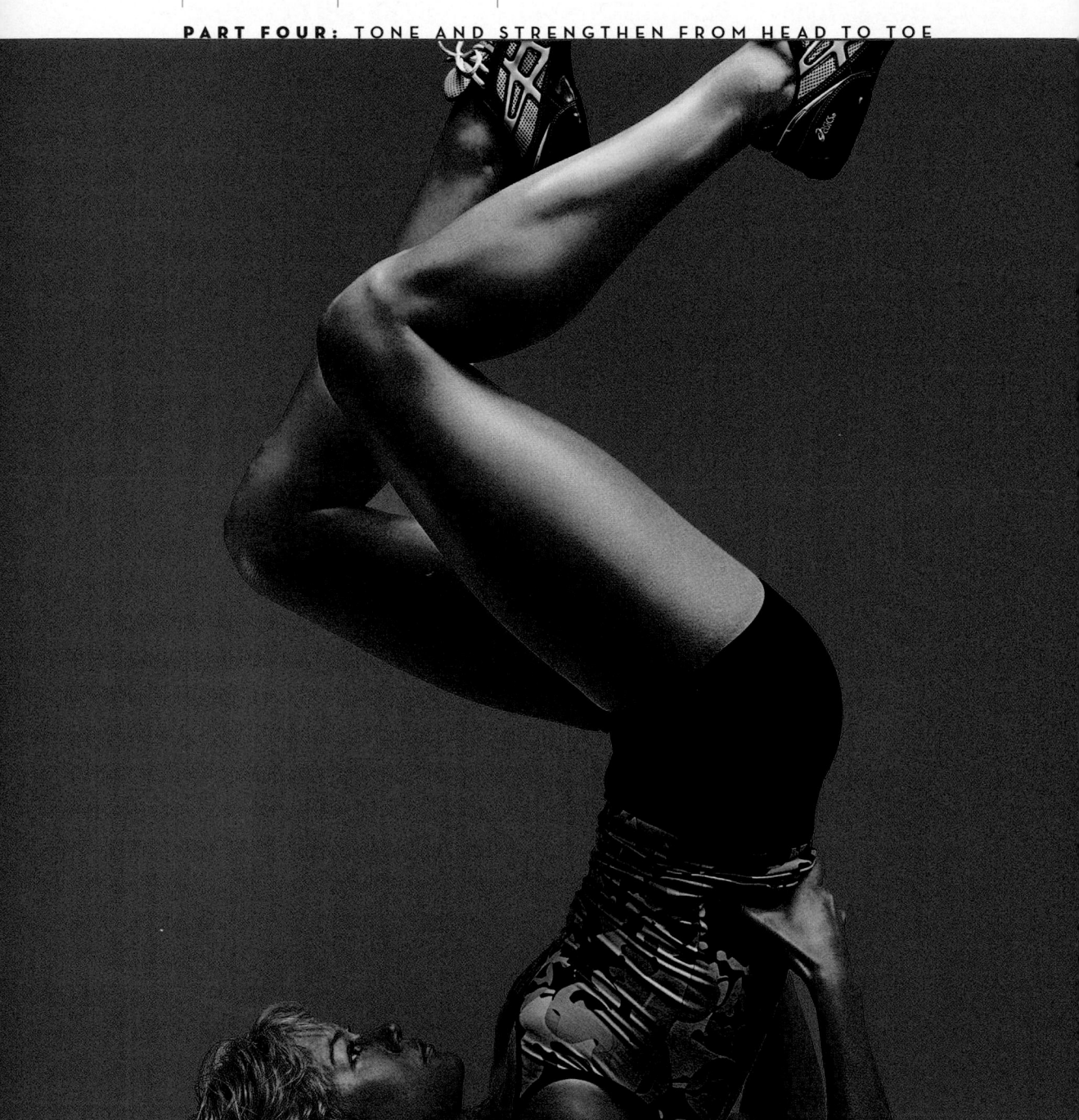

CHAPTER NINETEEN

ALL THE RIGHT MOVES

THE BEST EXERCISES FOR EVERY INCH OF YOUR BODY ARE MORE BASIC THAN YOU'D THINK.

DESPITE THE THOUSANDS OF CHOICES on Shoes.com, you probably have no trouble finding the perfect pair: Search for black patent-leather heels under $100, talk yourself into the $200 Prada look-alikes, click on Checkout—done! But choosing the best exercises isn't nearly so easy. There seem to be countless options, each just slightly different from the rest, all promising you the abs—or shoulders, or legs—of your dreams. No wonder you sometimes throw up your hands and resort to the eeny-meeny-miny-moe method.

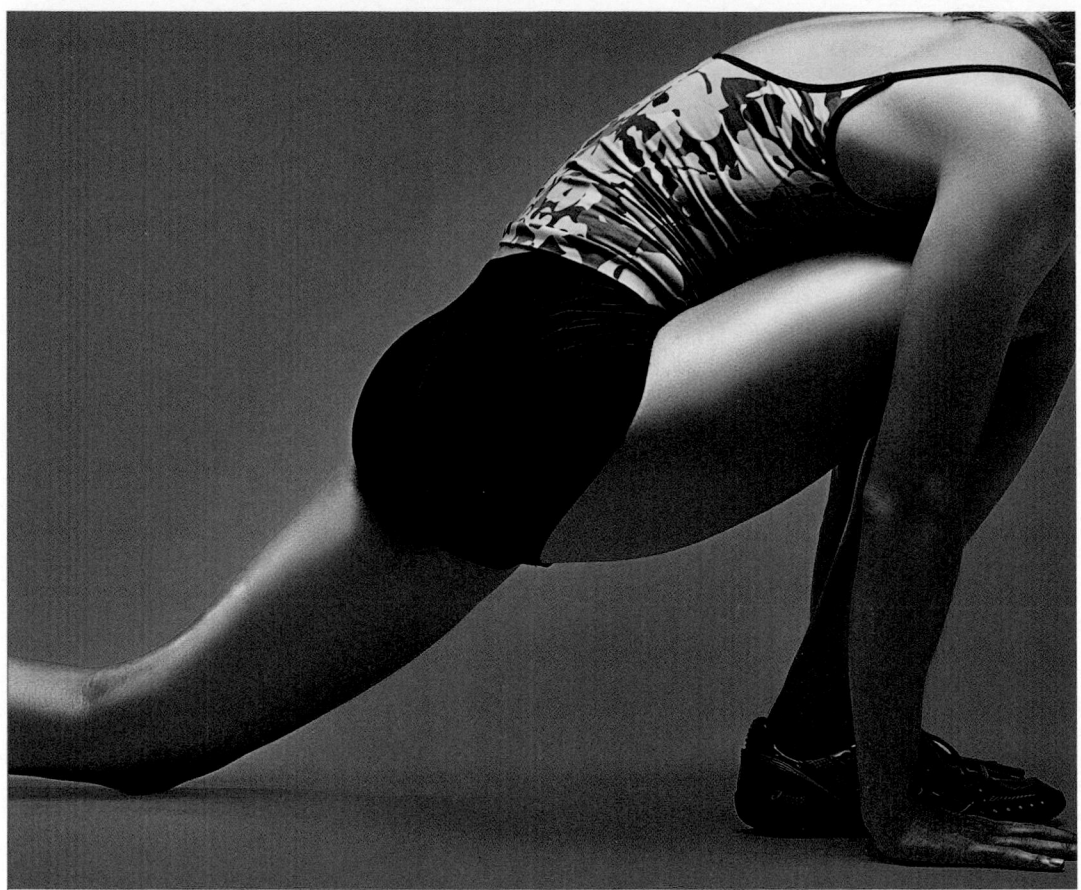

But random acts of exercise are hardly the best way to tone and hone your body. So we consulted the experts and sorted through the scientific studies to answer one simple question: What's the absolute best move for every key body part, from flabby arms to jiggly thighs? The 10 winning exercises, it turns out, are surprisingly basic—forget those complex gyrations that tax your mind more than your muscles.

What's more, these terrific 10 "involve compound movements, which target multiple muscles," says Lori Incledon, C.S.C.S., author of *Strength Training for Women*. Muscles work in tandem, she explains, so strengthening the core of one has peripheral benefits that radiate to the surrounding tissue. Done right, these moves will give you better tone and overall strength in just 2 weeks—and a whole new body in a couple of months. For a new pair of shoes to go with it, you're on your own.

INSTRUCTIONS

»» The only equipment you'll need is a set of dumbbells, an exercise bench, and a chinup bar.

»» Unless otherwise specified, do three sets of 8 to 10 reps of each exercise with a weight that feels challenging by rep 8.

Triceps

THE BEST EXERCISE DIP

The problem with the most popular arm move, the pushup, is that it works the chest first and the triceps second. "The best triceps exercise is one that uses it as the prime mover during the exercise," says Stephanie Barclay, C.S.C.S., director of fitness and wellness at North Park University. The dip does just that.

How to do it: Sit on the edge of a flat exercise bench and place your hands, fingers facing forward, next to your thighs. Place your feet on the floor in front of you, knees bent. Keeping your arms straight, scoot forward so your butt is hovering in front of the edge of the bench (**A**). Inhale, bend your arms, and lower your butt (**B**), stopping when your upper arms are parallel to the floor. Exhale and push yourself back up, straightening your arms.

Also works: Chest

Add a twist: To make the move even more challenging, extend your legs straight in front of you.

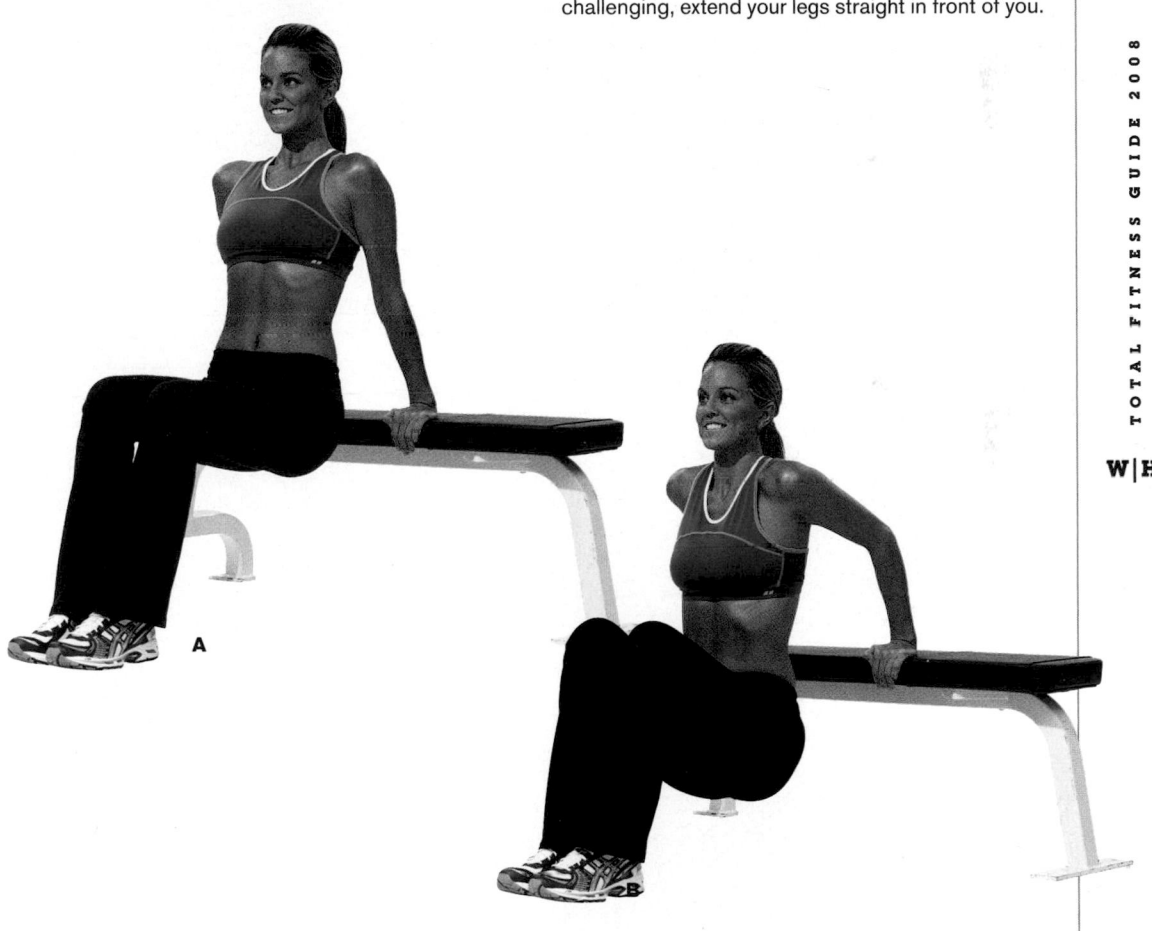

Biceps

THE BEST EXERCISE CHINUP

The chinup gets a bad rap as a simple exercise that simpleminded guys use to prove their super-manliness. But those meatheads are actually on to something. "You can load your biceps with a lot more weight on a chinup than you can on a curl," says Mike Mejia, a New York–based strength and conditioning specialist.

How to do it: Using a wide, underhand grip (palms facing you), hang from a bar with elbows straight, knees bent back, and ankles crossed (**A**). Pull yourself up until your chin clears the bar (**B**) and slowly lower yourself back to start. Do as many as you can.

Also works: Shoulders, triceps, lower arms, upper back, lower back

Add a twist: We won't lie—chinups are tough. If you can't manage one yet, have a workout partner help you raise yourself by placing her hands beneath your ankles.

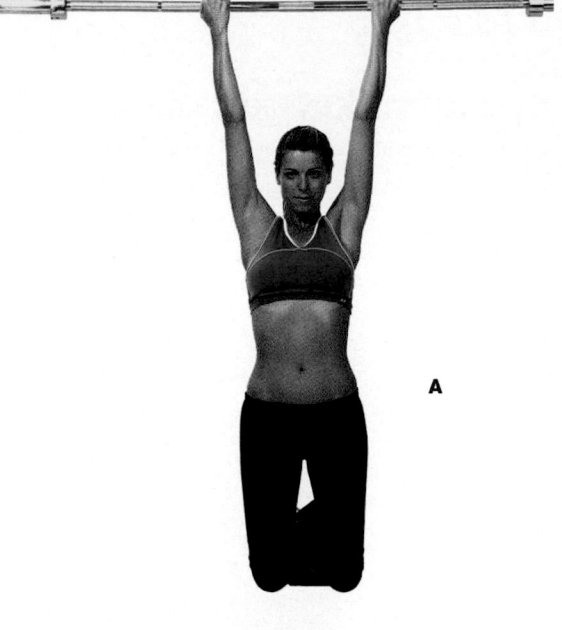

A

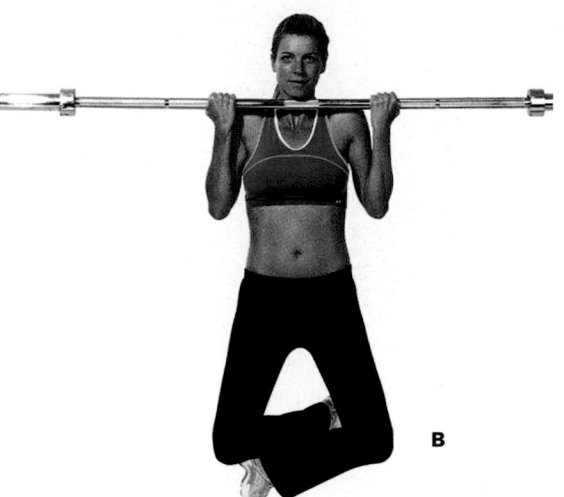

B

SMALLEST MUSCLE: Stapedius (which is inside the ear)

Shoulders

THE BEST EXERCISE
DUMBBELL MILITARY PRESS

Your job might not require heavy lifting, but that's no reason to ignore your shoulders. The military press gives your upper body tone and helps you hoist weighty objects without much trouble. "And using dumbbells allows more freedom of movement than the traditional barbell press," Mejia says. That means less strain on your shoulders.

How to do it: Sit on a bench with your feet hip-width apart. Using an overhand grip, hold a set of dumbbells at your shoulders (**A**). Press the weights straight up, focusing on control (**B**). Slowly lower them back to start.

Also works: Biceps and triceps

Add a twist: To engage your core, turn your torso as you push the weights overhead. Alternate sides.

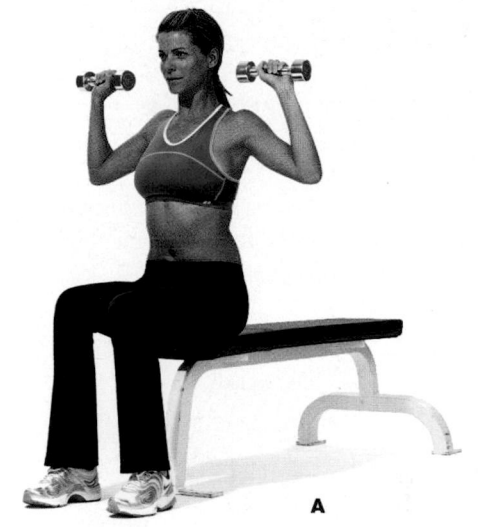

A

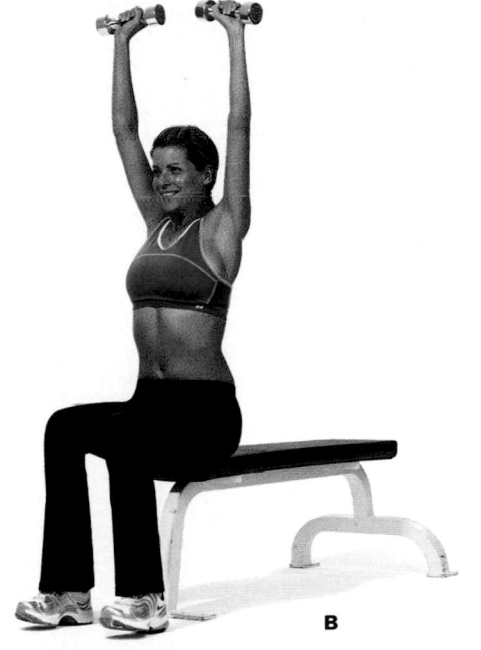

B

Upper Back

THE BEST EXERCISE DUMBBELL ROW

Rows work the major muscles of the upper back and midback more effectively than other gym or at-home exercises, Mejia says.

How to do it: Position your right knee and right hand on a workout bench (a large chair can substitute nicely) so your back is parallel to the floor (**A**). With your left hand, lift the dumbbell straight up to torso level, keeping your elbow in and pointing slightly toward the ceiling (**B**). Hold for 1 second. Slowly lower the weight to a dead hanging position and repeat. Switch sides between sets.

Also works: Triceps

Add a twist: Try it without a bench, which will test your balance as well. Bending over till your torso is parallel to the floor, stand on one leg with your other leg bent behind you and do one set of rows. Switch legs.

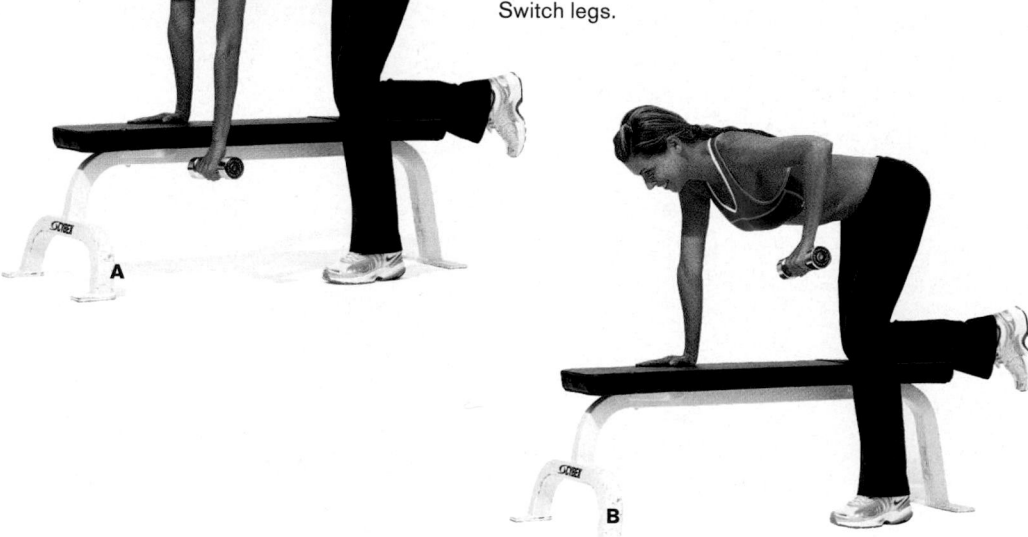

Abdominals

THE BEST EXERCISE REVERSE CRUNCH

It's one-stop six-pack shopping. A study from the University of Nebraska Medical Center found that the reverse crunch works all three visible abdominal areas—upper abs, lower abs, and obliques—at once.

How to do it: Lie on your back, knees bent (**A**). Bring them in to your chest and back down (**B**).

Also works: Obliques

Add a twist: To strengthen your obliques even more, twist your legs to one side as you raise them, alternating sides.

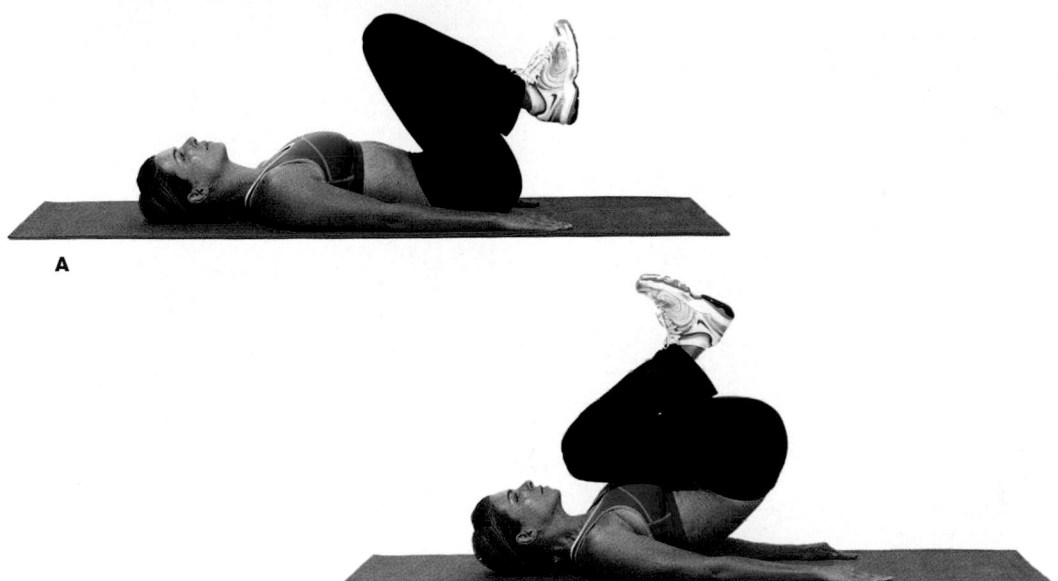

A

B

TOTAL FITNESS GUIDE 2008

W|H

Lower Back

THE BEST EXERCISE
ALTERNATING SUPERWOMAN

Your power, balance, and stability all come from your core, and while ab work is important, without an equally strong lower back to control every movement, a six-pack is all but worthless. A 2005 study in the *Journal of Strength and Conditioning Research* found that the so-called superman (in this case, superwoman!) exercise is the most effective at honing the neglected half of your core.

How to do it: Lie facedown on the floor with your arms out in front of you (**A**). Lift your right arm and left leg off the floor (**B**), hold for 10 seconds, then lower them and switch sides.

Also works: Glutes and hamstrings

Add a twist: Increase the difficulty by lifting both arms and both legs off the floor at the same time.

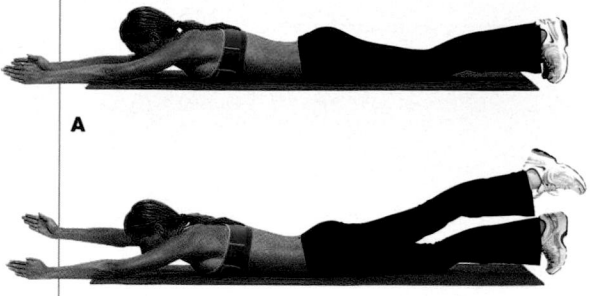

Chest

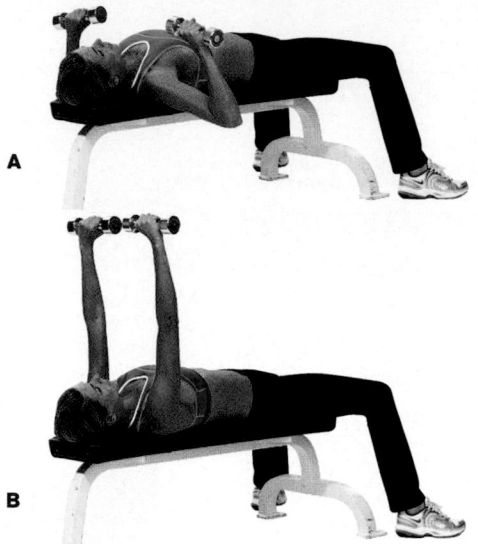

THE BEST EXERCISE
DUMBBELL CHEST PRESS

Even if the chest press weren't the single smartest way to perk up your pecs–a 2005 study from Truman State University found that the bench press activates chest muscles longer than the fly–you should do it anyway. Because nothing makes you feel more like a weight-lifting badass than lying on your back and pumping iron.

How to do it: Lie on your back on a flat bench, letting your elbows and shoulders drop. Hold a dumbbell in each hand on either side of your chest (**A**). Lifting both weights at the same pace, push them straight up until your arms are fully extended (**B**). Hold them there for 1 second, then return to start.

Also works: Shoulders, triceps

Add a twist: To improve muscle tone, concentrate on contracting your chest throughout the exercise, not just while you're lifting.

Calves

THE BEST EXERCISE
TOE RAISE

Strong calves can defeat a frequent runner or walker's worst enemy: shin splints. If you choose only one exercise to strengthen your calves (and sculpt fantastic-looking legs), make it the toe raise, Mejia says.

How to do it: You can do a toe raise on pretty much any step or curb. Stand on a step with your feet slightly apart, drop your heels down below it (**A**), then push straight up onto your tip-toes (**B**). Slowly lower your heels and repeat. Squeeze your calves at the top of the exercise to get the most benefit.

Also works: Quads and hamstrings

Add a twist: Hold a pair of dumbbells at your sides, but not more than 10 pounds total—calf muscles can tear easily.

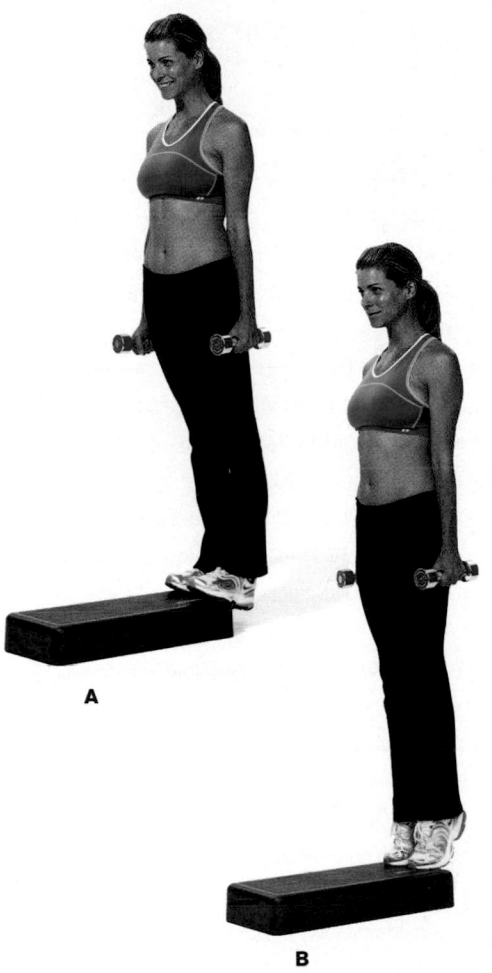

A

B

TOTAL FITNESS GUIDE 2008

W|H

Quadriceps

THE BEST EXERCISE
DUMBBELL SQUAT

Several studies over the last decade comparing squats with leg presses have found that squats are the safest and most effective way to work your quads. Gym rats will tell you to use the Smith machine (the large rack that holds a straight bar), but most women are better off sticking with dumbbells to avoid injury. "Most of these types of machines were built for a 5'10", 185-pound man," Incledon says.

How to do it: Stand, holding a dumbbell on each side with arms hanging straight down (**A**), and bend your knees until your thighs are just past parallel to the floor. Your back should be at roughly 45 degrees, your eyes looking straight ahead (**B**). Extend your legs, straightening back up to return to standing.

Also works: Glutes

Add a twist: Combine squats with upright rows: From the standing position, lift the dumbbells to chest height by raising your elbows. Lower the weights slowly then immediately perform a squat. Repeat.

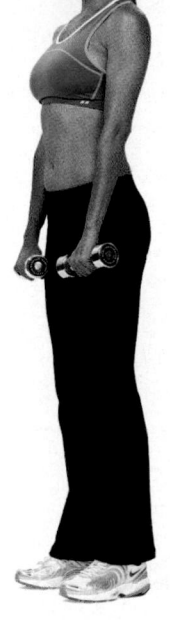

A

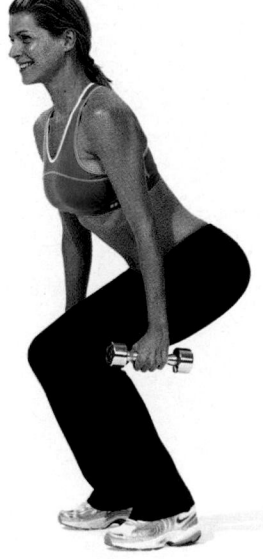

B

FASTEST MUSCLE: Orbicularis oculi (which closes the eyelid and contracts in 1/100 second)

Butt

THE BEST EXERCISE
ROMANIAN DEADLIFT

This move can give you the lean shape of an Eastern European supermodel. "It combines two of the most often neglected but vitally important movements–hip and spinal extension," Mejia says.

How to do it: Stand with feet hip-width apart, knees slightly bent, and back straight. Hold a dumbbell in each hand, arms hanging straight down (**A**). Bend from your hips and lower the weights, keeping your neck in line with your spine and your hips back (**B**). Contract your glutes and hamstrings and return to start.

Also works: Hamstrings

Add a twist: Do the move on one leg at a time. Keep your balance by extending your nonworking leg out behind you.

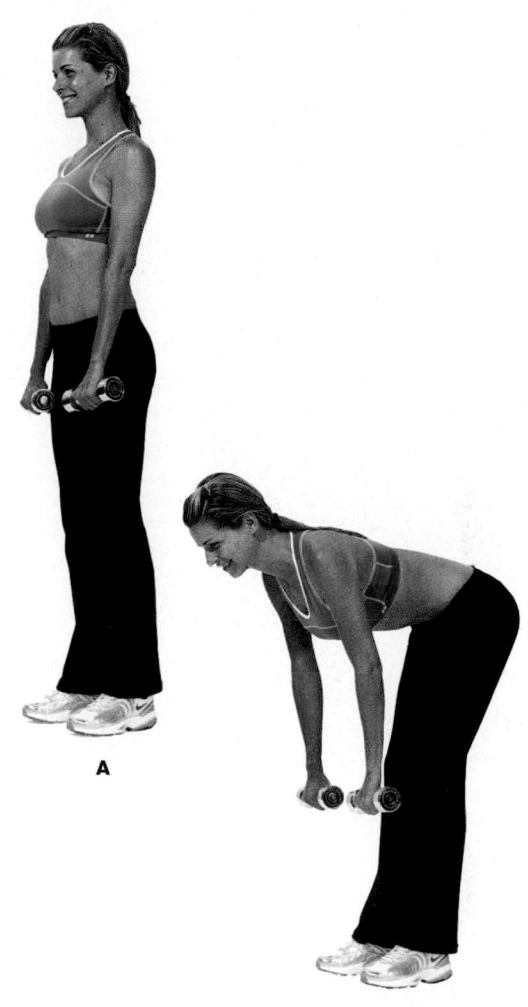

A

B

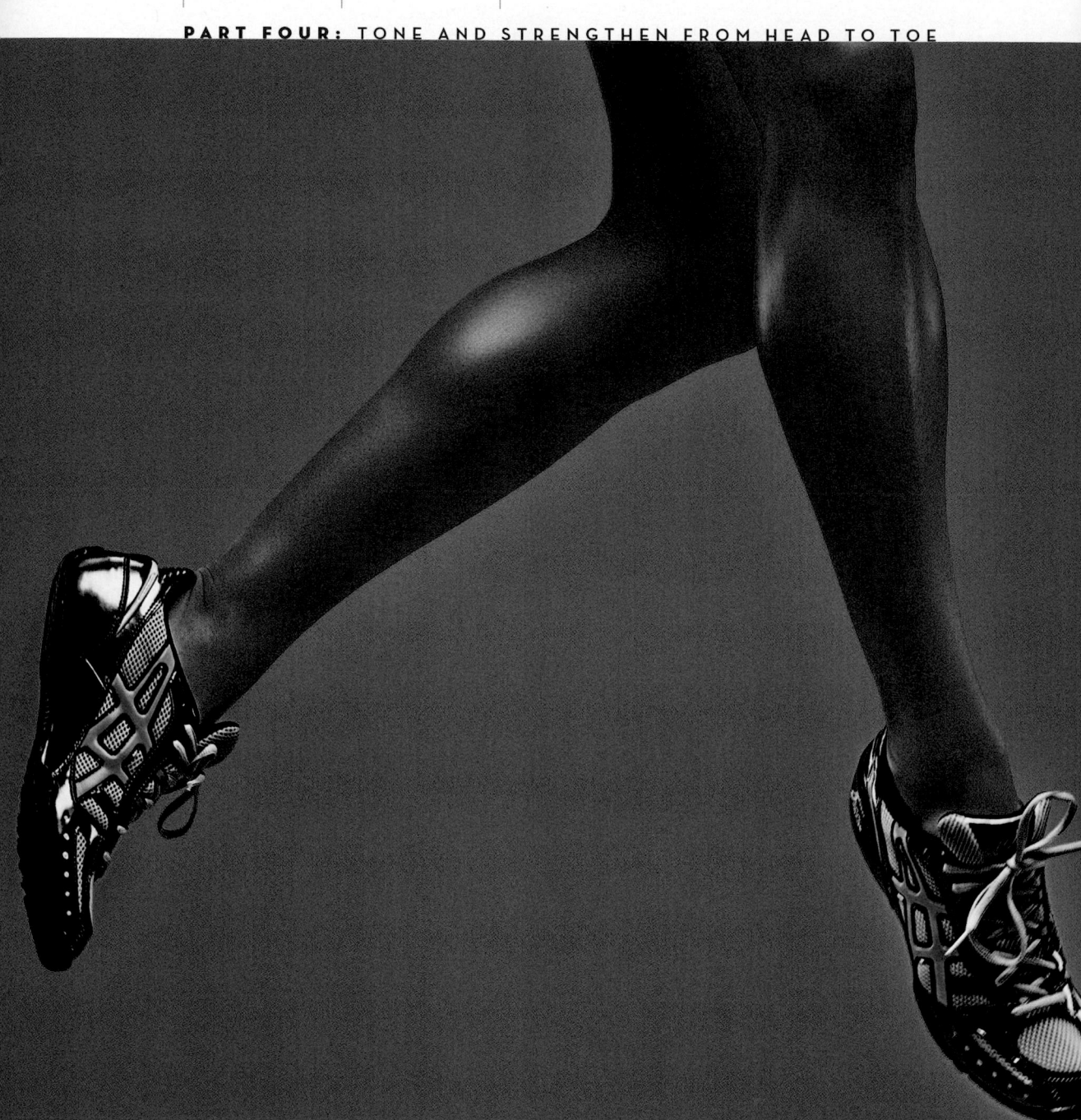

CHAPTER TWENTY

DON'T MISS A MUSCLE

FOUR MOVES FOR YOUR MOST COMMONLY MISSED AREAS.

YOUR ABS AND BUM get plenty of workout TLC, but your calves, chest, lower back, and rear deltoids are likely getting the shaft, according to Ellen Barrett, a personal trainer and owner of the Studio, a Pilates and yoga center in New Haven, Connecticut. Eliminate these weak spots by adding the following moves to your regular strength workout once a week and you'll prevent muscle imbalances that can lead to injury. Do each move until you can't do another rep with perfect form.

Calves

WHY WORK 'EM: TO PREVENT KNEE INJURIES
AND SHIN SPLINTS.

FORGET-ME-NOT MOVE:

PLIÉ HEEL LIFT

Stand with your heels touching, toes turned out.
With straight legs, lift both heels up off the floor.
Keeping heels lifted, plié by bending both knees
slightly (**A**). Next, drop your heels down to the floor
(**B**) and roll them back up, still in the plié. Continue
lowering and lifting your heels at a steady pace
until fatigued.

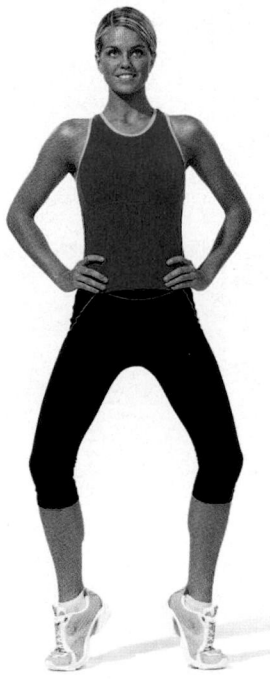

A

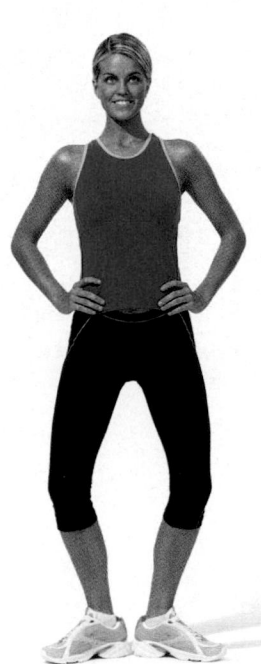

B

Chest

WHY WORK IT: TO TAKE PRESSURE OFF YOUR MORE DELICATE SHOULDER JOINTS.

FORGET-ME-NOT MOVE:

SCOOP HOLD

Grab a 3- to 5-pound dumbbell in each hand. Sit with your knees bent, feet together flat on the floor, and arms extended outside your knees (**A**). Raise your feet 6 to 12 inches and lift the weights with straight arms to at least shoulder height (**B**), pressing them together at the top. Hold here until fatigued.

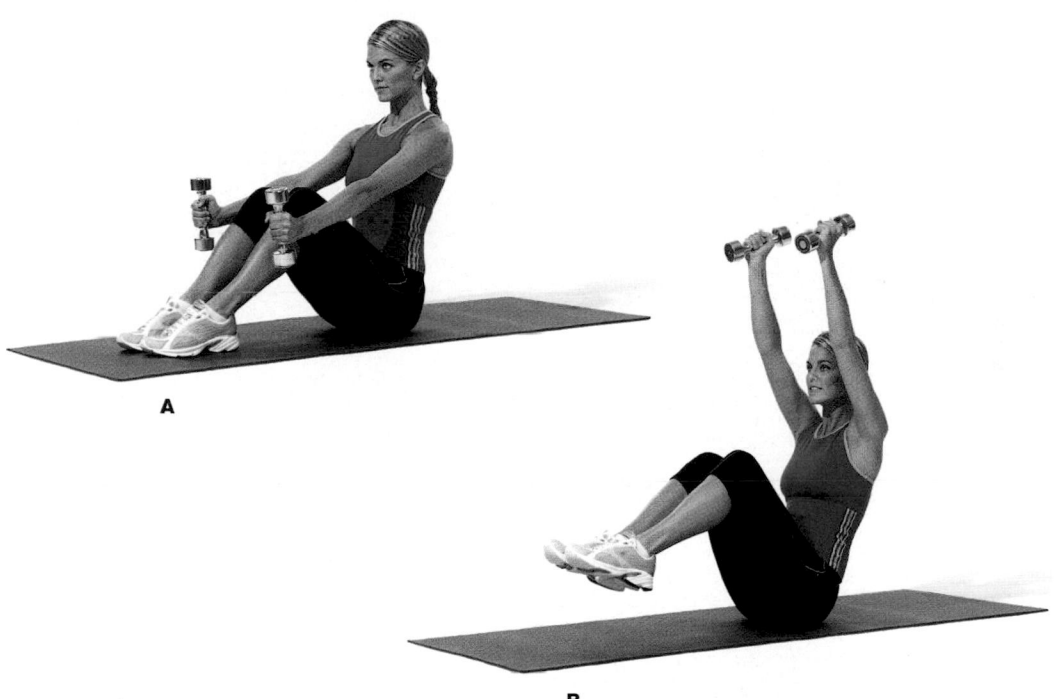

A

B

Lower Back

WHY WORK IT: WHEN YOU HAVE STRONG ABS BUT A WEAK LOWER BACK, YOU'RE MORE LIKELY TO STRAIN THE MUSCLES THAT SUPPORT YOUR SPINE.

FORGET-ME-NOT MOVE:

SWIMMING

Lie facedown, with arms extended. Lift your arms and legs a few inches, so only your hips are on the floor. Lift your right arm and left leg as high as possible (shown). Repeat with your other arm and leg. Alternate until fatigued.

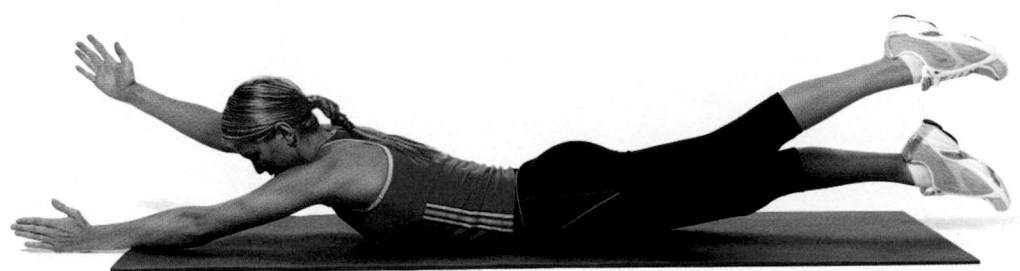

Rear Deltoids

WHY WORK 'EM: THE STRONGER THESE SHOULDER-SUPPORTING MUSCLES ARE, THE MORE OVERALL LIFTING STRENGTH YOU HAVE.

FORGET-ME-NOT MOVE:

REVERSE FLY

Grab a 3- to 8-pound dumbbell in your left hand. Place feet wider than shoulders and turn toes and torso to the right. Lean foward, with your right hand on your thigh (**A**). Lift the weight out to the side to shoulder height (**B**), then lower. Continue until fatigued. Switch sides.

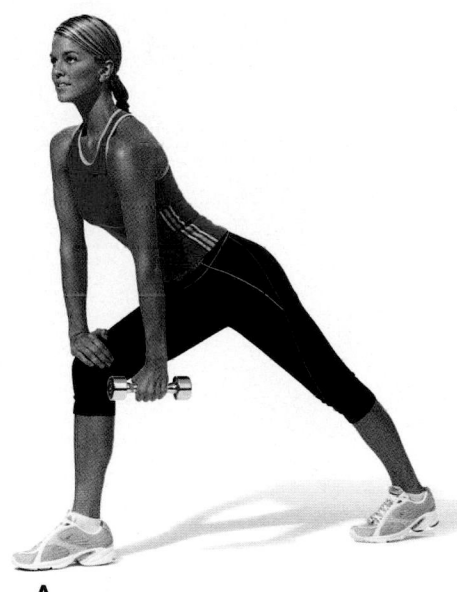

A

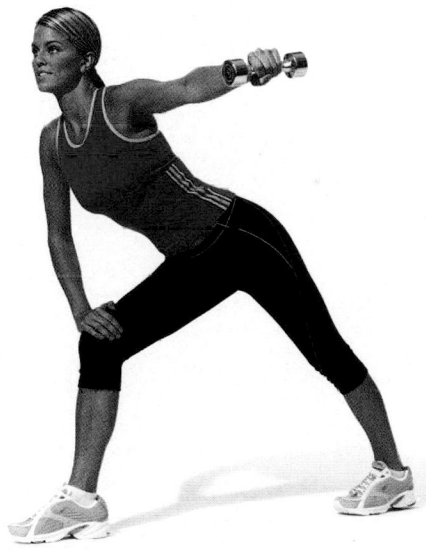

B

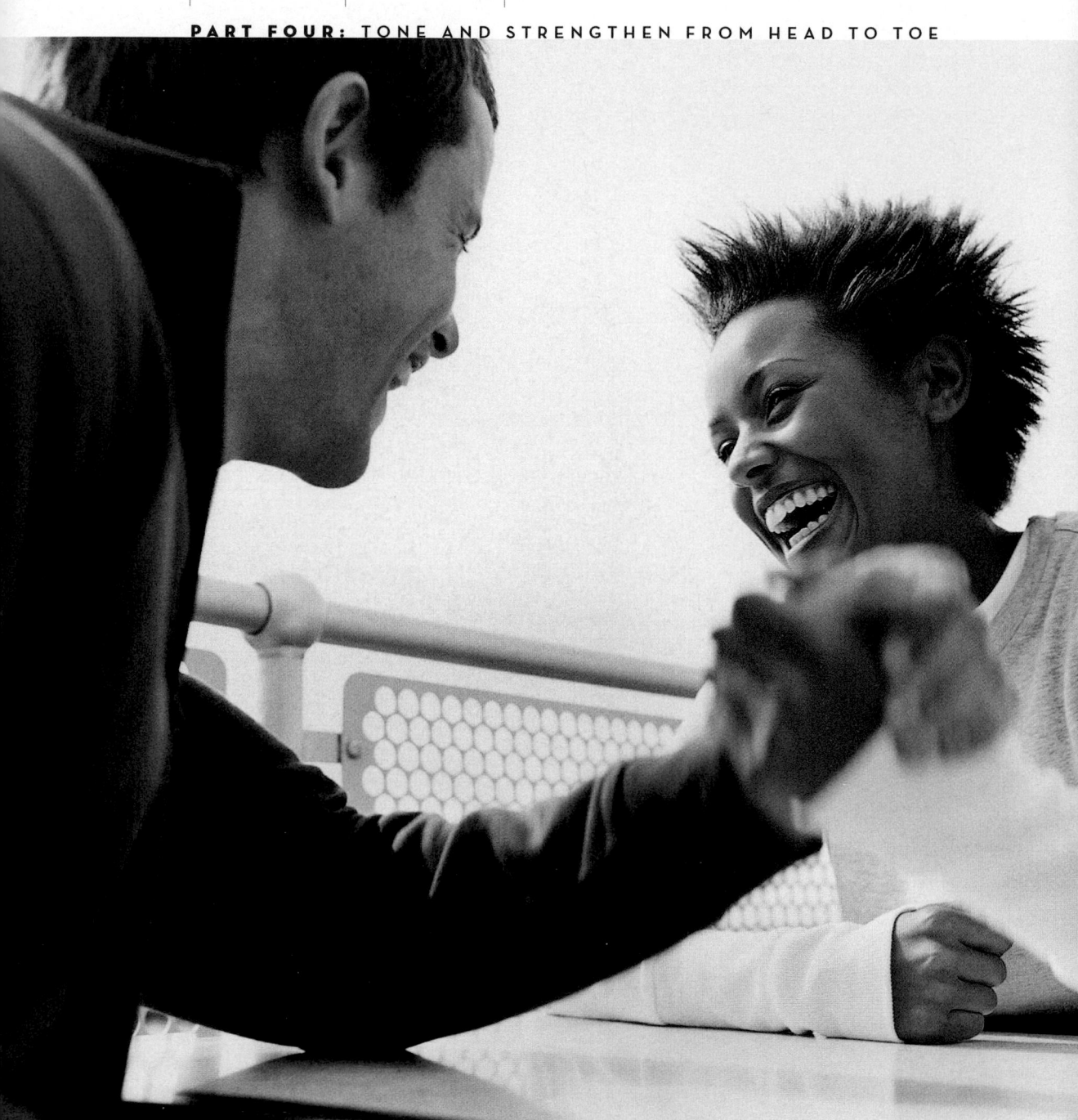

CHAPTER TWENTY-ONE

WE CAN WORK IT OUT

TURN YOUR GUY INTO THE ULTIMATE EXERCISE BUDDY–NO MATTER HOW DIFFERENT YOUR FITNESS MENTALITIES MAY BE.

BY KATE ASHFORD

YOU DON'T NEED SCIENTIFIC RESEARCH to tell you that dragging your man to Anthropologie to help you pick out the perfect new party top is a colossal waste of time. Some endeavors, however, are worth a team approach. Consider this: A University of Pittsburgh study showed that women who work out with a partner lose a third more weight than those who go it alone. And then there's this: Exercise increases blood flow throughout your body—including down there. So yeah, working out with him is a pound-shedding, sex drive-revving option you should take advantage of—pronto.

SPOT ON
HOW TO MAN HIS BENCH EVEN WHEN HE'S LIFTING TWICE YOUR BODY WEIGHT

Get hands on. Spotting is nine-tenths psychological—just the fact that you're touching him or the weights can help him eke out a few more reps, says Los Angeles-based trainer Mike Curry. If he's lifting a barbell, put your palms lightly on the underside of the bar inside his hands (no help, though). If he's got dumbbells, put your hands under his wrists, not his elbows, to avoid throwing him off balance at a critical moment.

Don't be intimidated. If he's struggling, get him over the hump by boosting just 5 to 10 percent of the weight for him. So even if he's hefting 80-pound dumbbells, you're only lifting 4 to 8 pounds with each hand. You can handle it.

Find your stance. Be prepared to act if he needs some assistance by standing with your knees bent and your feet slightly wider than your shoulders. Position yourself close enough to the weight that you won't have to lean forward to help him lift it.

Be alert. He may need your help for either part of the exercise: the lifting or the lowering. It's important to be aware that people can get injured during the relaxation phase if they put weights down too quickly, says exercise physiologist Sheila Kalas. Make sure you're paying attention the whole time so you can help him guide the weight back to the rack safely.

Which is great advice if you can use it, but few couples are matches made in fitness heaven. (Him in your Cardio Capoeira class? Um, no.) Don't despair, though: Even if the only "gym" in his life is a stick of mystery meat called Slim, you can still benefit from working out together, no matter what your exercise personality or goal. Try these tricks from leading trainers, physiologists, and fitness pros to get your butts moving together in no time.

You . . . love to work out

He . . . hasn't broken a sweat since high school

DO-IT-TOGETHER STRATEGY Your best plan of attack: motivation. "Men are goal-oriented," says Eleanor Cole, Ph.D., a psychologist in New York City, "so set up rewards for meeting small goals." (Kinda like when you bought yourself that new Stella gym bag.) It takes about 4 weeks—or, say, 12 trips to the gym—for exercise to become a habit. Get him addicted by offering a small incentive after every four workouts, like an Amazon.com gift card for a pair of weight-lifting gloves or movie tickets for *Blades of Glory,* the Will Ferrell figure-skating flick. (Warning: Be prepared for 2-plus hours of Ferrell in spandex. On ice.) After he makes it to week 4, cement his new habit with the 0.55-ounce, 1-gig iPod Shuffle, the world's smallest MP3 player ($79, apple.com).

If the gym isn't his thing, look for a coed sports team, says Kate Hays, Ph.D., a Toronto-based sports psychologist, to provide a steady play date on the field or court. Check active.com to find athletic leagues in your area. "Ideally, pick something different than what you're already good at," Hays says. If you play tennis Sharapova-style, he may start to lose motivation when he can't even return your serves.

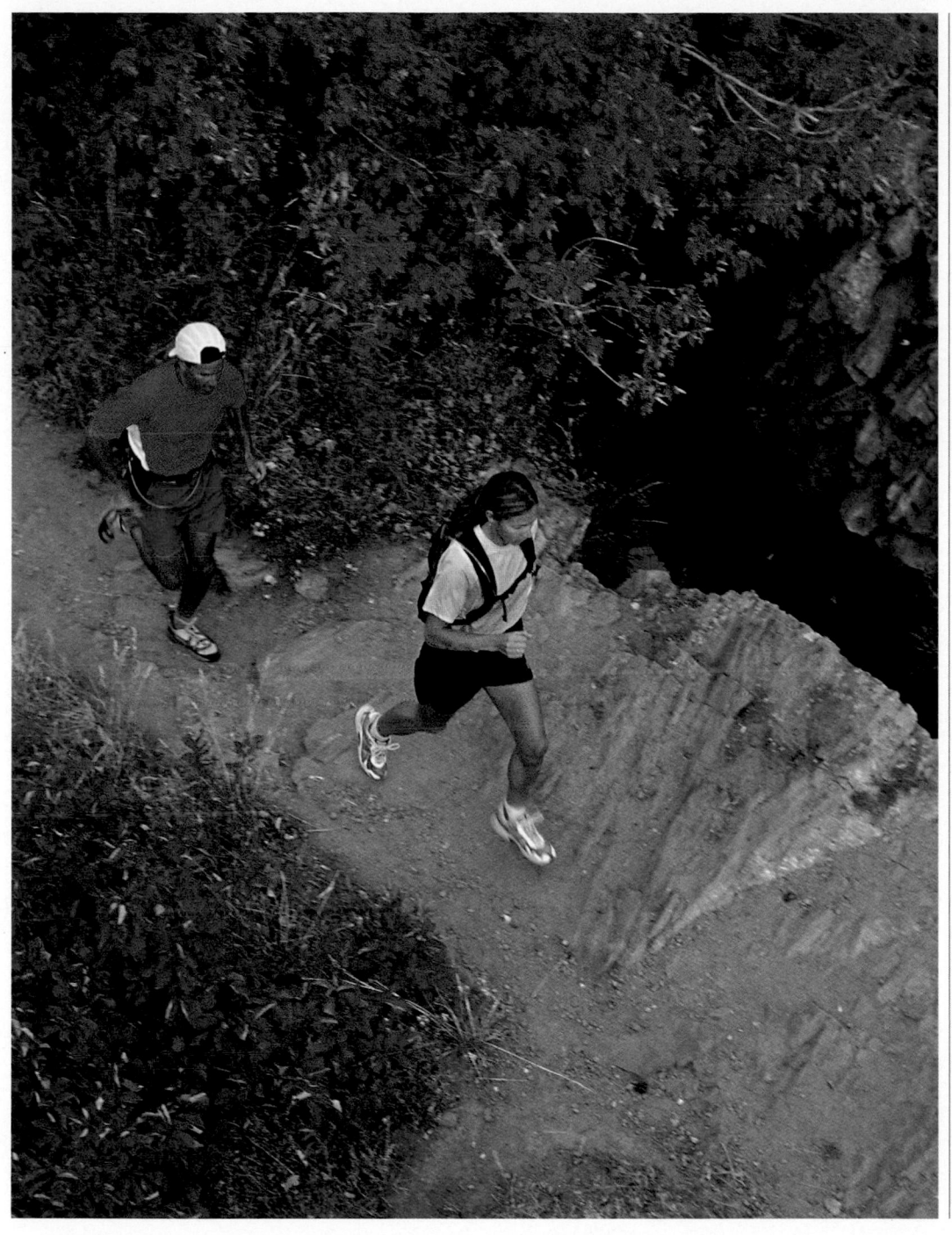

You . . . want to tone up

He . . . wants to bulk up

DO-IT-TOGETHER STRATEGY Lifting weights isn't going to turn either of you into a bulging muscle freak—unless you want it to. It's all in the approach. To get lean and strong with weights, work large muscle groups, such as the back, chest, and legs. "They burn the most calories," says Sheila Kalas, an exercise physiologist at the University of Kentucky and owner of Fitness Plus in Lexington.

So join your man on days when he's doing the following fat-obliterating exercises: squats, leg extensions, and leg curls for the lower body; chest presses, flies, lat pulldowns, and rows for the chest and back (visit womens*healthmag.com to learn the moves). To tone up and kill calories, do one to three sets of 12 to 15 reps, using enough weight that your muscles are fatigued (but not completely spent) when you get to the last rep. To build mass, he should do three to five sets of 8 to 10 reps, using enough weight that by the end of the last set, he can't do one more rep. Sick of waiting around for your turn on the machine? Finish your session with a few time-saving, calorie-busting tandem moves like the three on these pages from Michael Curry, owner of Stronghold Fitness in West Los Angeles.

You . . . play to win

He . . . plays to annihilate

DO-IT-TOGETHER STRATEGY Okay, so you're both cutthroat maniacs. No worries. In a 2002 study, researchers at Penn State University found that when women anticipate competition they get a surge of testosterone, which boosts the libido—you do the math. Use this to your advantage by choosing a workout strategy that plays off your it-doesn't-matter-how-much-I-love-you-I'm-going-to-whoop-your-sweet-ass nature—without killing each other in the process.

If you're all about the weight room, you can keep his Schwarzenegger-size ego in check with this trick: Figure out what percentage of your respective body weight each of you is hoisting, suggests Rachel Cosgrove, C.S.C.S., who owns a gym in Santa Clarita, California, with her husband and workout partner, Alwyn. Simply divide the number of pounds you're lifting by your body weight and, voilà, suddenly the playing field is level.

If you're more about cardio, run or bike together three times a week. On day 1, he chooses the route. On day 2, you devise the workout plan. And on day 3, play Simon Says: Do intervals, alternating who gets to set the time, distance, and style (here's your chance to see him make a fool out of himself skipping or high-kneeing to the next streetlight). "Our bodies love routine, but that gets us into a rut," Curry says. Mixing it up this way "shocks the muscles, and you start burning major calories again."

PARTNER SQUAT

WORKS CORE AND ENTIRE LOWER BODY

Stand back to back with legs hip-width apart, leaning against each other, arms at your sides (**A**). Slowly lower your hips together until your thighs are parallel to the floor (**B**). When you've both reached that point, push back up to standing at the same time. Do three sets of 10 to 12 reps, resting 30 to 60 seconds between sets.

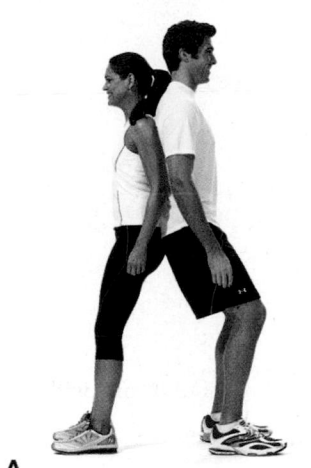

A

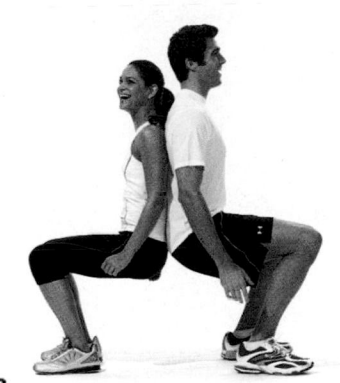

B

PARTNER ROW

Stand facing each other, with 5 to 10 feet between you, each holding an end of a set of bands. With feet hip-width apart, extend your arms to shoulder height, with bands slightly taut (**A**). Pull your elbows back until your upper-back muscles contract (**B**). Return to start—that's one rep. Do three to five sets of 20 to 30 reps, resting 30 to 60 seconds between sets.

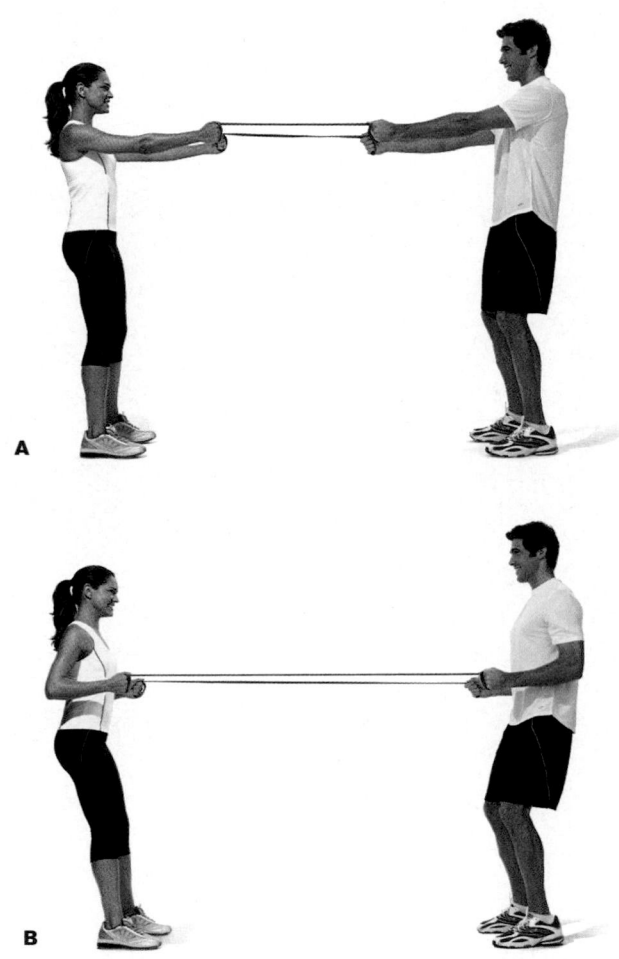

PARTNER CHEST PRESS

WORKS CHEST, CORE, SHOULDERS, AND TRICEPS

Stand facing away from each other, holding a set of exercise bands. Walk forward until bands are taut. With feet hip-width apart, hold hands at chest height with elbows bent 90 degrees (A). Together, push your arms straight out (B). Take 2 seconds to extend and 4 seconds to get back to start. Do three to five sets of 20 to 30 reps, resting 30 to 60 seconds between sets.

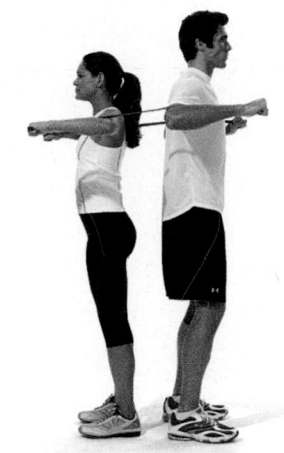

A

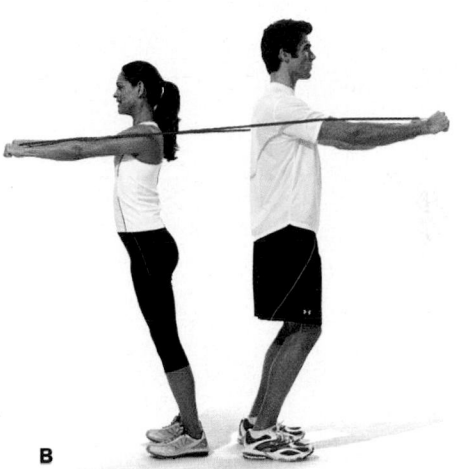

B

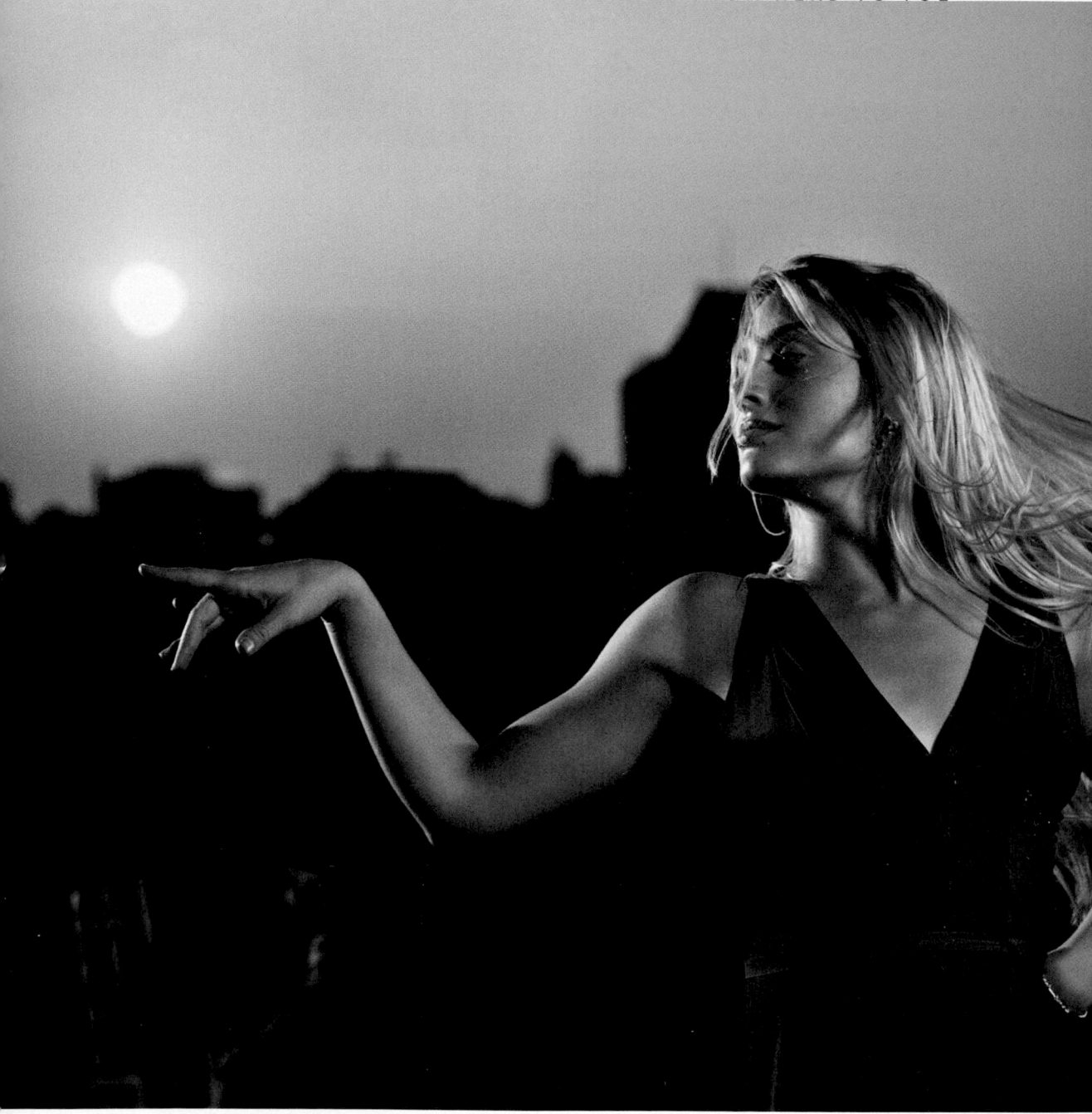

CHAPTER TWENTY-TWO

BUST A MOVE!

FOUR WAYS TO GET YOUR STYLISH GROOVE ON.

BY LARA MCGLASHAN

TOTAL FITNESS GUIDE 2008

W|H

SHOUTS OF JOY are as common on the treadmill as they are on C-SPAN. "People are sick of doing cardio this ol' way; they want to move," says Carol Espel, the national director of group fitness for Equinox Fitness Clubs. That's why dancing for fitness—big movements that fry calories and build major strength and flexibility—is making a comeback. We tapped dozens of fitness and dance gurus to find the four biggest trends. Take our crash course, then get out of the gym and onto the dance floor.

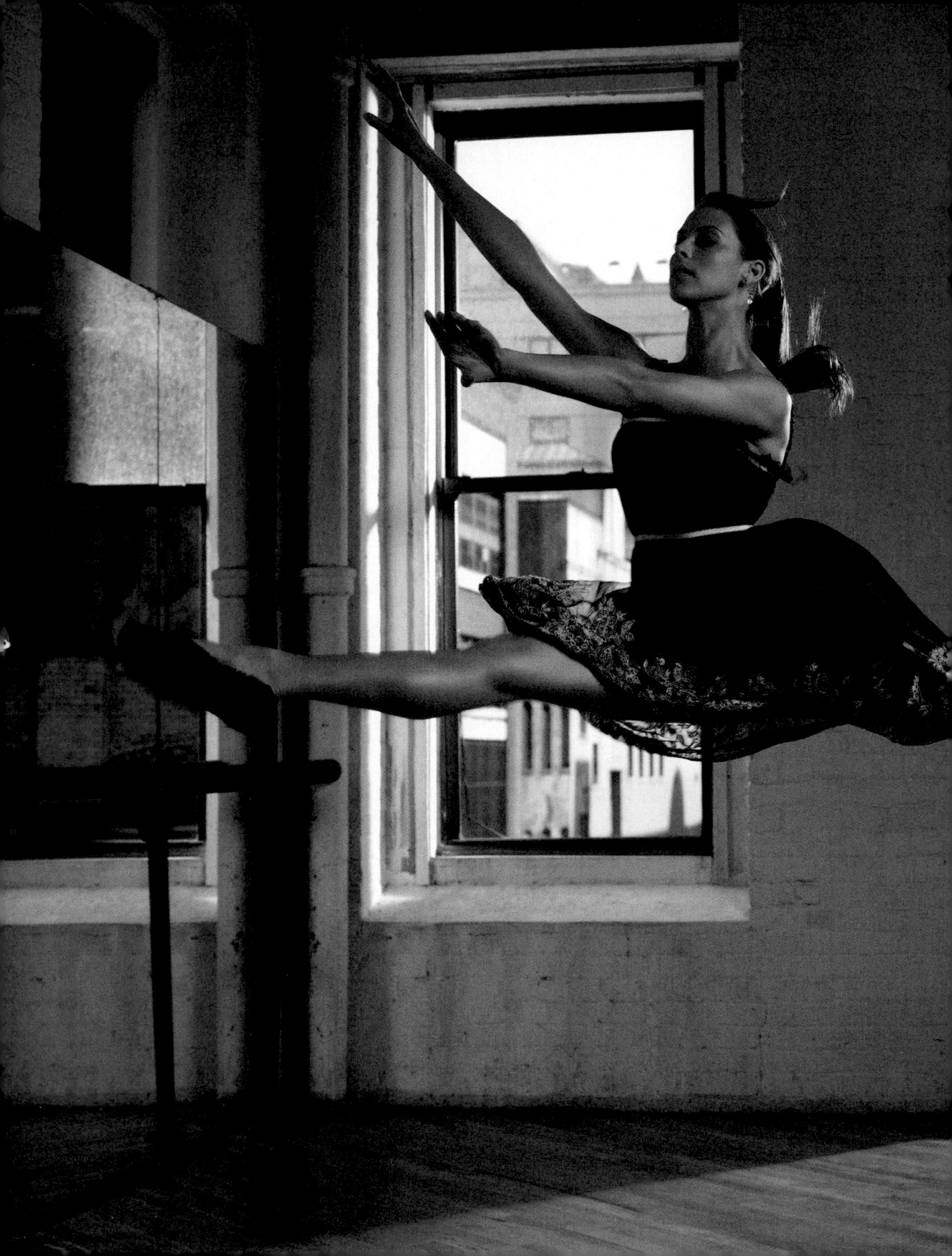

Ballet

THE 411

Influenced by the balance and fancy footwork required for fencing (the 15th century equivalent of Monday Night Football), ballet developed as a form of entertainment for Italian royalty. Later, French king Louis XIV, a ballet dancer himself, opened the Académie Royale de Danse to establish the technical standards and techniques still in practice today.

THE LOOK

Waiter, come back! Show off this knockout dress while you leap (gracefully) for the shrimp. Made of the same micromesh as a ballerina's tutu, the outermost layer features delicate embroidery and satin piping. With all that stylish action, no one will even notice if you drip a little cocktail sauce. Future Paradise tulle party dress ($275, 914-723-9058); Seychelles black fringed satin flats ($65, nordstrom*.com); Jools gold wire earrings ($61, jools.us).

LOOK-LIKE-A-PRO MOVE
GRAND JETÉ

Do it Turn your right foot out 90 degrees and place your left toe on the floor 2 feet behind your right heel. Keep elbows slightly bent, fingertips pointing toward each other (A). Kick left leg forward and fall onto it so it's turned out 90 degrees and your right toe is pointed a few inches off the floor behind you (B). Fall forward onto your right foot, dragging your left toe on the floor. Push off your right foot to do a split leap, left leg leading. Reach your left arm up toward the ceiling and your right out in front of you (C).

BODY BENEFITS

There's nothing better for posture and flexibility. "People gravitate toward ballet for the same reasons everyone piles into Pilates classes: They want that long, lean look," Espel explains.

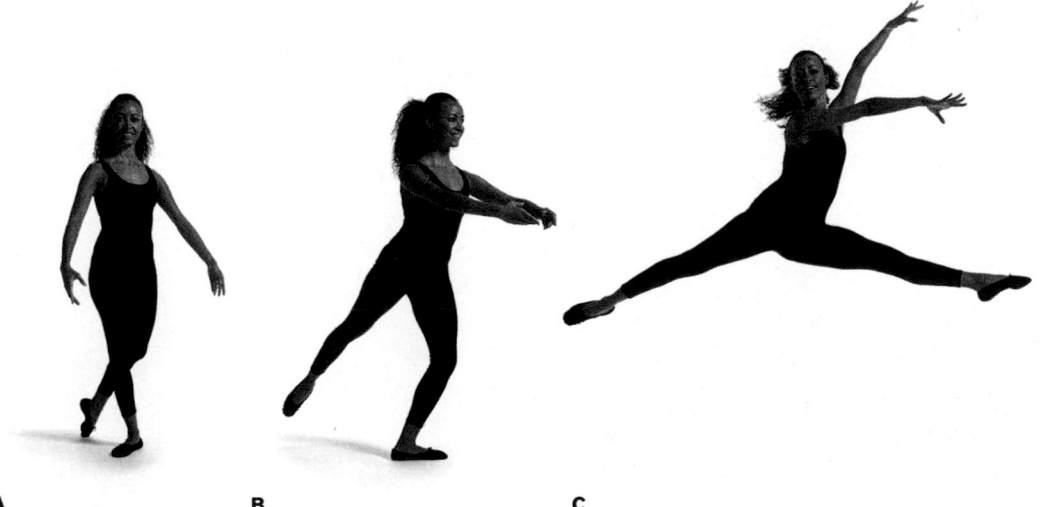

A   B   C

African

THE 411

This tribal dance has gone from the Discovery Channel to MTV, catapulted into the mainstream—and into gyms nationwide—by artists like Beyoncé, Busta Rhymes, Ludacris, and TLC. Traditional moves depict and celebrate war, childbirth, funerals, and other rites of passage, according to Nzingha Camara, who teaches West African dance in Los Angeles. Try a class at your local gym or visit nzinghacamara.com to find out when Camara will be teaching in a city near you.

LOOK-LIKE-A-PRO MOVE
KUKU

A popular West African party dance. These basics will get you going.

Do it Stand with your feet hip-width apart, knees bent 45 degrees (A). With elbows slightly bent, throw your arms front to back, following the motion with your head (B). As your arms circle back, kick your right heel up toward the ceiling behind you

THE LOOK

Different drummer. Each sequin on this satin-lined dress dangles from its own tiny piece of thread, generating some super-high holiday wattage. But don't let the delicacy mislead you: Our model danced hard for an hour without sending a single sequin to its maker. Tadashi sequin fringe dress ($308, tadashi.com); Mark Have a Ball silvered hoop earrings ($12, meetmark.com); White House Black Market Debut bangles ($48, whitehouseblackmarket.com).

Bonus: It makes the most of your ripped quads.

(C). Repeat, lifting your left foot. Land with both feet in the original position (D), then throw your head back as you straighten your arms out at shoulder height. Repeat steps C and D. Continue from the top, following the music's rhythm.

BODY BENEFITS

The low, grounded stance works your thighs and glutes, and the big, sweeping arm movements increase range of motion in your shoulders.

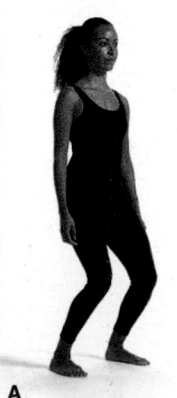 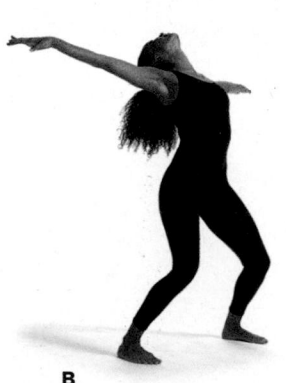 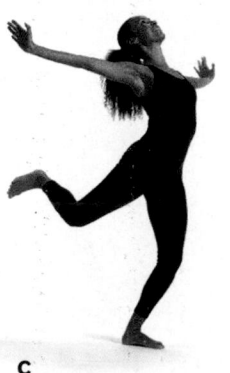 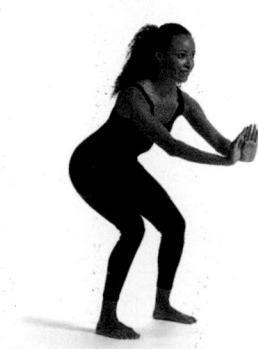

A B C D

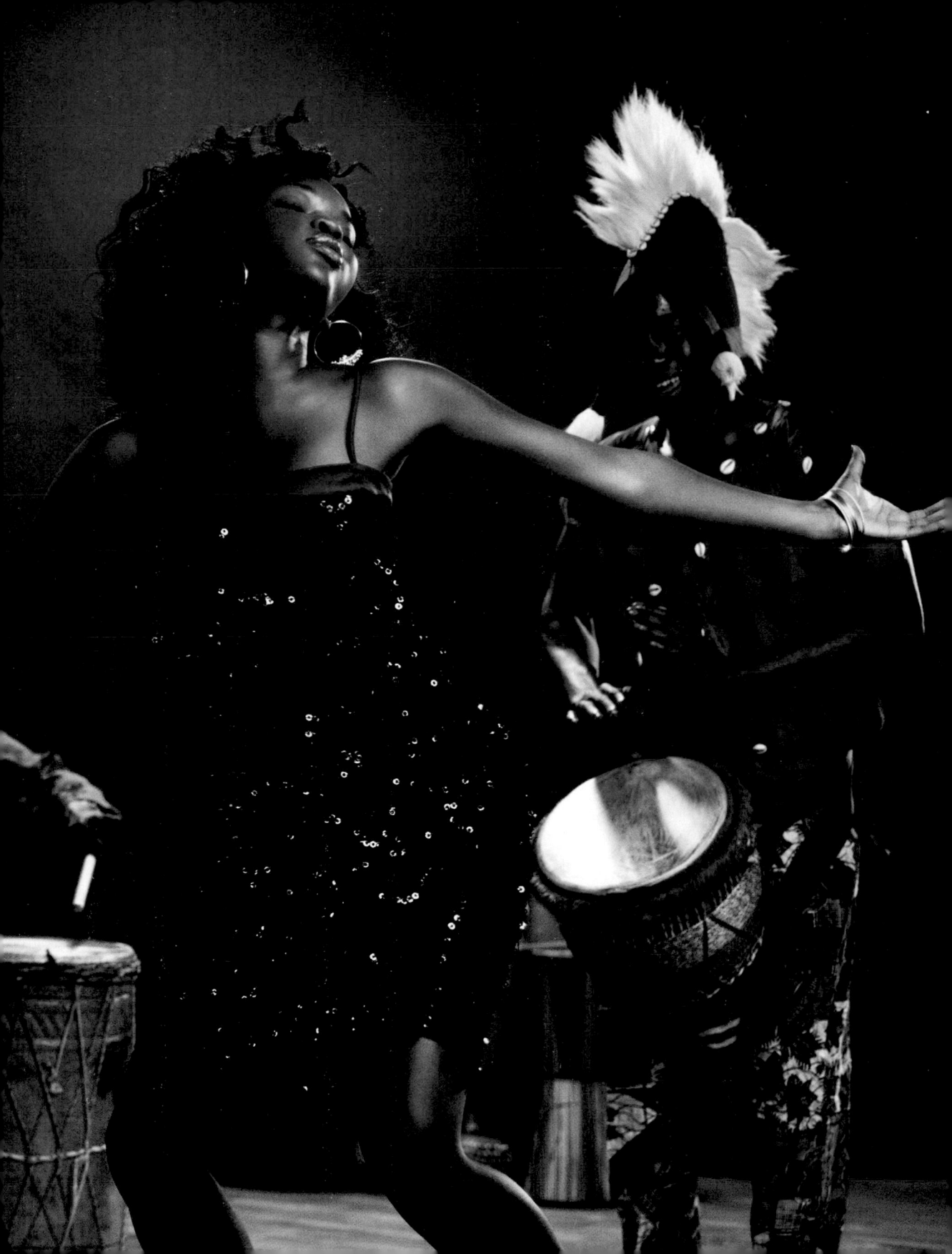

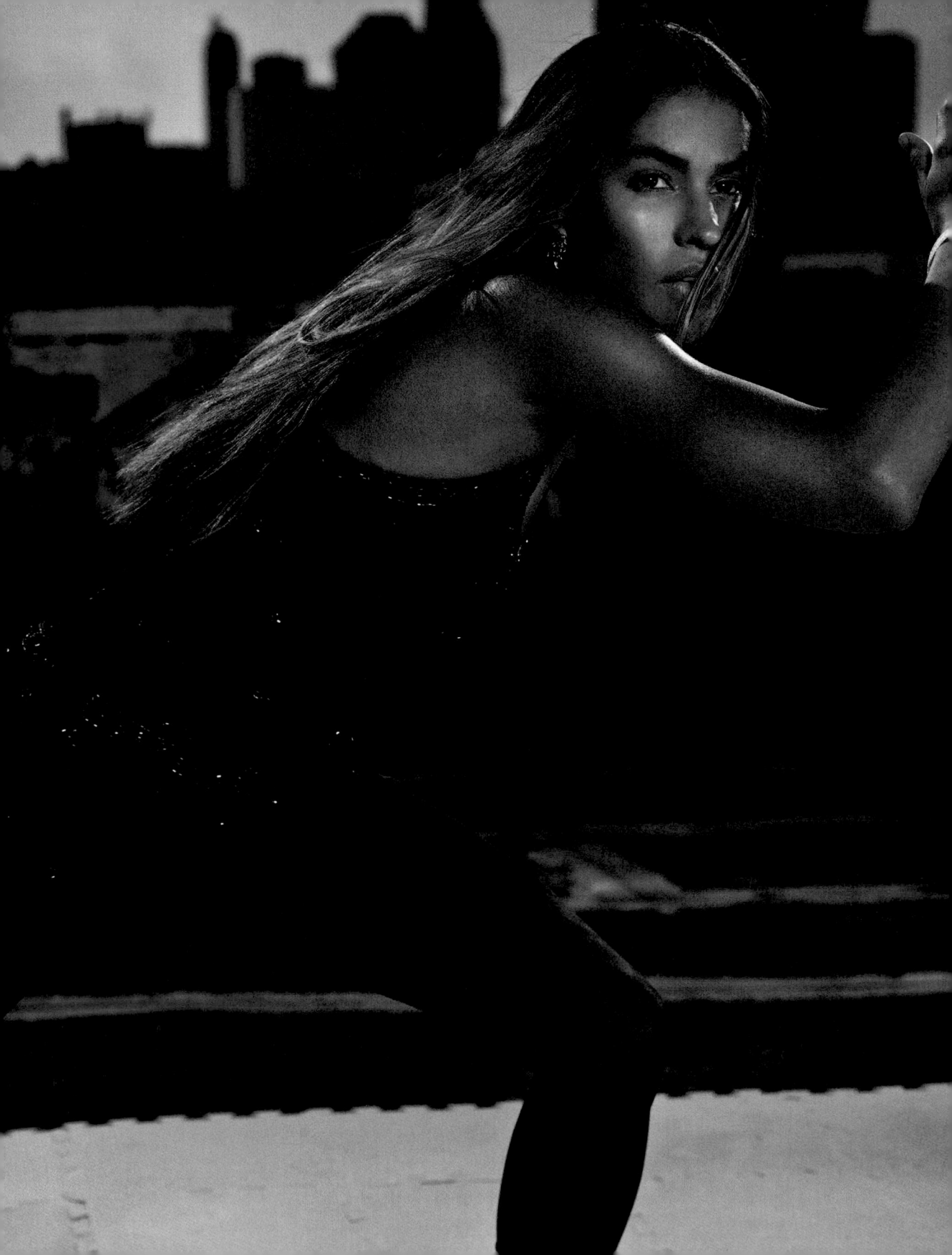

Capoeira

THE 411

In the 1500s, African slaves in Brazil were forbidden to practice martial arts because their owners feared that fighting would lead to revolt. Only by disguising their defensive kicks and dodges as dance moves could they continue to train. To find a class near you—and stir up a little fairy dust during the holidays—visit capoeirista.com.

THE LOOK

Punch it up. Pair this spaghetti-strapped, tunic-style mini with leggings for one of the season's hottest looks. Embellished with black glass beading, this little number will really flash your martial arts mojo. Anjali Kumar beaded minidress ($242, anjalikumar.com); Wendy Culpepper Isabella silver earrings ($125, wendyculpepper.com); Whiteflash.com diamond bracelet and ring (whiteflash.com).

LOOK-LIKE-A-PRO MOVE
ESQUIVA

Do it Stand with your feet wider than your hips, arms at your sides (A). Take a big step back with your right foot and place your left palm flat on the floor outside your left foot, bending your right arm 90 degrees and raising it to mouth level (B). Staying low, lift your left arm off the floor and pivot your feet (and rotate your hips and torso) 90 degrees to your right, raising your left arm to mouth level (C). Pivot to the left so you're in position B, but with your left arm straight out at shoulder height behind you. Step your right foot forward so it's even with the left and you come to a center squat position (D). Repeat on the opposite side by stepping back with your left foot.

BODY BENEFITS

The moves are both aerobic (dance demands endurance) and anaerobic (martial arts require short bursts of speed and strength), so you're getting a perfectly balanced cardio workout, says Corey Hoey, a private capoeira instructor at Equinox in New York City.

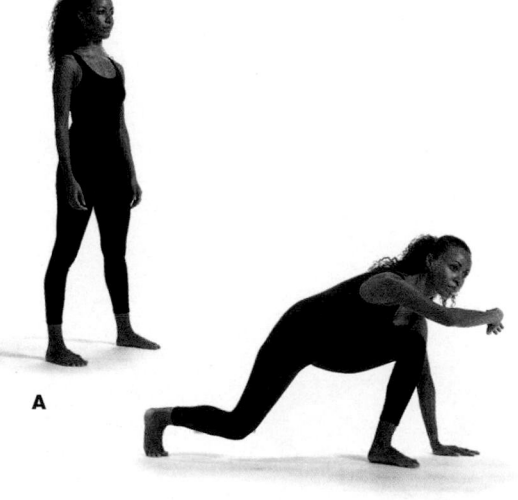

A

B

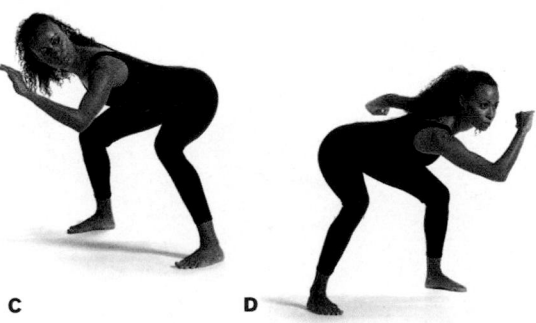

C

D

Hip-Hop

THE 411

Hip-hop is like tofu—it's always taking on different flavors. The Sugarhill Gang is most often credited with coining the term back in the 1980s, but this constantly morphing dance style takes its cues from genres as diverse as African, funk, and disco. Current styles include krumping (similar to moshing) and booty popping (insert your own junk-in-the-trunk joke here).

THE LOOK

Cue it up. Flaunt your chiseled waist in this jersey-knit frock; the shirred panel and skinny satin ribbon belt will play up your midsection. And the full-cut skirt flows easily whenever you get funked up. Theory black viscose Carlissa dress with pleated front and satin ribbons ($415, theory.com); Nina Vespa T-strap sandals ($70, ninashoes.com); Whiteflash.com diamond earrings and bracelet (whiteflash.com).

LOOK-LIKE-A-PRO MOVE
KICK IT

Do it Kick your right heel and then your left heel forward, crossing your arms to make an "X" with each kick (**A**). Step your right foot forward into a lunge position and push your arms out to the sides at shoulder height, wrists flexed (**B**). Bend elbows and cross your wrists while pushing off the right foot to spin to the left, dragging your right toe around your body in a full circle (**C**). Once around, land in a wide plié squat, punching fists toward the floor (**D**). Then jump, tucking your knees to your chest (**E**).

BODY BENEFITS

Explosive jumps work your quads, calves, and hip flexors, according to Shaun Thompson, a hip-hop instructor in Los Angeles.

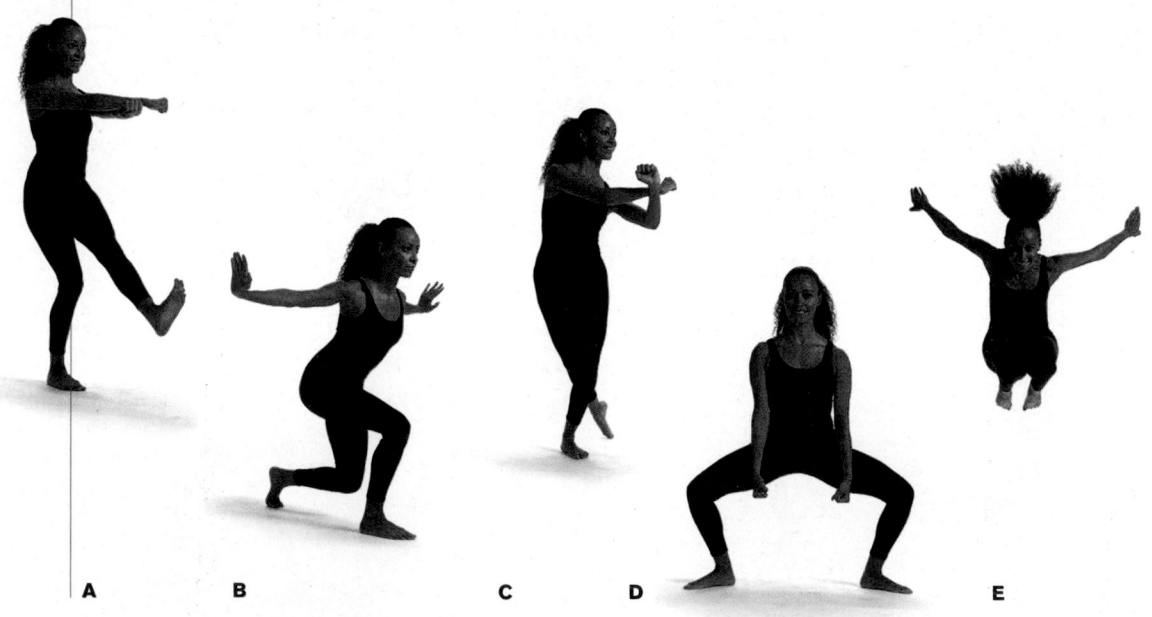

A   B   C   D   E

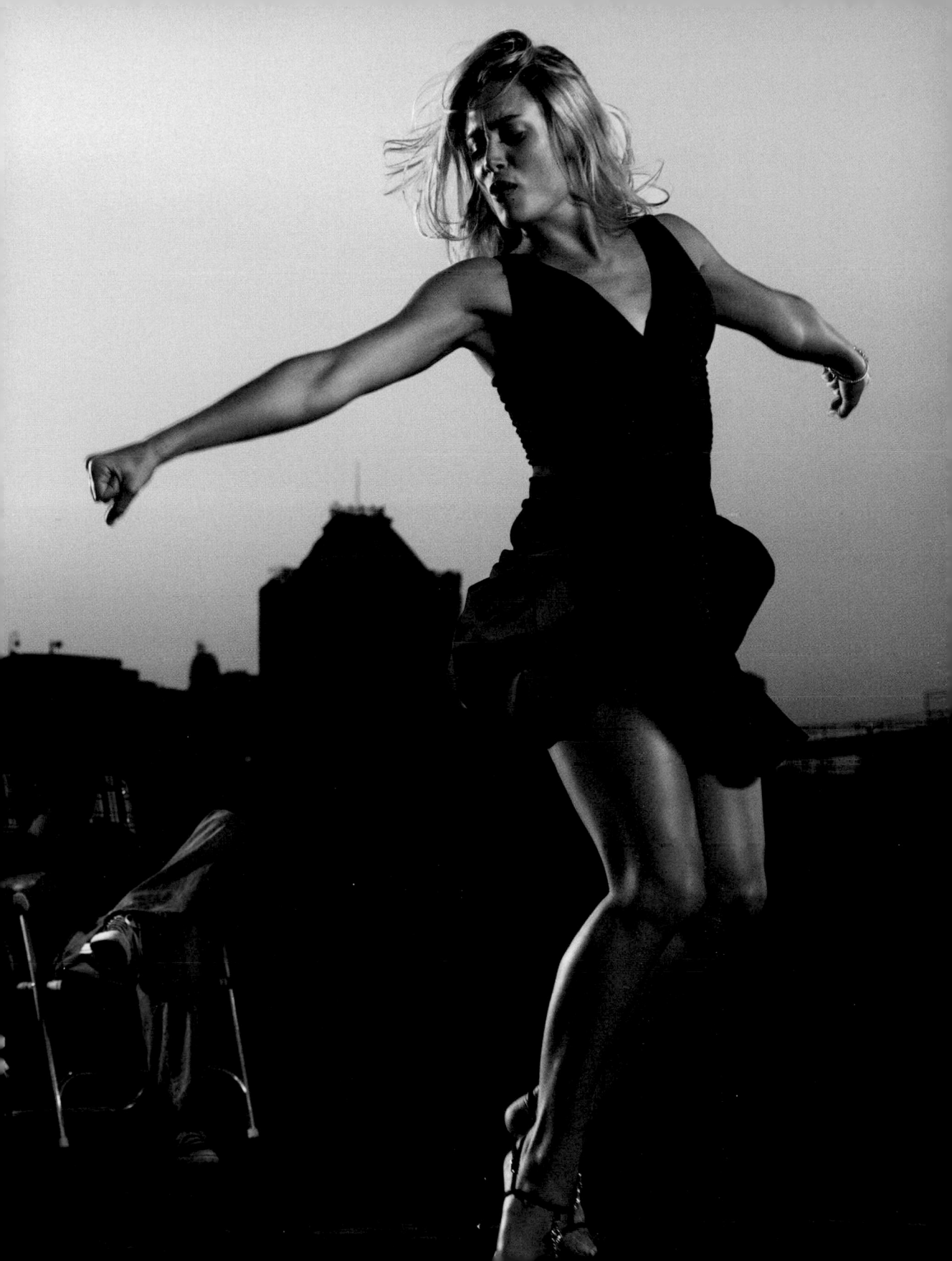

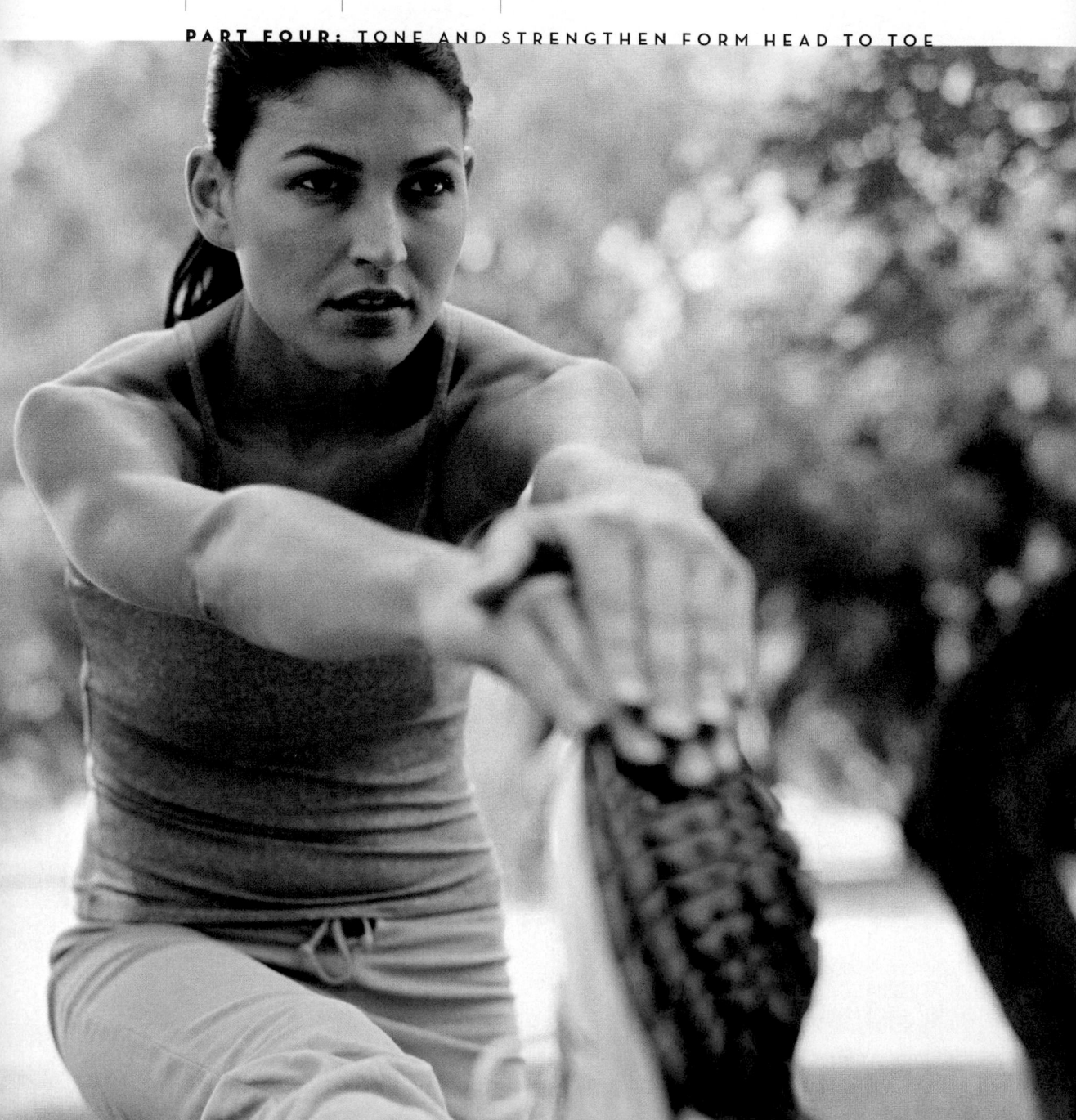

CHAPTER TWENTY-THREE

GET FIT IN ANY TIME

WHETHER YOU HAVE 10, 20, 30, 45, OR 60 MINUTES, YOU CAN MAXIMIZE YOUR WORKOUT—AS LONG AS YOU KNOW THE BEST WAYS TO GET TIME BACK ON YOUR SIDE.

BY LARA ROSENBAUM

IN AN AGE WHEN free time could be an exhibit at a history museum, there's nothing worse than wasting precious minutes in such frustrating clock-crushers as traffic jams, dial-up connections, and restroom lines. Fortunately, when it comes to fitness, you can benefit from exercise sessions of any length, whether you have 1 minute or 60 of them—but that's only if you know the best ways to maximize your time and organize your workouts. Even if you exercise for 1 minute every day for a few weeks, you'll see results, because your body naturally responds to stimulus, says Juan Carlos Santana, owner

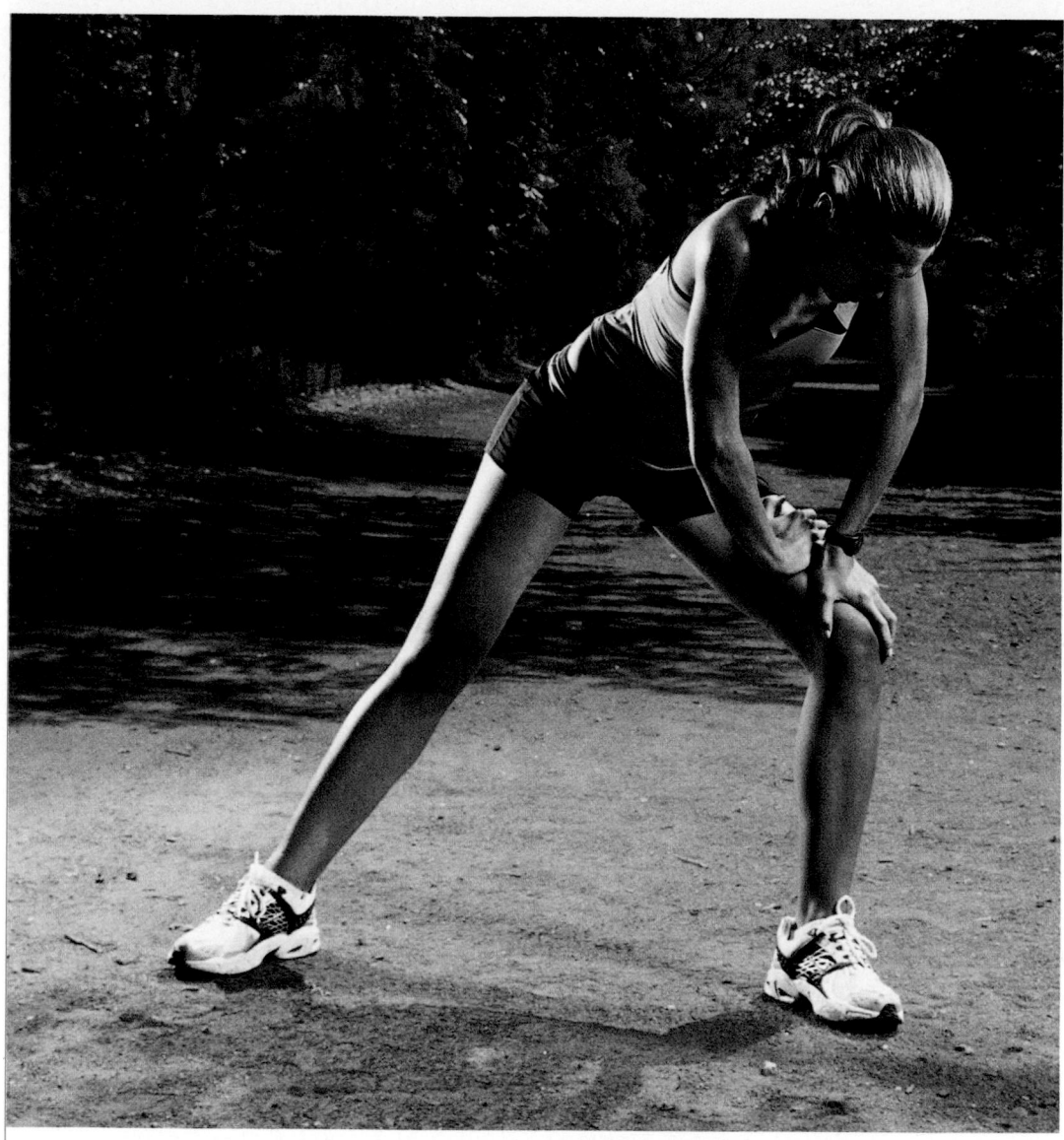

and director of the Institute of Human Performance in Boca Raton, Florida. That's why we asked top fitness experts to help you figure out what to do when, depending on the open slots in your schedule. That way you can get the body you want in the time you have.

10 Minutes

BUILD YOUR BASICS

A 10-minute workout is a fitness quickie. It's so fast it might not seem worth the effort, but you can still get satisfying results if you know what you're doing. While it's not enough time for a great fat-burning workout, 10 minutes will help you build a solid fitness foundation if you develop a strong core and sense of balance. "You can tone up key areas and work on stabilizing the spine, which will help you to avoid future injuries," says Chere Schoffstall, a trainer at the National Academy of Sports Medicine in Calabasas, California.

Option 1: Stretch and Strengthen

Start your 10-spot with dynamic stretches, which are body-weight exercises that utilize your range of motion. They'll keep you flexible and work your core at the same time. Do two or three sets of 12 deep squats and walking lunges so you can warm your muscles as you stretch. Next, twist at the waist as you walk your lunges and do a set of 10 to each side. For core work, do three sets of eight full-range, slow situps to work the length of your core. "Keep your feet unanchored because it will force you to use your abs instead of relying solely on your hip flexors," says Mike Mejia, a strength and conditioning specialist in New York City. "You'll have to focus and control your movement to pull yourself up and keep your feet on the ground."

Option 2: Get Balanced

Balance work trains your small proprioceptive muscles to improve reaction time and strength and help prevent injuries. "It's also important to work your glutes, because that's where balance comes from. It's the bottom of your core," Schoffstall says. For core stability, do three sets of the plank (pushup position with elbows on the floor, using the length of your abs to keep your body flat and still), 20 seconds each. Then do three sets of bridges (see page 242). Finally, perform two sets of 10 to 12 repetitions of both single-leg squats and side lunges. When you press up from the side lunge, balance on your standing leg.

20 Minutes

MAX OUT

In the same amount of time it takes to wait for your skinny mocha latte, you can get the most out of your muscles. A 20-minute workout gives you enough time to push yourself as hard as you can without feeling like you just scaled Mount Kilimanjaro. When you only have a short amount of time, the trick is to increase your intensity to get results, says Adam Ernster, a celebrity trainer in Los Angeles. The reason it works? You'll speed your metabolism so you can burn even more calories after your workout.

Option 1: Change Your Muscle Circuit

Build muscle to burn calories. "For every pound of muscle you gain, you burn on average about 50 calories a day maintaining it," Ernster says. (Don't worry, though: Those extra pounds of muscle look a lot smaller on you than fat.) To build muscle in less time, Ernster suggests changing the order of your exercises. It will keep your body from adapting and make it work harder, he says. You can also make exercises more complicated to make your muscles work harder. For instance, perform standing moves on an unstable surface like a foam pad or a Bosu ball to challenge your core-stabilizing muscles, or add complex exercises like squat shoulder presses to work more muscles (in this case, your whole body) at once. When you perform the shoulder press, use one arm at a time to make it even more intricate. "The added bonus with moves like these is that when you work large muscle groups, you burn more calories in the same amount of time," says trainer Nancy Cummings, Ed.D.

Option 2: Up Your Cardio Intensity

By increasing the friction between the treadmill belt and your feet, you can make a cardiovascular workout much harder—and more effective. Try this killer butt-toning trek from Gregory Joujon-Roche, owner of Holistic Fitness in Los Angeles. Walk on a treadmill for 2.5 minutes, gradually increasing your speed to 3 mph. Next, raise the treadmill to its steepest incline and set your speed to a walking pace that's almost jogging (about 3.8 mph). Keep your body low and extend your stride, flicking your back foot up at the end. Keep your feet on the treadmill as long as possible to create friction, and focus on feeling your glutes. Hold the handles of the treadmill, and use your ab muscles to control your body. Keep this going for 15 minutes, then reduce your speed and incline to cool down for 2.5 minutes.

30 Minutes

BURN FAT

Your choice: Spend 30 minutes watching another *Friends* rerun, or boost your heart rate to burn more fat and calories. "You really need 30 minutes to start dipping into your fat stores," says Ellen Barrett, owner of the Studio at Buff Girl Fitness in New Haven, Connecticut.

Option 1: Blitz Your Body

You can get a total-body workout with five basic exercises and no exercise equipment at all, says Kathy Kaehler, author of *Kathy Kaehler's Celebrity Workouts*. Start with jumping jacks to warm up. Then do these five exercises for 1 minute each

without stopping: chair squats (squat in front of a chair and sink down until your butt just touches the seat), lunges, pushups, crunches, and jumping jacks. Do the circuit four times; for more of a burn, pick up the pace. "It doesn't have to be fancy, but treat fitness like you're trying to catch the train," Barrett says. To add variety, mix in leg lifts, side ab curls—any calisthenics—and do each as fast as possible for 30-second or 1-minute intervals. Do a 5-minute warmup (mix jumping jacks with some dynamic stretches) and a 5-minute cooldown (an easy walk and some static stretches), and go hard for 20 minutes in between.

Option 2: Superset Strength

If you normally work your upper body on one day and your lower body on another, maximize your time and calorie burn by doing both in the same workout. Simply superset your exercises by alternating moves in between sets—without taking more than 15 or 20 seconds of rest in between. If you do a set of squats, do a set of bench presses next. If you move on to lunges, superset with lat pulldowns or rows. "Even though your body is still being taxed and your heart rate is up, you're at least getting some moderate level of recovery," Mejia says.

Option 3: Play, Don't Think

Add intensity by forgetting about how hard you're working—in the form of tennis, volleyball, or anything competitive. "You're exercising, you're sweating, and that's when you really change your body. But you're also getting out of your head," Joujon-Roche says, which is a good thing. No opponent? Hit the basketball court. Every time you miss a basket, do sets of walking lunges, pushups, crunches, or full-court sprints.

45 Minutes

ADD EXTRAS

Whether you're in the kitchen or the bedroom, it's a lot easier to get creative when you have some time to work with. That's also true in the gym. With the extra 15 minutes from your normal 30-minute workout, you can not only burn more calories, but also fine-tune and amplify your workouts to develop the areas you typically neglect. "With 45 minutes you will have enough time to add that extra little something that can dramatically change the way your body looks and performs," Mejia says.

Option 1: Include Agility

Add agility drills to work on balance, skill, and coordination, which can help prevent injuries and improve sports performance. Ernster suggests running with quick feet through an agility ladder at the end of a workout. Go back and forth as fast as you can and keep your toes on the ground for as little time as possible. Next, side-step through it. If your gym doesn't have a ladder, make your own with sticks or tape, spacing the lines about 1 foot apart, or simply go through the motions for the same benefits. To keep your muscles quick, do 10 minutes of agility drills at the end of a 30-minute strength routine. Along with ladders, try grapevines (moving sideways, quickly whip the trailing foot around the front of the lead foot so that it lands slightly behind it) and 180-hops (hop and turn 180 degrees, and then turn back, jumping in both directions). Next, spend 5 minutes stretching and cooling down.

Option 2: Isolate

Add ancillary exercises to your strength workout, Cummings says. Once you work the large muscle

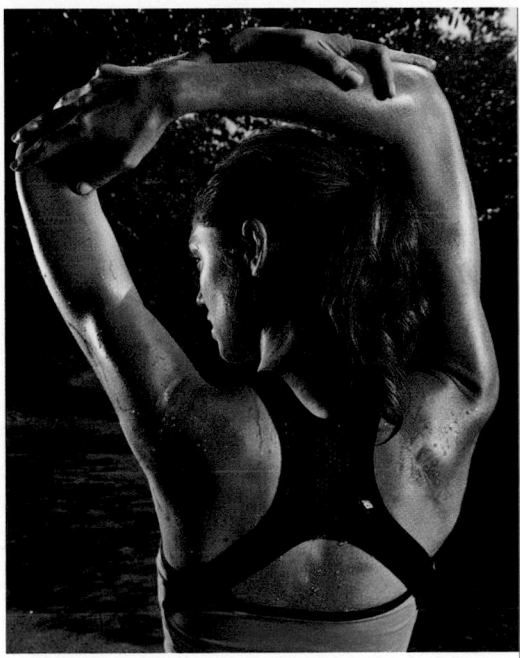

groups, work the smaller ones (like wrists and calves) to polish your shape and prevent injuries. For instance, work your rotator cuffs to help strengthen muscles that will help your tennis-swinging and kid-carrying. Lie on your right side with a light dumbbell in your left hand, elbow tightly at your side. Open your left shoulder slightly and swing your left forearm toward the ceiling, but keep your upper arm tucked to your body to create a short, controlled motion. Do 10 repetitions on each side.

Option 3: Add Cardio Bursts

At the end of a weights or cardio workout, do driveway (or gym) sprints to quickly speed your heart rate, Mejia says. The quick bursts will boost your metabolism, and the changes of direction work the small muscles and tendons around your ankles. Do a few sets of jumping jacks to warm up, since they'll help prepare your ankles and knees for the quick stops and starts. Place a marker at the end of your driveway or gym (a shoe, rock, or cone) and sprint out to it, touch it, and sprint back (remind you of middle school P.E.?). Repeat 5 to 10 1-minute intervals and see how many passes you can make during each minute, going for more speed each time.

60 Minutes

DO IT ALL

It may feel like a luxury to have an hour to work out, but it's what the American College of Sports Medicine recommends for maintaining optimum fitness, 3 to 5 days a week. On the days you can steal an hour, use it to work your cardiovascular and muscular strength. "It's enough time to stress your muscles and include a proper warmup and cooldown," Santana says. "And when you exercise for an hour, it will also help you burn more fat postexercise—up to 8 hours."

Option 1: Train Circuits

If you have a lot of energy and are up for a challenge, Schoffstall suggests creating a six- to eight-move circuit that combines strength, cardio, and stretching. After a 10-minute warmup that includes dynamic flexibility (see Option 1 in the 10-minute workout) and core work, begin your circuit working from the chest down. Work your chest, back, shoulders, biceps, triceps, and legs in that order. (To start with basics, try chest presses, back rows, shoulder presses, biceps curls, triceps kickbacks, and then side lunges.) Then complete a set of jumping jacks or jog in place for 5 minutes. If you do some of the standing moves with one leg or on an unstable surface, it's good to work your legs last, because they're a big muscle group and can better endure fatigue, Schoff-

stall says. And when you switch from one opposing muscle group to another, you're actively stretching one muscle while strengthening another. For instance, when you do a bent-over row to strengthen your back, you're actively stretching your chest. Aim to complete three sets of the circuit in an hour.

Option 2: Advance Your Circuit

For the more advanced, increase the intensity of your circuits by doing a minute of cardio in between each exercise. Your whole workout morphs into a giant cardio session, since your heart rate will be raised throughout. The short cardio bursts can actually enhance your aerobic endurance and help prepare you for everyday life. "After all, life is a series of intervals," Santana says, "because you do everything in bursts."

Option 3: Listen to Your Heart

Weekends are great for slow, long-distance cardio, Cummings says. Not only will you relieve stress, but you'll burn fat. "These days are usually the most beneficial for fat-burning, because when you're working in your low-aerobic threshold, your body burns carbs and fat for fuel. They're sustained energy sources," Cummings says. Do a 5- to 7-minute dynamic warmup, go for your 45-minute excursion, and then stretch for the next 5 to 7 minutes. Shoot for a pace that allows you to talk, or check your pulse and aim for 60 percent of your maximum heart rate (220 minus your age). Then add a short abs routine. Try four-way abs to work them from all angles: Do 25 reps each of regular, oblique (both sides), and reverse crunches. Next, flip over and do 10 Supergirls: Clasp your hands under your chin and lift your shoulders off the floor a few inches, then release.

BOTTOMS UP

Whatever your schedule, you can still work your butt off. By strengthening the largest muscles in your body—your glutes and thighs—you'll burn more calories. Trainer Mike Mejia designed this program to shape your glutes from every angle. Choose the moves based on your time frame.

> **10 MINUTES: Do the moves in group A to work the largest amount of muscles and build your strength base.**
> **20 MINUTES: Do group A and group B to work balance and core stability.**
> **30 MINUTES: Do group A, B, then C to hone and shape your glutes.**

A1 OVERHEAD BROOMSTICK (WOODEN BAR) SQUAT

Hold the stick above your head and squat, keeping the stick in line with your hips and heels. Use your core to stabilize your body as you sink down and press up. Do three sets of 10 reps, and when that gets easy, use a barbell or Body Bar to add weight.

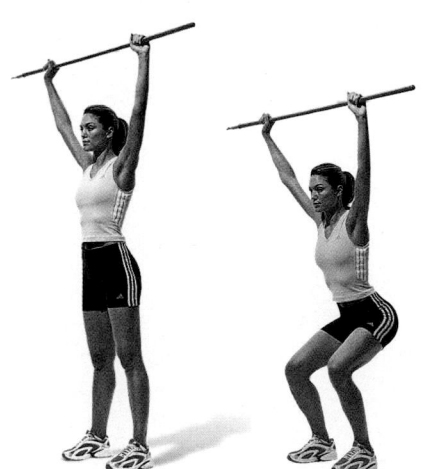

A2 REVERSE FLARED KNEE HYPEREXTENSIONS

Lie face down on a Swiss ball and tilt forward, placing your palms on the floor. Bend your knees 90 degrees and flare them out, keeping your feet together. Next, squeeze your glutes to lift your hips, and then release and lower them. Do three sets of 10.

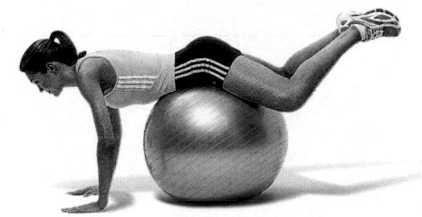

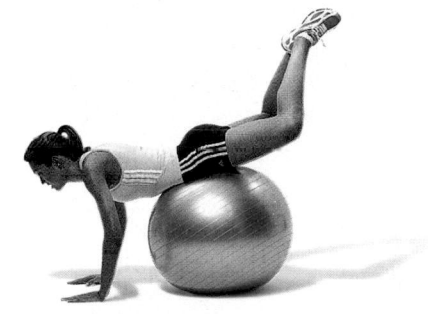

B1 SINGLE-LEG ROMANIAN DEADLIFT

Grab a pair of light dumbbells and balance on your left leg with knee slightly bent and aligned over your middle toes. Keep your right leg raised and close to your body as you slowly bend at the waist without rounding your back, and lower the weights toward the floor. Next, squeeze your glutes and hamstrings to pull yourself up and return to start. Do three sets of 10 on each leg.

B2 BRIDGE ABDUCTION

Lie on your back with your knees bent and press your hips up into a bridge, creating a 90-degree angle with your knees. Next, extend left leg and bring it out to the side while keeping your hips up. Go for three sets of 10 reps, then switch legs. If your hips start to dip to the side or fold, stop and rest for a few seconds.

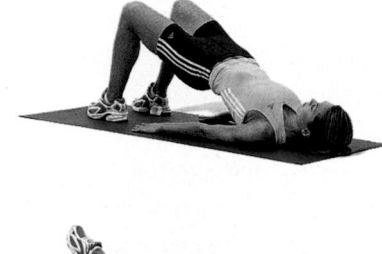

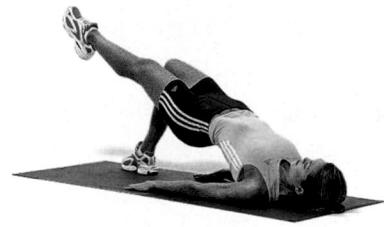

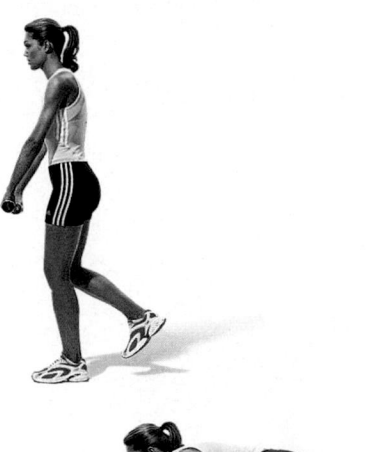

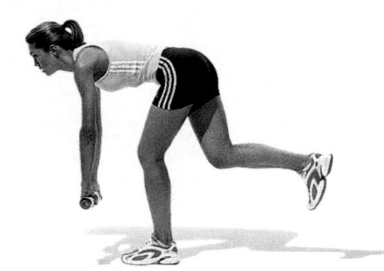

C1 BALLET SQUAT

Stand with your feet wide apart, toes turned out, and press up onto the balls of your feet. Keeping your heels up, slightly roll your pelvis under and squat down, maintaining a straight line from your tailbone up your spine. Press up to start while keeping your heels off the floor and repeat for three sets of 10. Try these without weights first to nail your form, and when you add weights, hold them at your hips.

C2 CURTSY LUNGE

Grab a pair of dumbbells and hold them at your hips. Step back about 3 feet with your right foot and cross it behind your left foot. Sink your weight down, keeping your torso upright and your hips and shoulders as flat as possible. Press up and sink back down for 10 reps, then switch sides. Do 3 sets.

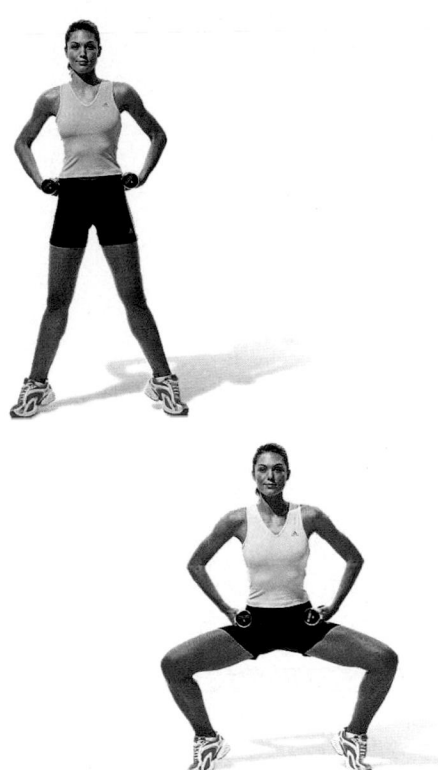

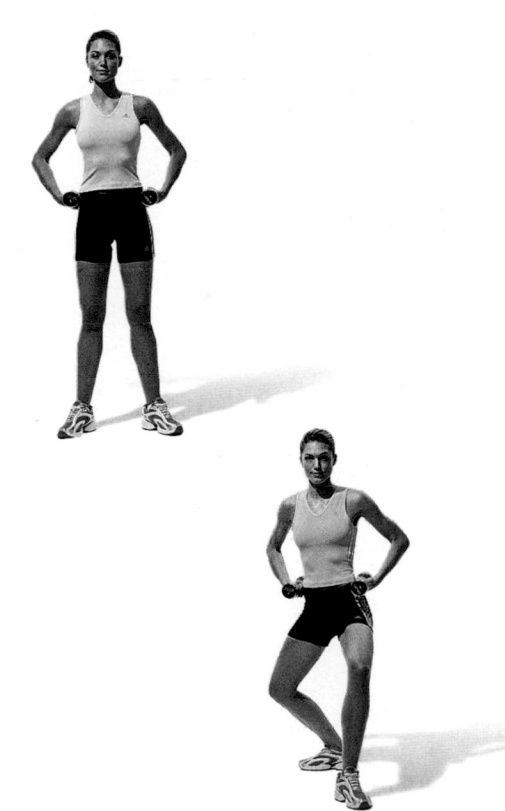

THE 1-MINUTE WORKOUT

"Something is better than nothing" applies to more than just IRS refunds. It's also true for fitness. Only a minute to work out? Then use it. "You won't burn tons of calories, but you'll be able to increase muscle tone, strength, and power," trainer Juan Carlos Santana says. The only thing you'll need is your body weight, so you can do either of these two moves–and burn roughly 10 to 20 calories–anywhere, anytime.

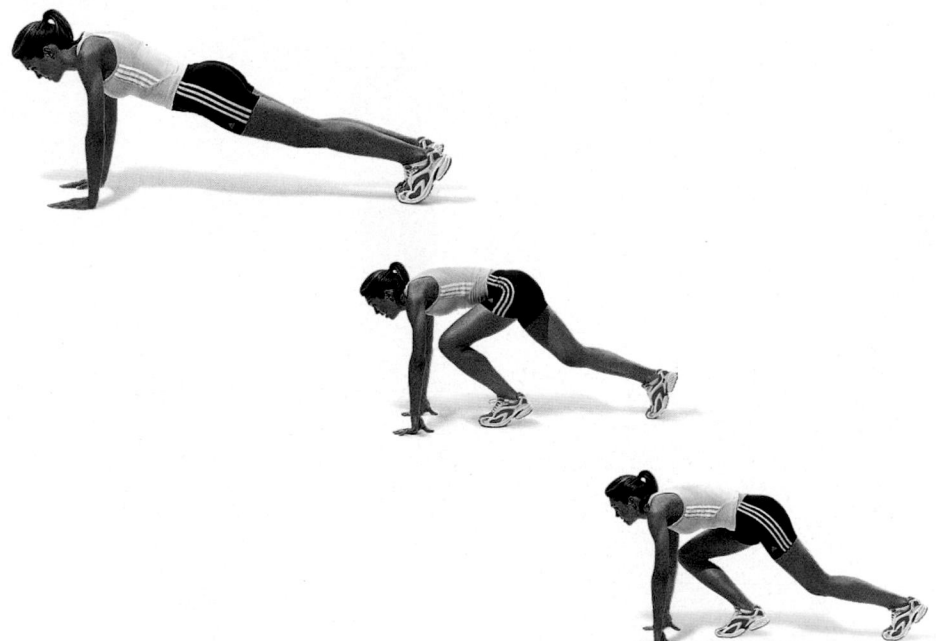

MOUNTAIN CLIMBERS T

They not only tone just about every muscle, but they also can improve your speed. Start in a pushup position and jump your left knee to your chest, placing the left foot beneath your stomach while keeping your right leg straight back. Next, quickly switch feet and repeat as fast as you can for 1 minute.

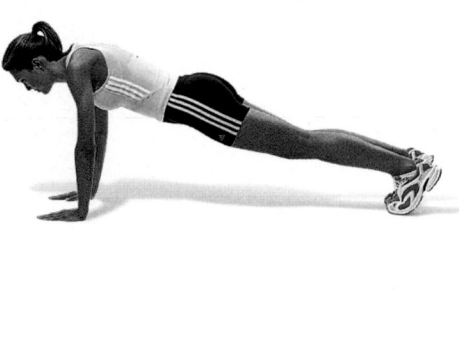

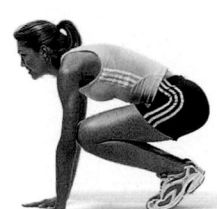

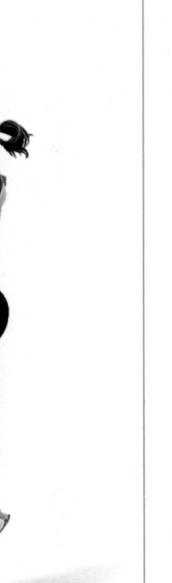

BURPEES

Don't let the name dissuade you: This move is one of trainer Chere Schoffstall's favorites. Start in a pushup position, and squeeze your abs and glutes. Lower your body into a pushup and press up to start. Next, quickly jump your feet forward into a squat, and jump up as high and as smoothly as you can. After you land, place your hands on the floor and jump your feet back into a pushup. Repeat the sequence as many times as you can in 1 minute.

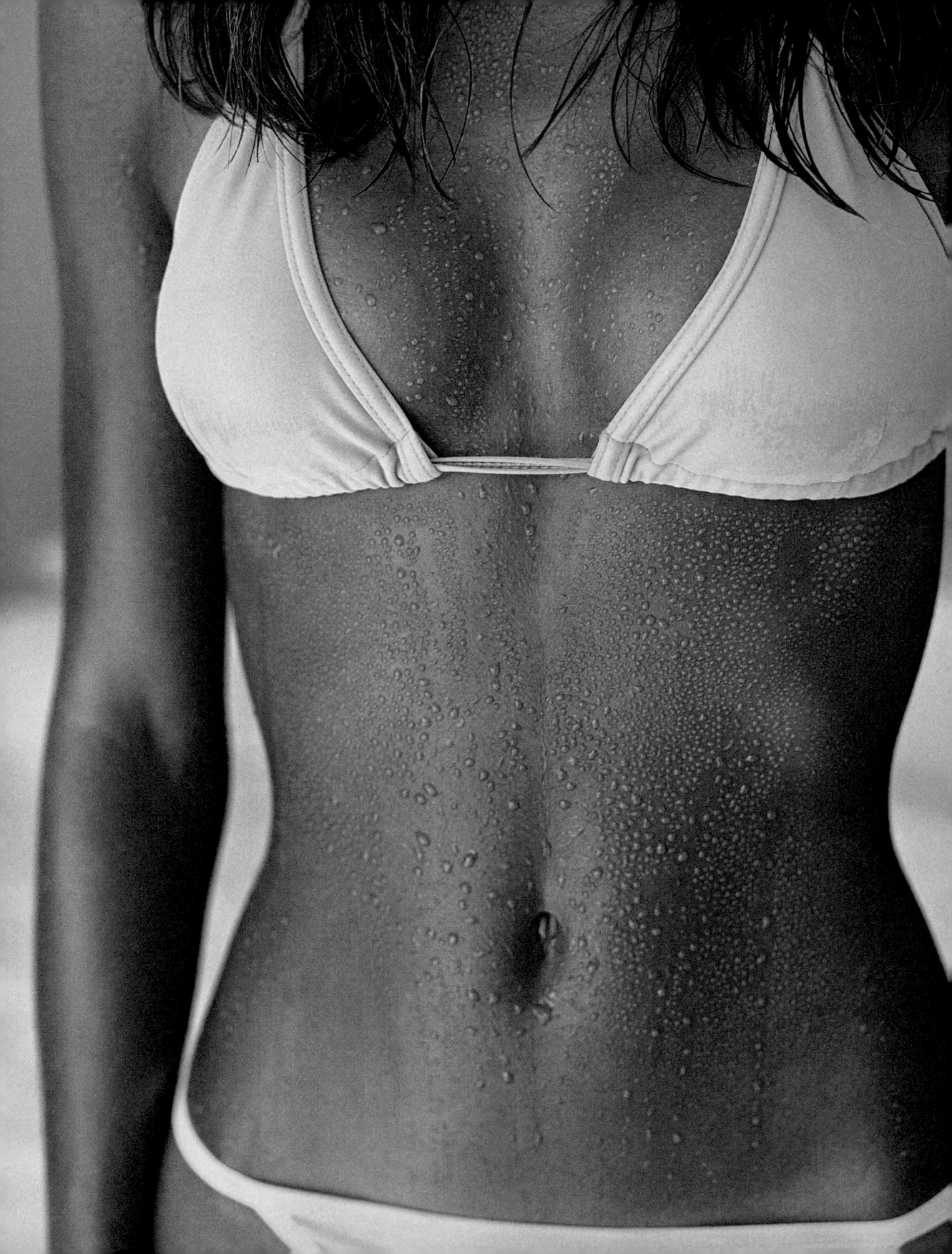

PART FIVE

target practice

You are greater than the sum of your parts, no matter how big those parts are. But let's face it—a flat belly, an awesome set of guns, and a butt like a ripe peach would take us over the moon! Read on to discover how to tone and strengthen all of your beautiful parts.

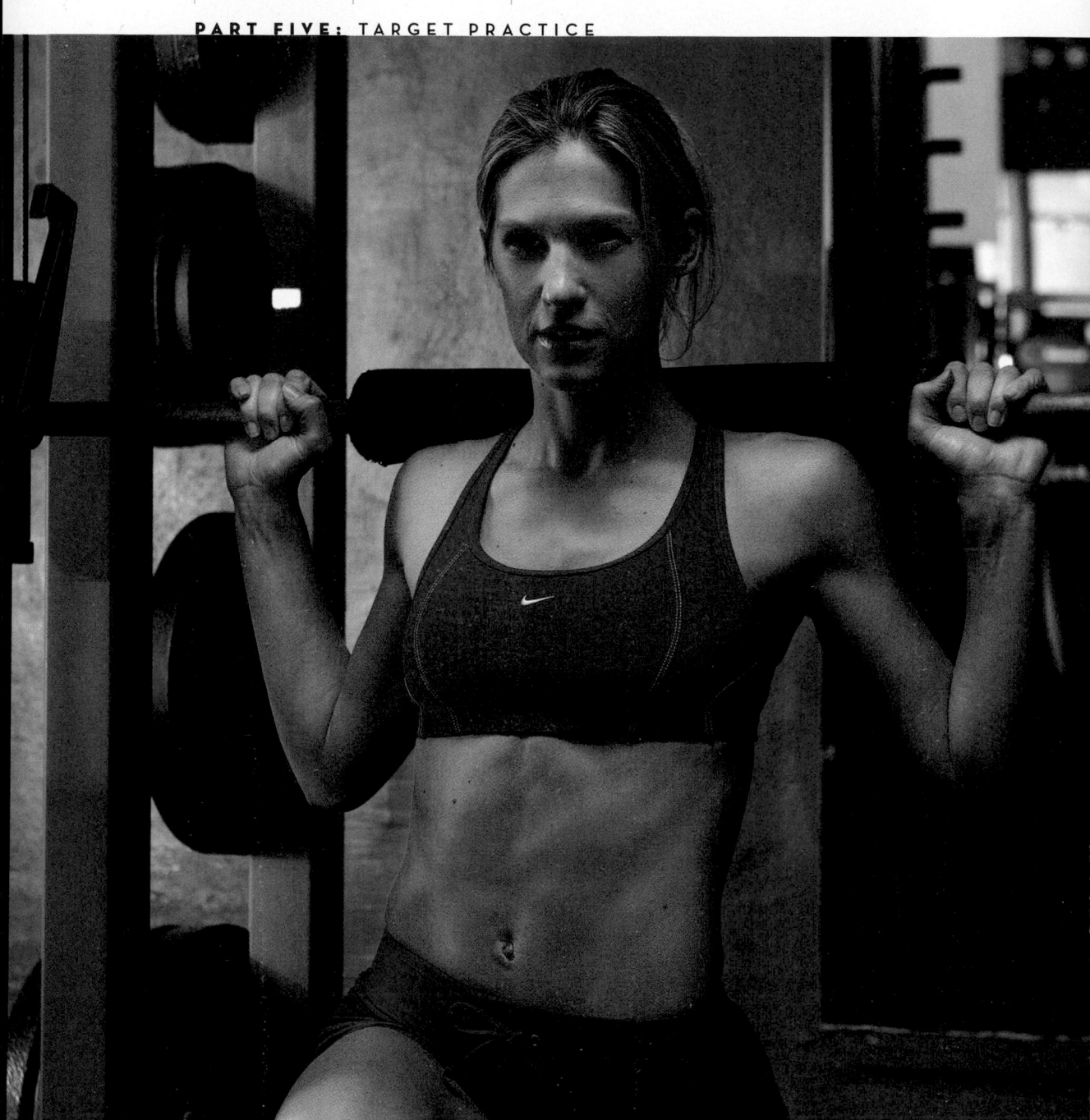

CHAPTER TWENTY-FOUR

SLEEK AND STRONG

BUILD A TONED UPPER BODY BY USING THE SAME OLD EQUIPMENT IN ALL NEW WAYS.

BY LARA ROSENBAUM

SOME THINGS IN LIFE should only be used the way they were intended (prescription medications and nail clippers come to mind). But the beauty of a Swiss-Army-knife society is the allure of multipurpose products like duct tape, Worcestershire sauce, and silk scarves. Unfortunately, it seems that ever since the day Gustav Zander opened the first gym in 1865, we've been treating gym equipment like the ladies' room: We use it exactly the same way every day. It's difficult to make progress in your workout program—and see changes in your body—when your workout repeats itself like a scratched CD. That's because your metabolism plateaus when your body and muscles adapt to doing the same exercises over and over. To keep your body constantly challenged—and ultimately burn more fat—we asked top trainers for ways to get the most from your equipment to build the tight and toned upper body that you want.

1 | Smith Machine

TRADITIONAL USES: BENCH PRESS FOR YOUR CHEST AND ARMS.

TRY INCLINE PUSHUPS

Hook the bar onto the third rung from the floor and place your hands on it about shoulder-width apart. Move your feet back into a pushup position (A). Lower your chest to the bar and return to the starting position (B). Do 10 reps. Drop the bar to the second rung and do 10 more pushups, then do the last 10 with the bar on the first rung. These pushups work your arms, shoulders, and chest muscles from different angles, says Gunnar Peterson, author of *G-Force: The Ultimate Guide to Your Best Body Ever.* If you can easily perform reps on the bottom rung, make the move more advanced by putting your feet on the bar and your hands on the floor.

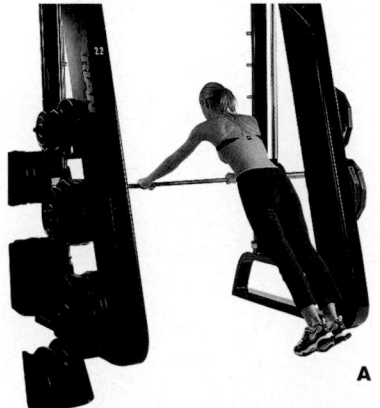

A

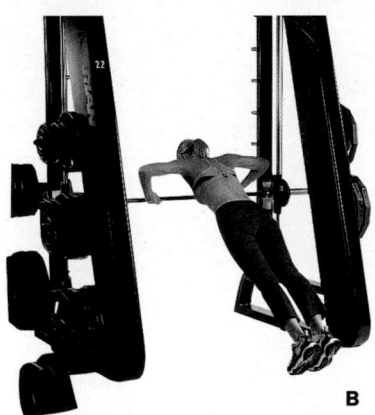

B

2 | Lat Machine

TRADITIONAL USES: PULLDOWNS TO WORK YOUR UPPER BACK AND BICEPS.

TRY STANDING V-PULL

Stand facing the machine and grab the bar with your hands just outside the curves, palms down. Step back about 2 feet (**A**). Keeping your arms straight, pull the bar down to your hips (**B**). Do two sets of 10 reps. This works the length of your lats and helps shape your back into a V from your shoulders to your waist, says trainer and physiologist Tom Holland. Plus, you'll contract your abs and work your core while trying to keep your body still. Use a light weight (about 20 pounds) to allow your back—and not your arms—to pull the bar. As a change, try lowering the weight even more, turning to the side, and pulling the bar with one hand down to your hip.

3 | Bench

TRADITIONAL USES: BENCH PRESS, WHICH WORKS YOUR CHEST AND TRICEPS.

TRY INCLINE PULLUPS

Lie on the bench keeping your body straight and slide back a few inches so your thighs can rest on the bench. Grip the bar with your palms facing your head and slightly wider than shoulder-width apart (**A**). Pull your body up until your chest meets the bar (**B**). Tighten your core to keep your body straight and perform 10 to 12 reps. "You'll work your arms, shoulders, chest, and back, making this the perfect all-in-one upper-body exercise," says trainer Nancy Cummings. It's also easier than a regular chinup. When 12 reps become easy for you, Cummings recommends doing as many as you can in one set.

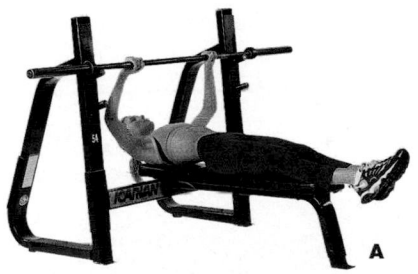

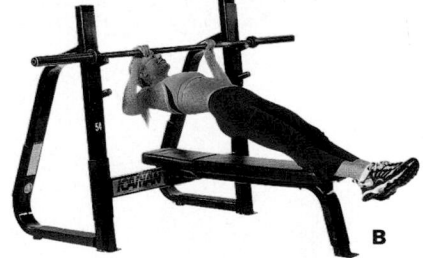

W|H

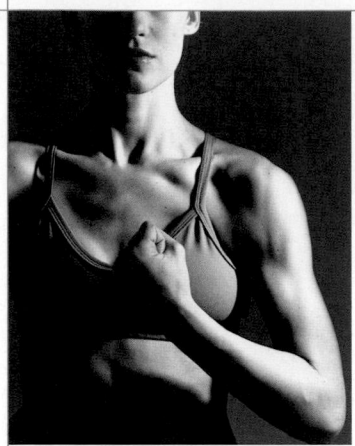

WELL-ARMED

A QUICK WORKOUT TO ADD TONE TO ALL SIDES OF YOUR ARMS

Though your arms can hide under sweaters and coats during some part of the year, the season of tank tops is never that far off. Try this arm-and-shoulder workout by Jan Wyche, a personal trainer at Chelsea Piers in New York.

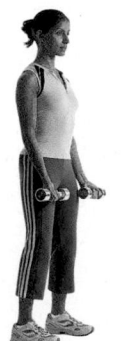
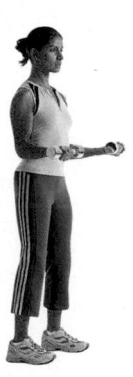

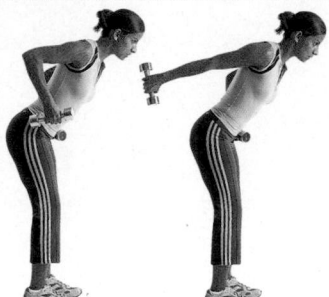

ONE-ARM ROW KICKBACK

UPPER BACK AND TRICEPS

Bend forward slightly at the hips. With your left hand at your side, hold a dumbbell in your right hand, palm facing in and arm extended toward the floor. Pull the dumbbell up to your waist, keeping your arm close to your body. When your elbow hits 90 degrees, straighten your arm behind you so that it's parallel to the floor. Perform 10 reps, and repeat on the other side.

21'S

BICEPS

Stand with a dumbbell in each hand, palms forward. Curl until elbows hit 90 degrees, then lower to start; do seven reps. Follow immediately with seven more curls, this time bringing the dumbbells to your armpits, then lowering until your elbows reach 90 degrees. Finish with seven complete curls, lowering the dumbbells to your hips and curling them all the way up.

LATERAL RAISE

SHOULDERS

Stand with feet shoulder-width apart with a dumbbell in each hand, palms facing each other, arms in front with elbows slightly bent. Raise arms until parallel to the floor. Return slowly and do two sets of 10 reps.

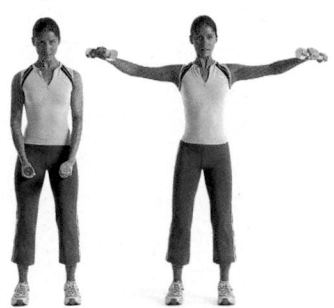

WALKOVER PUSHUP

WHOLE UPPER BODY

With a medicine ball that's big enough for you to place both of your hands on, get into a pushup position. Place your left hand on the ball and your right hand on the floor, and do a pushup. At the top of the exercise, walk your right hand onto the ball, place your left hand on the floor, and do another pushup. Do five reps on each side. (If you're a beginner, try these on your knees.)

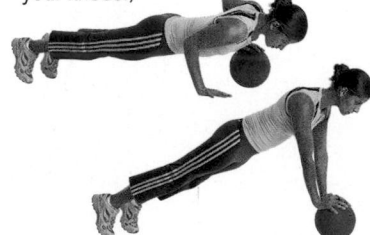

4 | Cable with High-Rope Attachment

TRADITIONAL USES: TRICEPS PUSHDOWN, WHICH ISOLATES THE BACK OF YOUR ARMS.

TRY SEATED HIGH ROW

Grab the rope and sit on the floor with legs straight out in front of you and knees slightly bent (A). Tighten your abs and lean back 45 degrees. Pull the rope to your chest by bringing your elbow behind you (B). Perform three sets of 10 reps. "This move is phenomenal—it works your back, shoulders, and arms, but it also hits your core, since you need to hold yourself still," Cummings says. Start with a light weight (about 20 pounds) to focus on form; when it's easy to hold your body at the 45-degree angle, increase the resistance.

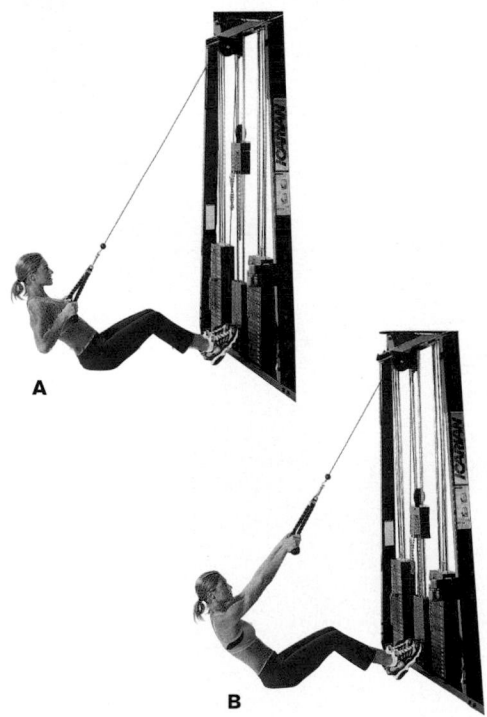

5 | Chinup Bar

TRADITIONAL USES: UNDERHAND CHINUPS, WHICH WORK YOUR BACK AND ARMS.

TRY HANGING SIDE CRUNCHES

Hang from the bar, holding it with your palms facing forward, and bring your knees up so that your thighs and torso form a 90-degree angle (A). Next, pinch at your left side, curling your left hip up toward your left shoulder (B). Use your core to keep yourself from swinging, and repeat to the right. Continue alternating sides for 20 reps. This is one of Cummings's favorite moves because it strengthens all of your core. "It's really hard to get the very sides of your abs," she says, "and you really need these muscles for everything you do—even walking." To make it easier, use a machine that allows your elbows and arms to support your body weight, or use straps on the chinup bar to add support.

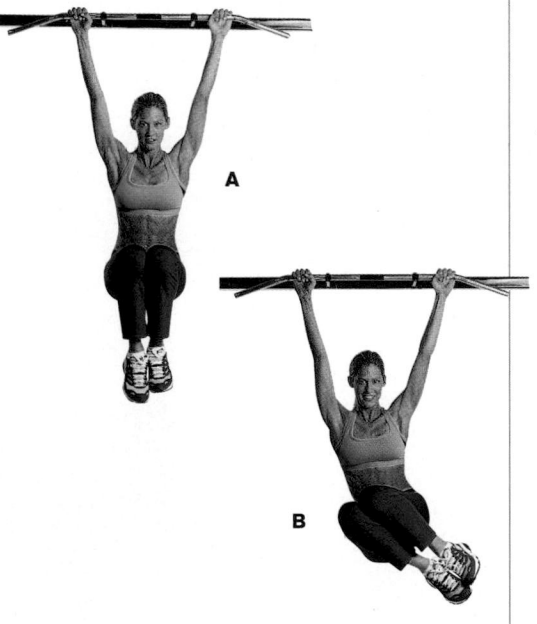

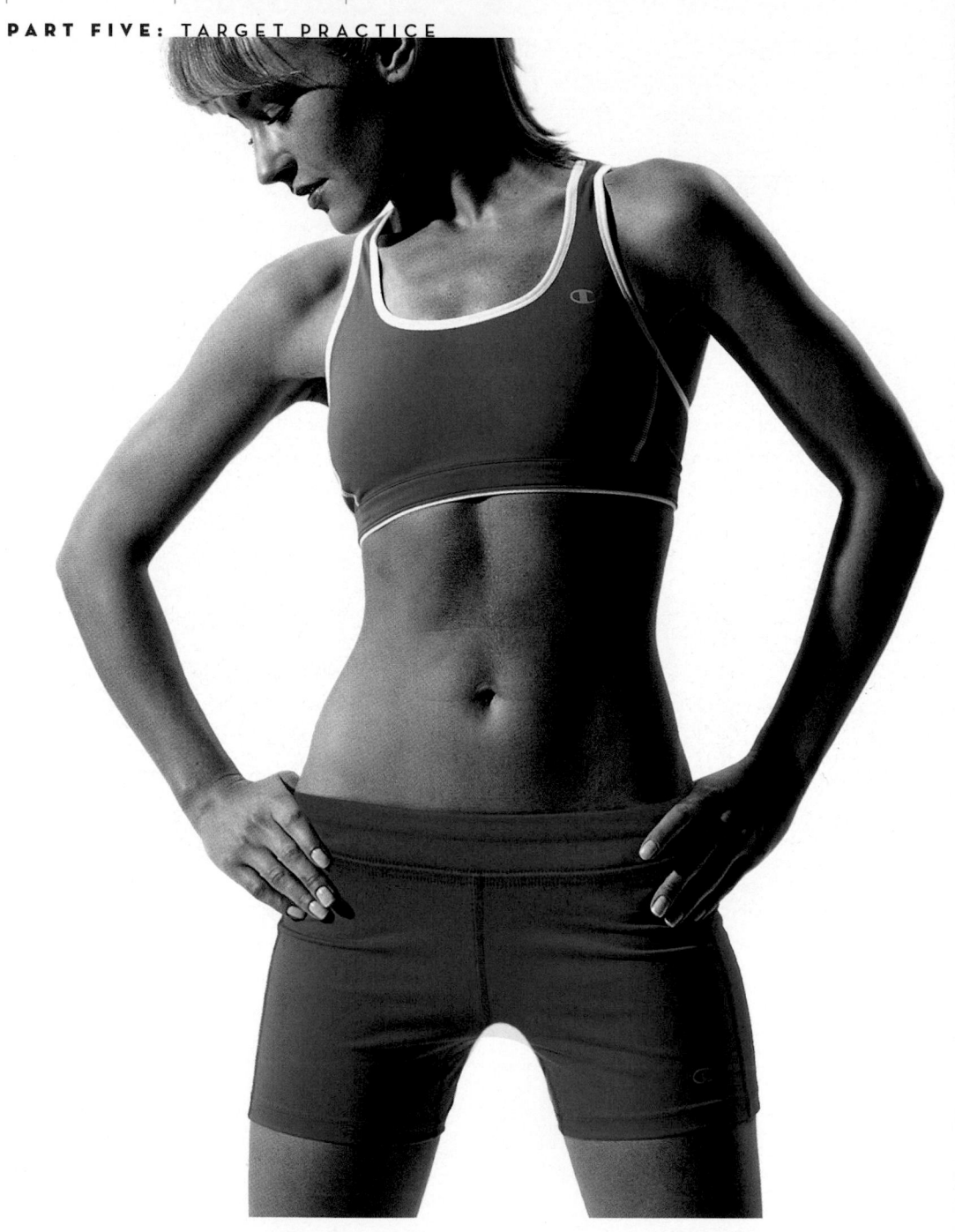

CHAPTER TWENTY-FIVE

AT-HOME ABS

SCULPT YOUR STOMACH WITH THESE SIMPLE MOVES.

BETWEEN THE GIANT INFLATABLE BALL, circuit weight contraption, and occasional balancing act—your ab routine is starting to look like Cirque du Soleil. Unless you plan to take that show on the road, it's time to get back to basics with our at-home workout. No, this doesn't involve sweating through 250 of the same old situps—these six moves will work your core from every angle, hitting all abdominal muscles (including obliques) and your primary back muscles (erector spinae). You can do these moves from Kurt, Brett, and Mike Brungardt, authors of *The Complete Book of Core Training*, as a stand-alone core workout or incorporate them into your total-body routine.

TOTAL FITNESS GUIDE 2008

W|H

Mainline moves

PICK FOUR EXERCISES, AND UNLESS OTHERWISE NOTED, PERFORM TWO OR THREE SETS OF 8 TO 20 REPS.

SUN SALUTE WITH CROSS

WORKS WHOLE WAIST AREA

Stand with legs slightly more than shoulder-width apart, arms extended overhead with hands just touching. Bending forward at the waist, reach down and touch your right foot, keeping your torso straight and moving as one unit. Straighten back to start. Repeat on the opposite side to complete one rep.

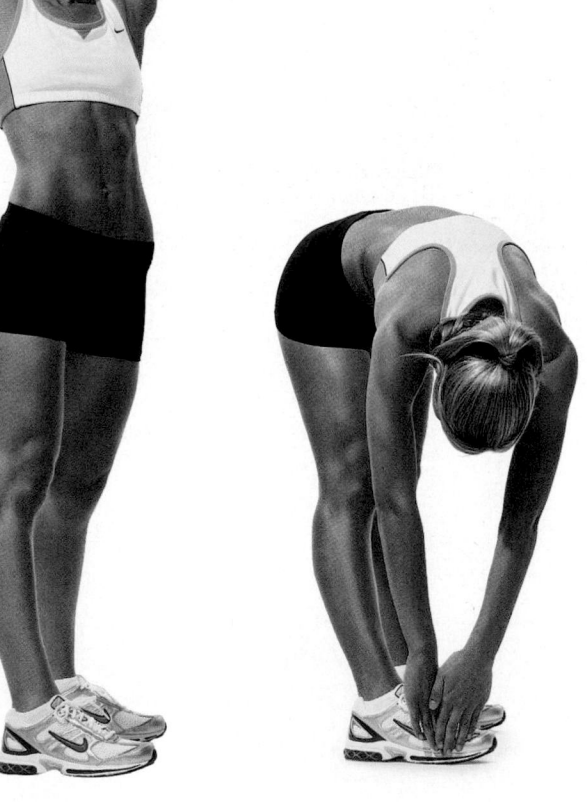

ANKLE REACH

WORKS BACK

Lie on your belly with legs straight and toes touching the floor. Bend your arms with palms on the floor in line with your ears. Reaching both arms back and up, bend your right leg, reaching your heel toward your butt as you touch your hands to your right ankle. Slowly lower your arms and leg to start. Repeat with your left leg to complete one rep.

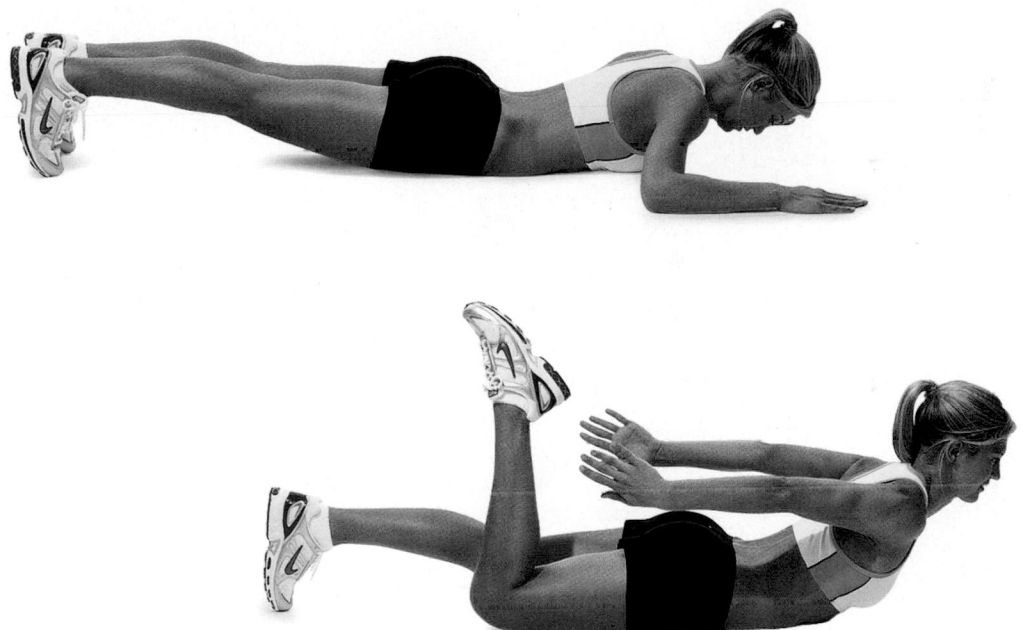

TOTAL FITNESS GUIDE 2008

W|H

DOUBLE-SIDE JACKKNIFE

WORKS OBLIQUES

Lie on your left side, your legs stacked and straight.
Wrap your left arm in front of your torso, placing it on
your right hip, and put your right hand behind your
head. Simultaneously raise your torso and legs,
bringing your head toward your hips. Return to start in
a controlled motion and repeat for all reps, then
switch sides and repeat reps to complete one set.
Too hard? Start by lifting just your legs.

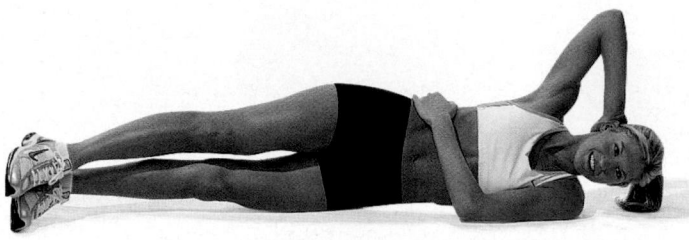

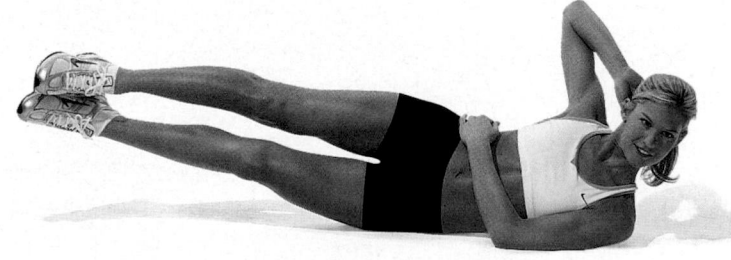

DYNAMIC V-CRUNCH

WORKS UPPER AND LOWER ABS
AND OBLIQUES

Lie face up with your legs straight—in line with your hips and perpendicular to your torso. Extend your arms in front of you, keeping them in line with your shoulders. Contract your abs and lower your legs so they're at a 45-degree angle with your hips. Then reach toward your left leg, simultaneously raising it and bringing it in line with your hips. Lower your left leg. Repeat with the right leg to complete one rep.

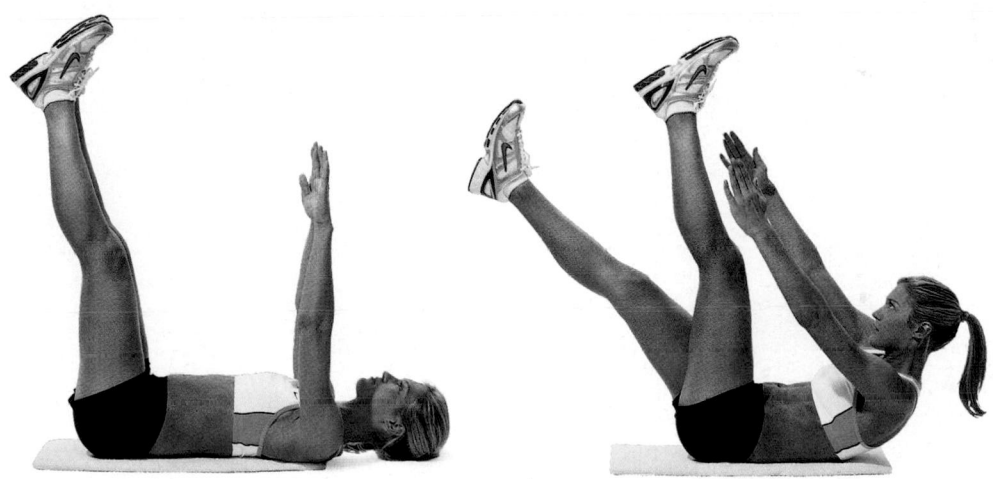

W|H

RAISED-HIPS CRUNCH

WORKS UPPER AND LOWER ABS

Lie face up with knees bent and feet flat on floor, hands behind head, and fingers unclasped. Press your hips off the floor into a bridge position, keeping your hips level. Maintaining the bridge, contract your abs and then raise your head, neck, and shoulders off the floor as one unit. Pause, then lower, and repeat. For more of a challenge, lift one foot slightly while you perform half of your reps, then lift the other foot off the floor for the other half.

SIDE DOUBLE CRUNCH

WORKS OBLIQUES AND UPPER AND LOWER ABS

Lie balanced on your right buttock, with legs straight but not locked, arms straight, palms up. Simultaneously crunch your legs and torso together, bending your knees toward your chest while still balancing on your right buttock. Return to start and repeat for all reps, then switch sides and repeat to complete one set.

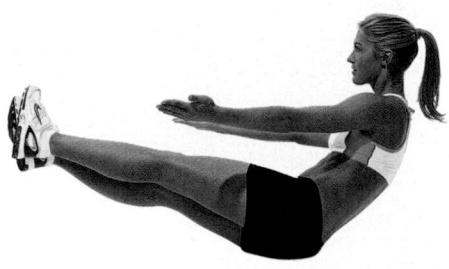

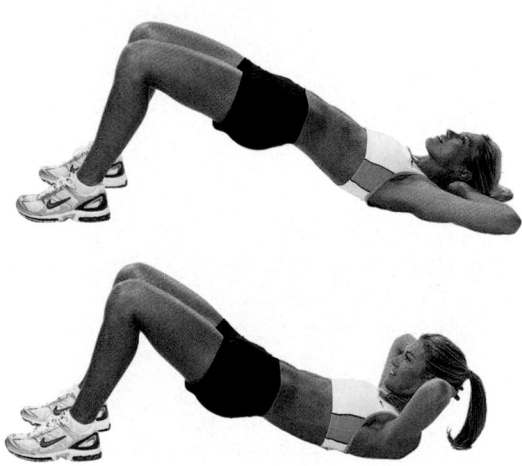

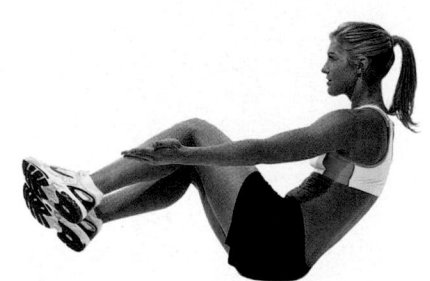

The Perfect Crunch

CIRCLE CRUNCH

WORKS UPPER AND LOWER ABS
AND OBLIQUES

These crunches work your abs from every direction, and the continuous motion forces you to isometrically hold your core tight, adding extra burn. The best part: They're totally doable—and you get a complete abs workout with one move.

Lie face up with your knees bent and feet flat on the floor, hands behind your head with light fingers. Lift your shoulders off the floor until you feel a tight contraction, and curl your torso around in a small, clockwise circular motion (starting from 6 to 9 to 12 to 3 and back down to 6). For the next rep, repeat in the opposite, counterclockwise direction.

MAKE 'EM HARDER Raise your legs with knees bent at 90 degrees, calves parallel to floor, as you perform each set.

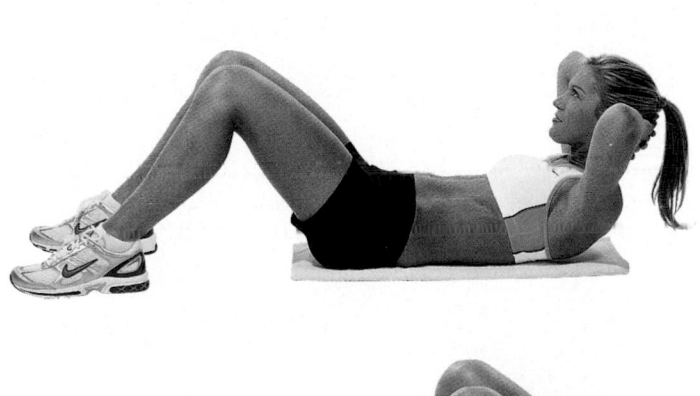

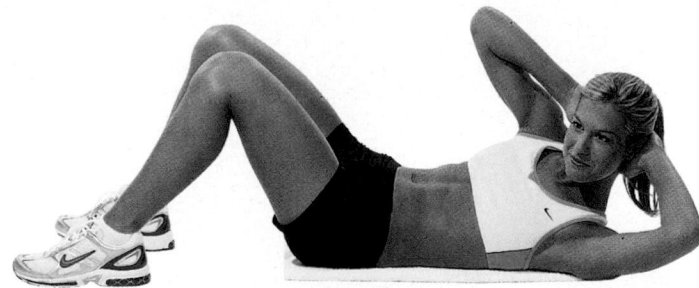

W|H

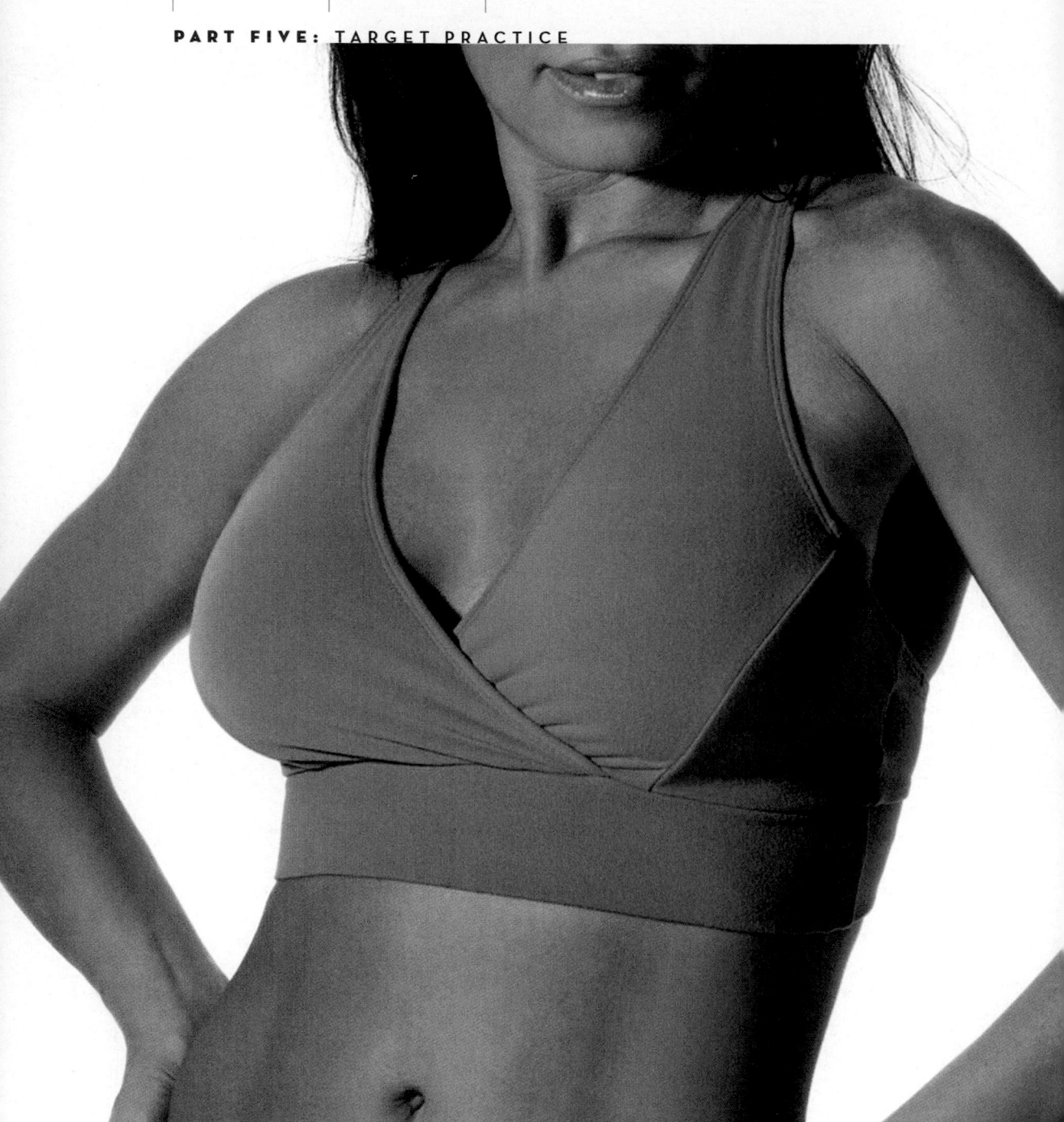

CHAPTER TWENTY-SIX

BELLY-BUSTING YOGA

CALM DOWN. A STRONGER, TRIMMER CORE IS AROUND THE CORNER.

YOGA IS YOUR SECRET WEAPON against belly fat. Soft and slow in pace, yoga can help relieve stress and still give you a challenging enough routine to burn calories, tone your abs, and improve flexibility. Less stress means two things: less unhealthy, nerve-induced snacking and fewer stress hormones to signal your body to store fat in your middle. A stronger, more flexible core means:

BETTER POSTURE. When your core is strong, those muscles can help brace and protect your spine and keep you properly aligned. Of course, when your spine is lined up and you move correctly, you're less likely to fall and injure other parts of your body.

BETTER DIGESTION. "When your abs hold you correctly, your digestive system can function more efficiently because you're not compressing your intestines," says Ana Forrest, creator of Forrest Yoga and *The Pleasure of Strength* DVD.

MORE ENERGY. More oxygen means more energy. "Strengthening your core improves your respiratory efficiency because proper alignment allows you to breathe deeply and therefore maximize your oxygen intake," says holistic health practitioner Paul Chek, founder of the Chek Institute in San Diego.

CLEARER HEAD. Mechanically, when you don't have solid core strength, especially in your chest and upper back, your neck will tilt back and pinch, which can cause headaches and even foggy thinking, Forrest says. "But at an even deeper level, when you're connected to your core, your ability to have gut feelings and instincts are stronger. You're physically and mentally more centered."

LOOK LEANER. Okay, this isn't a medical issue per se, but the better you look, the better you feel, right? "When you properly work your core, you can create more space between your vertebrae and stand half an inch to an inch taller," says Mimosa Gordon, principal Pilates instructor at re: Ab Pilates studio in New York City.

The Workout

You can begin to improve your core strength, shape, and flexibility with the following yoga-inspired exercises. Practice each of the following pairs of moves for a comprehensive workout, or add one from each group to your regular exercise routine.

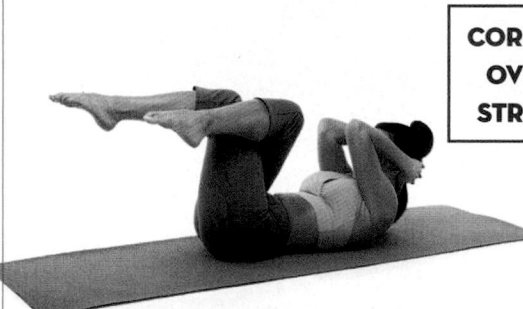

CORE GOAL: OVERALL STRENGTH

Lie on your back in traditional situp stance—with your hands clasped behind your head, feet on the floor, and knees bent. Then cross your right knee over your left knee, and try to interlock your right ankle with your left ankle. Next, inhale and curl your head and chest up. Exhale and curl your pelvis and thighs up, pulling your abs in toward your spine. Release and repeat three times. Next, place your hands on your left thigh. Push against your thighs as your thighs push against your hands. Hold for a breath and release, and then repeat the whole sequence with your legs switched.

TWISTED ROOT

"This strengthens your upper, middle, and lower abs, along with your inner thighs, all at once," Forrest says.

THE CURL (FUSION)

"Performing this move helps you build a brace for your back," says Elisabeth Halfpapp, creator of CoreFusion.

> **CORE GOAL: OVERALL STRENGTH**

Lie on the mat with your knees bent and your arms down at your sides. Roll your shoulder blades off the floor to form a large C from the top of your head to your knees, and let your hands slide up to the outside of your thighs. Tuck your pelvis up and under, and gaze beyond your knee. Hold for 30 seconds. Next, raise your arms up by your ears and hold for another 30 seconds. Return to start and rest for 30 seconds, then repeat for two more sets.

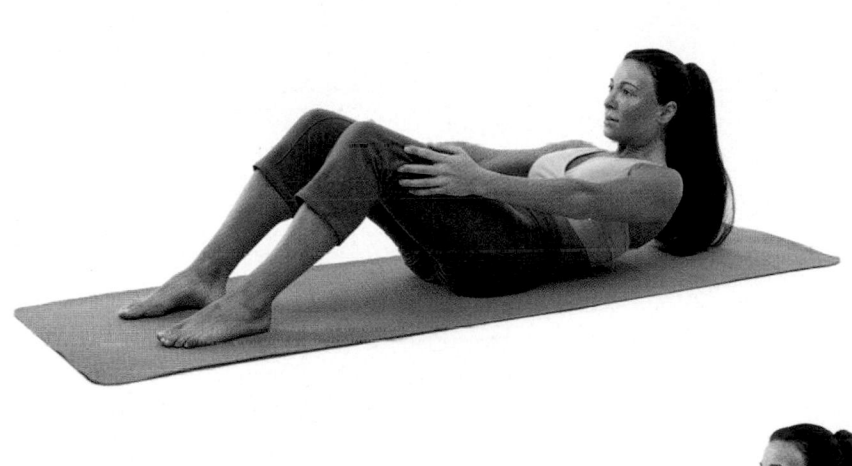

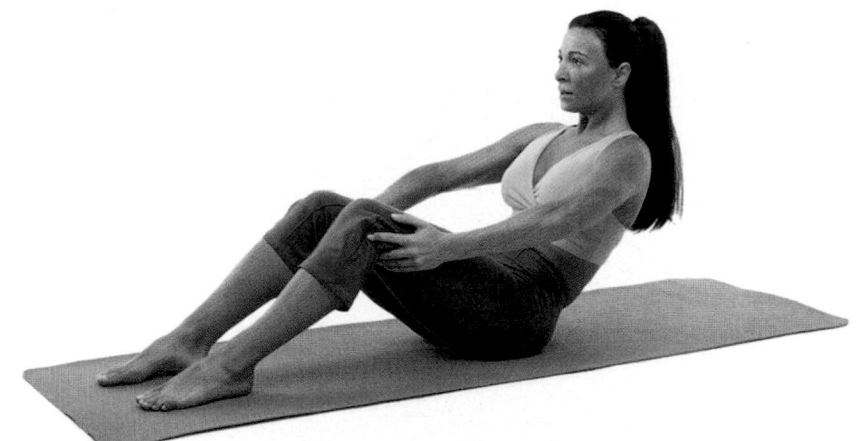

BRIDGE WITH ROLL

"This pose helps align your spine," Forrest says, "and it teaches you to properly use your buttocks, because you're pulling them away from your spine."

Place a foam roller (about $7 for a 12-inch version at exertools.com, or use a cylindrical bolster pillow or a rolled and doubled beach towel) between your thighs. Lie on your back with your knees bent and directly over your feet, and put your hands by your heels, palms up. Make your feet active by pressing your heels and balls of your feet into the floor with your toes up. Exhale and curl your tailbone toward the roll, and then using your abs and glutes, lift your hips and torso toward the ceiling. Hold for 5 to 10 breaths. Lengthen your ribs with each inhale, and focus on lengthening your back with each exhale. Lower down starting with your upper back and finishing with your lower back, keeping your pelvis tilted up.

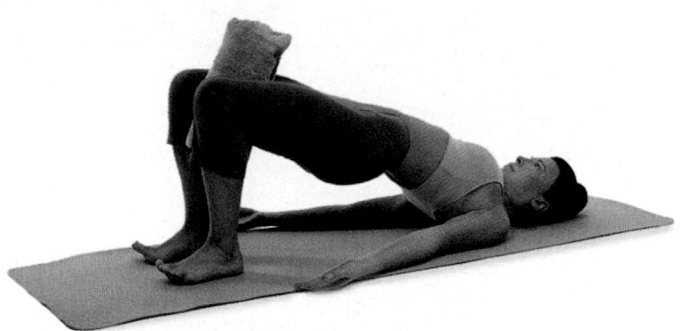

CAT-COW-POINTER SEQUENCE

"This puts your core through a wide range of motion," Halfpapp says.

Get on all fours and start this stretch by pulling your abs in and rounding your back upward into Cow pose. Hold for a few seconds, and then press your abs down toward the floor, arching your back into Cat. Repeat one more time. Next, raise your left arm in front of you, with your thumb pointing toward the ceiling, and extend your right leg out behind you. Hold this position for 5 seconds, then round your core, bringing your left elbow in toward your right knee. Hold this position for 5 seconds, then extend and bring in for one more set. Repeat with the other side for two sets.

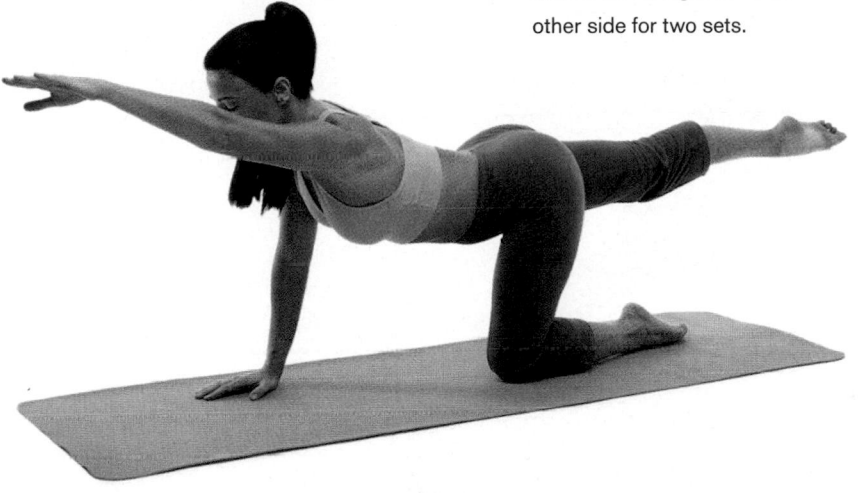

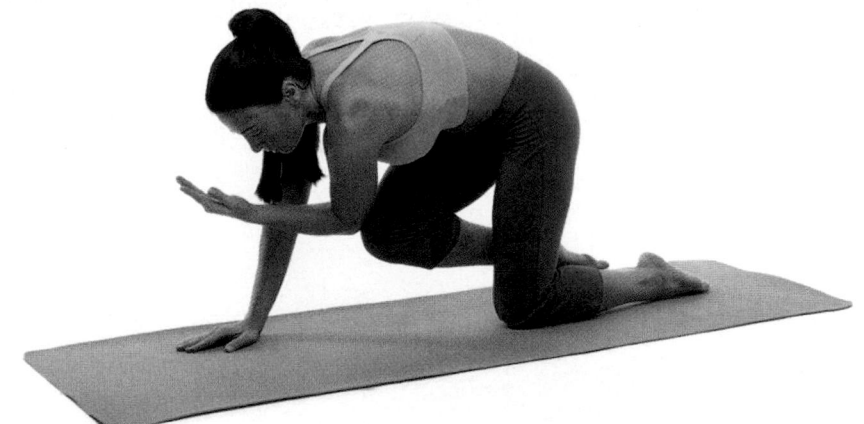

TWISTING WARRIOR

"You'll shape your obliques while decompressing your spine," Forrest says.

From a standing position, move into Warrior I, stepping your left leg forward, toes straight ahead, and your right leg back, toes turned out. Root your feet into the ground, engage your core, and twist at the waist, hooking your right elbow over your left thigh. Make a fist with your right hand and brace your left hand on it, lifting your torso up off your thigh and relaxing your neck. Hold for a few breaths, then repeat on the other side.

For more of a challenge, perform a bind by sliding your left arm down and around your thigh, clasping your hands behind your back.

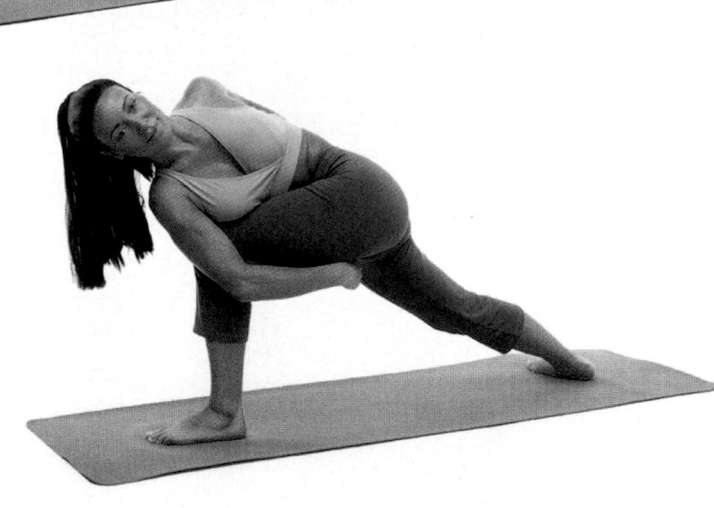

L-SEAT

Halfpapp's version of the L-Seat targets the lower abs, often the spot of the ominous "pooch."

Sit on the mat with your legs extended and feet flexed. Place your hands on the floor, just outside your thighs, and slightly round your torso downward, curling your abs. Next, pull your lower abs in toward your spine and use them to lift your hips off the mat. Your weight should be balanced between your hands and your heels. Hold for five counts and then release, repeating for three reps.

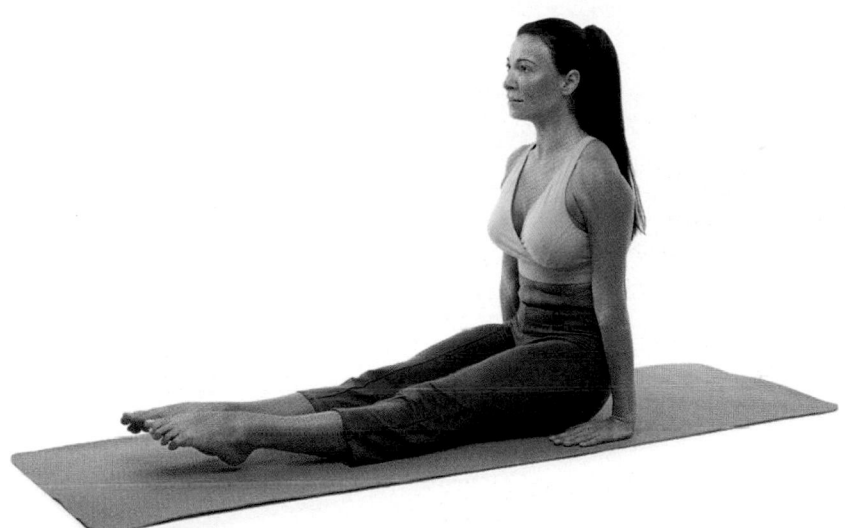

COBRA PUSHUP
WITH ROLL

"This pose strengthens your back as well as your glutes," Forrest says.

**CORE GOAL:
BACK
STRENGTH**

Squeeze a foam roll between your thighs and lie flat on your belly, tucking your tailbone toward the mat. Place your hands under your shoulders, with elbows up, and push the tops of your feet into the floor. Next, inhale and push up into Cobra, opening your chest and pulling your rib cage forward. Be sure to keep your shoulders down. Exhale and release, lowering yourself slowly and carefully, one set of ribs at a time. Repeat three times.

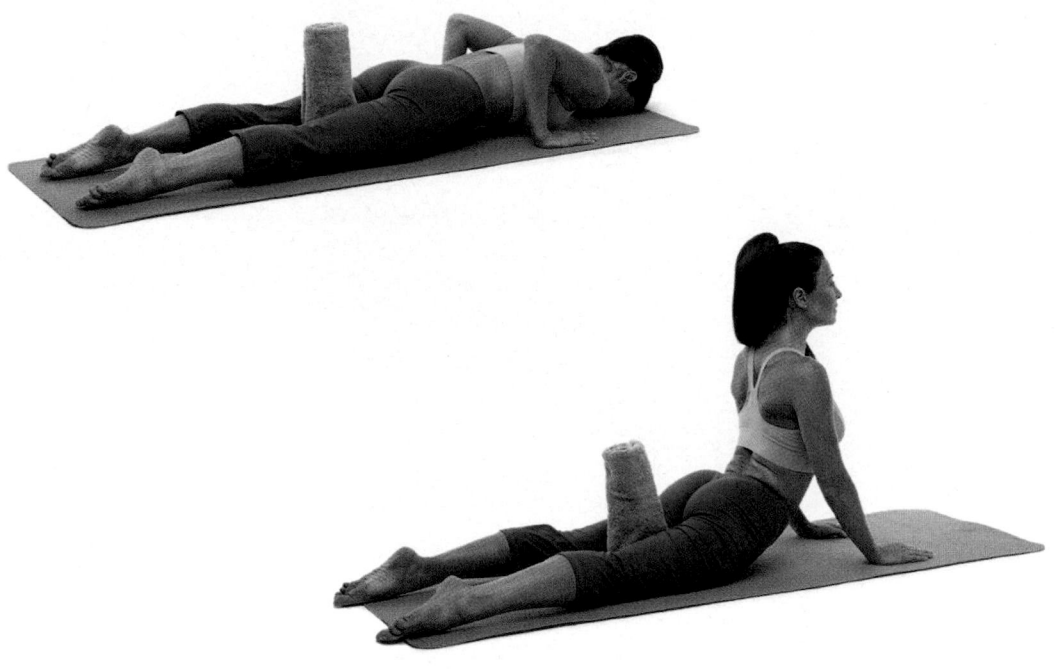

PRONE GLUTEALS

"This move tones your low back and glutes," Halfpapp says.

CORE GOAL: BACK STRENGTH

Lie facedown on the floor and place one forearm over the other, resting your forehead on both. Next, roll your pelvis slightly under and pull your abs up and in toward your spine. First raise your right leg a few inches off the floor, and then your left, keeping them about 1 foot apart, with toes slightly pointed. Squeeze your glutes and lower-back muscles, and pulse both legs up and down a few inches for 20 counts. Rest for 20 seconds and then repeat for a total of three sets. To work your mid-back, bring your heels together and slightly bend your knees, and repeat for one more set of 20 pulses.

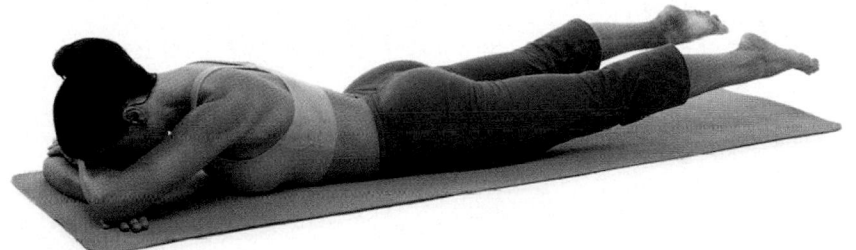

TOTAL FITNESS GUIDE 2008

W|H

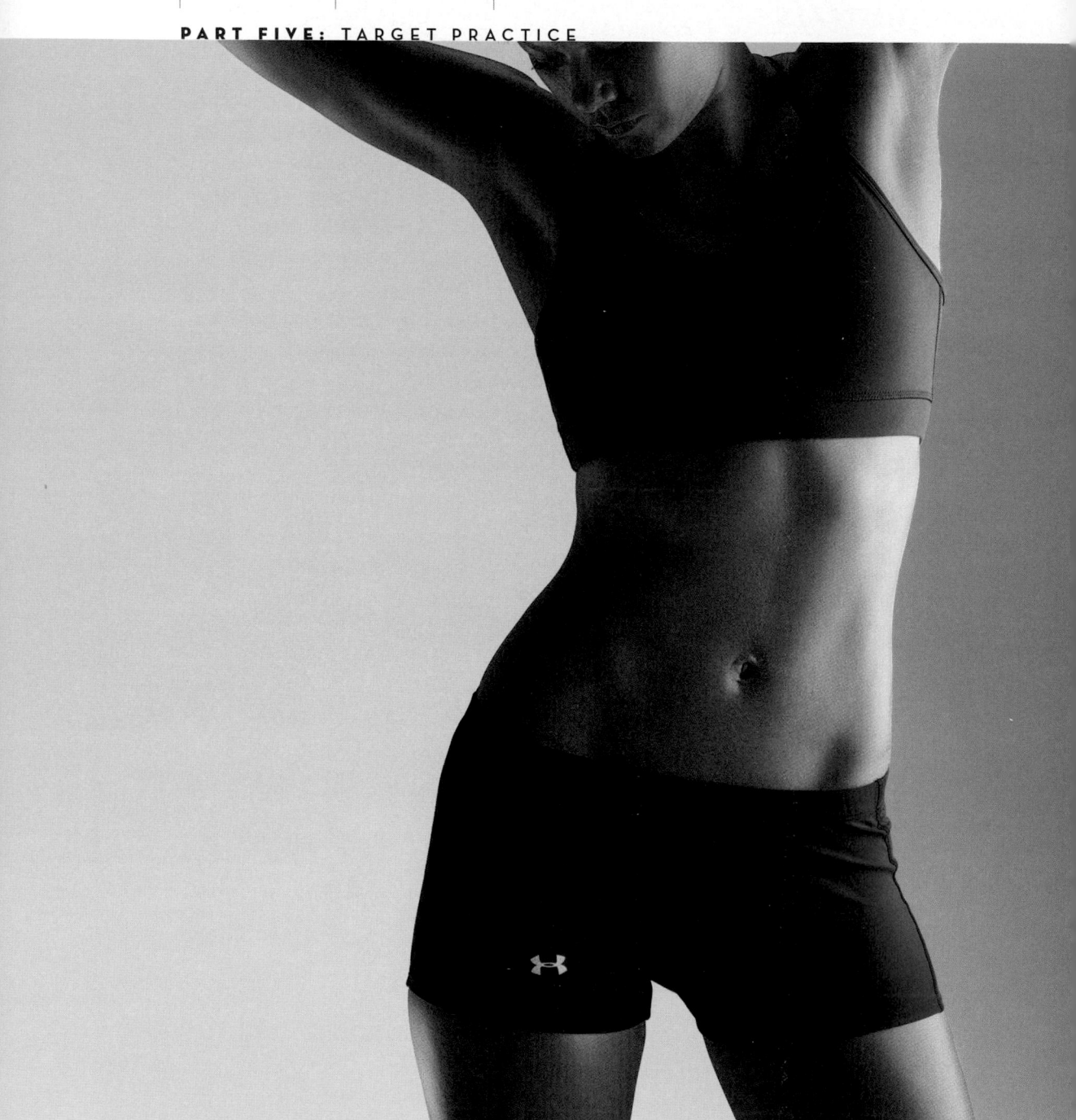

CHAPTER TWENTY-SEVEN

8 SMART SCULPTORS

FOR MAXIMUM MIDSECTION POWER, REPLACE THE DREADED CRUNCH WITH THESE UNCONVENTIONAL CORE MOVES.

CRUNCHES ARE LIKE THE BAD-BOY EX you've sheepishly stayed in touch with since college. It's been years and little good has come of the relationship, yet you keep going back for more. Need inspiration to move on? "A well-rounded core workout reduces your risk of back injuries and improves athletic performance," says Bill Hartman, a certified strength and conditioning specialist in Indianapolis. In fact, doing crunches by the truckload actually shortens the front of your abdominal wall and trains your body to move with limited motion. And because the move neglects the rest of your core, you're not developing your "powerhouse," the midsection muscles that help you move every which way—from twisting to reach a wine glass on the top shelf to stabilizing your body as you hurtle down a double black diamond. You can train your core to move in all directions with this 8-week, sequential program of midsection moves.

Function Junction

FOLLOW OUR HANDY COLOR-CODED KEY TO UNDERSTAND THE SCIENCE BEHIND THESE WACKY MOVES

TRAINER SAYS "Do this move and you'll see a huge difference in your spinal/hip extension."
TRANSLATION It lengthens the spine, which makes things like standing up after tying your shoes easier and safer.

TRAINER SAYS "Stick with this stabilization exercise, which works your transverse abdominis, and you'll have a perfectly neutral pelvis."
TRANSLATION Strengthening the muscles that stabilize your pelvis makes you less likely to take a nosedive when you trip over your labradoodle's bowl.

TRAINER SAYS "Training your spinal/hip flexion like this is crucial for overall core mobility."
TRANSLATION This exercise strengthens and increases the range of motion in the back and hip muscles that support your spine when you curve it—to pick up dropped keys or to haul yourself out of bed when your alarm blares.

TRAINER SAYS "Seriously, just do this and you'll have Gwen Stefani-caliber rotation."
TRANSLATION This move trains your obliques, giving you more strength and mobility when you twist your torso and hips—important for loading groceries into the trunk after you stock up at Trader Joe's.

TRAINER SAYS "Way to work your lateral flexion!"
TRANSLATION This move builds strength and sideways flexibility, so you won't pull a muscle hanging holiday decorations.

Hit More Core

To target your powerhouse from every angle, do this workout 2 to 3 days a week in addition to your regular routine or on off days. Following the order here, complete two full sets of each move, resting 30 to 60 seconds between sets. Most important: Never sacrifice form for reps. After 8 weeks, go back to week 1 but do the workout as a circuit. That is, perform the moves one right after another, with 30- to 60-second rests between each one. Complete the circuit twice. You should be done in about 15 minutes!

WEEKS 1 TO 4

● **Unilateral Romanian Deadlift**

● ● **Reverse Crunch to Modified Dragon Flag**

● **Side Bridge with Abduction**

● **Medicine Ball Rotation**

WEEKS 5 TO 8

● **Renegade Row**

● **Stability Ball Rotation**

● **Stability Ball Pass-Off**

● **Saxon Side Bend**

1 UNILATERAL ROMANIAN DEADLIFT

DO IT Grab a 5- to 10-pound dumbbell in each hand and stand with your feet together, arms at your sides (**A**). Extend your right leg behind you and lean forward from your waist until your torso is parallel to the floor and your arms are hanging straight down (**B**). Your body should form a straight line from your head to the heel of your right foot. Pause, then drive your left heel into the floor for balance as you raise your torso back to start. Do six to eight reps per side. **Tip: Keep knee slightly bent for balance.**

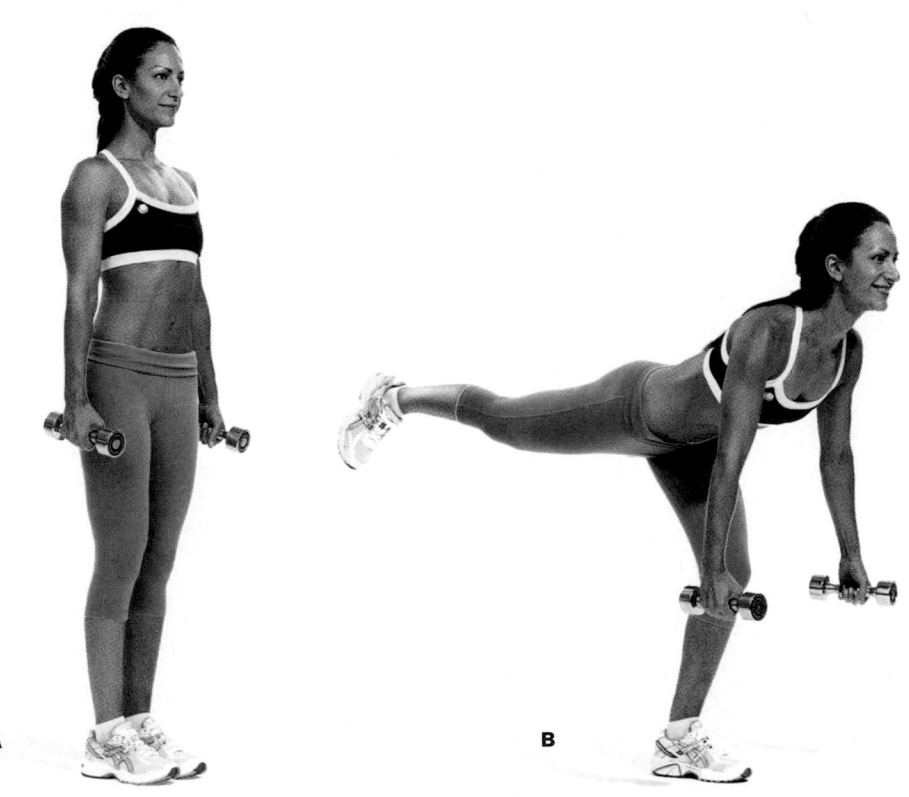

A

B

2 REVERSE CRUNCH TO MODIFIED DRAGON FLAG

DO IT Lie on your back on an exercise bench. Raise your legs and bend your knees to 90-degree angles over your hips. Grab the bench beneath your head (**A**). Curl your hips toward your chest, lifting your tailbone about 2 inches. Next, keeping your knees bent, raise your hips straight up so the bottoms of your feet face the ceiling (**B**). Slowly lower your body to the bench. Do five to eight reps.

Tip: Straighten then lower legs to make the move more challenging.

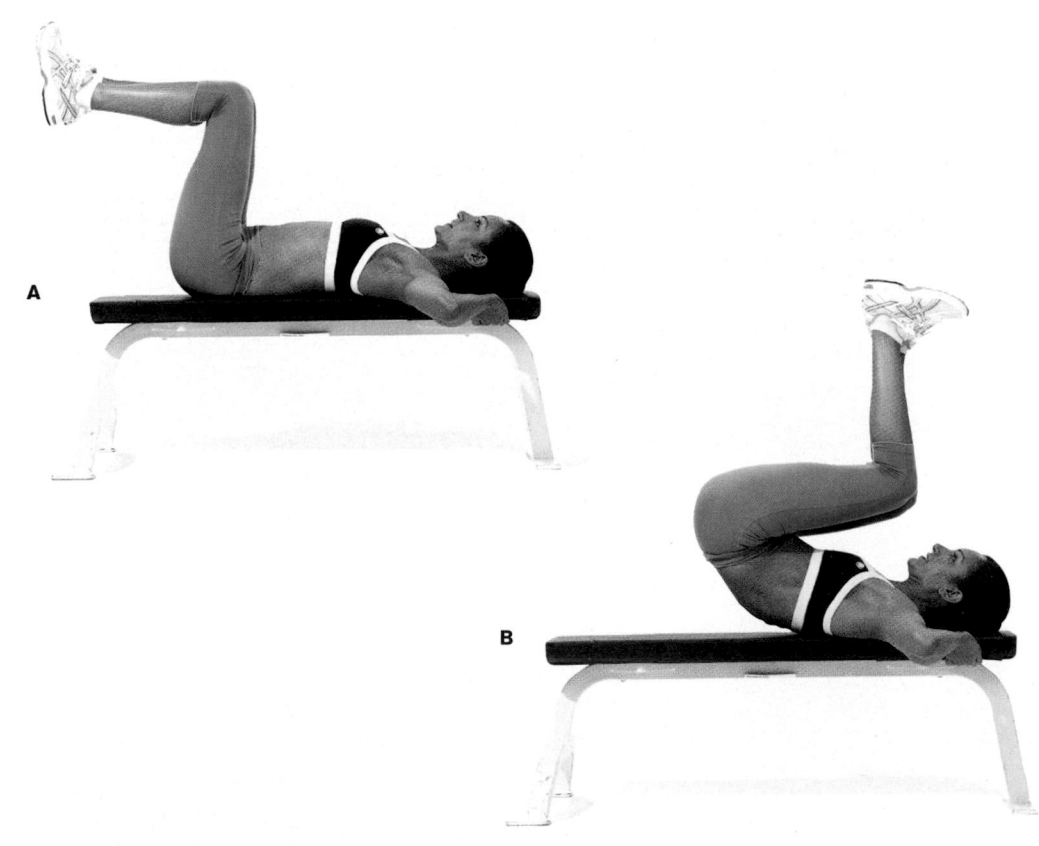

A

B

3 SIDE BRIDGE WITH ABDUCTION

DO IT Lie on your right side with your left leg on top of your right leg and your right elbow in line with your right shoulder. Keeping your lower back aligned naturally (with the same slight arch you'd have if you were standing up), lift your hips and torso so you're balancing on your forearm and foot. Your body should form a straight diagonal line from head to toe (**A**). Next, lift your left leg 45 degrees and hold it there for 5 seconds (**B**). Lower your leg first, then your hips and torso. Do 8 to 10 reps on each side.

Tip: If you can't raise your leg without losing form, keep it down until you build strength.

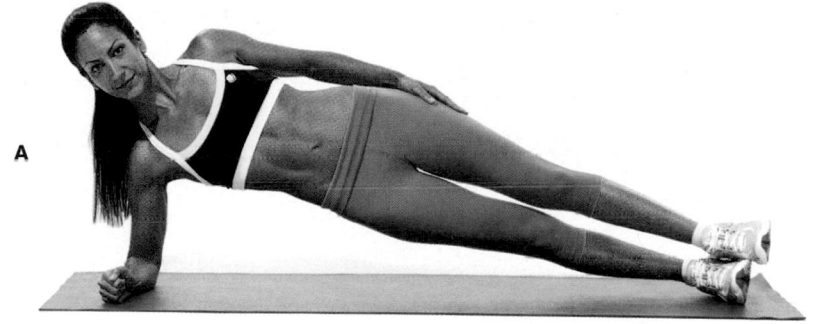

A

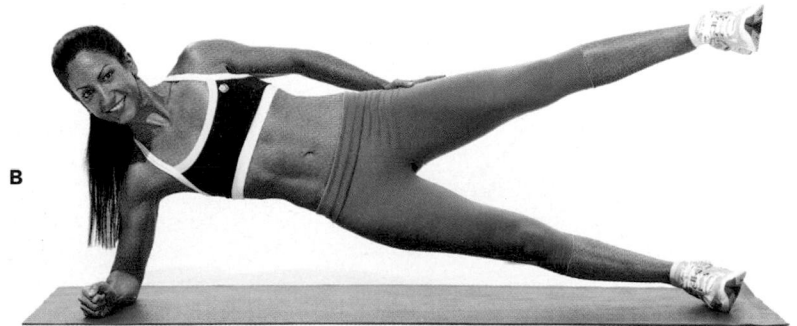

B

TOTAL FITNESS GUIDE 2008

W|H

4 MEDICINE BALL ROTATION

DO IT Hold a 4- to 8-pound medicine ball about a foot from your chest and sit on the floor with knees slightly bent. Lift your feet 3 inches off the floor so you're balancing on your butt. Cross your ankles and lean back 45 degrees (**A**). Maintaining this position, pull your belly button toward your spine and rotate your torso to the left, allowing your arms to follow. Touch the ball to the floor on the left side (**B**). Quickly twist to the right. Continue twisting until you've completed 8 to 12 touches on each side.
Tip: Turn your shoulders in the direction you're twisting.

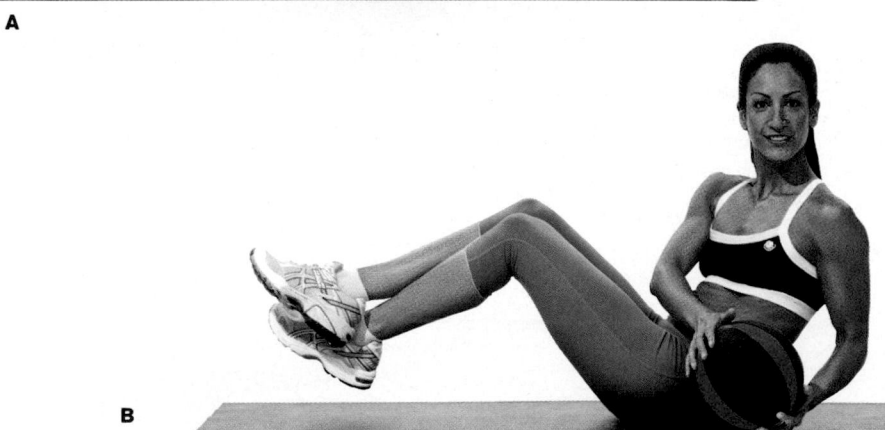

A

B

5 RENEGADE ROW

DO IT Grab a 2- to 5-pound dumbbell in each hand and get into plank position. Rest your hands on the dumbbells slightly closer than shoulder-width apart, palms facing each other (**A**). Brace your abs as you push the right dumbbell into the floor and pull the left one up until your elbow passes your torso (**B**). Hold for 2 seconds, then lower the dumbbell and repeat with your right arm. Continue alternating sides until you've completed six reps with each arm.

Tip: Don't rotate your hips or arch your back when you pull.

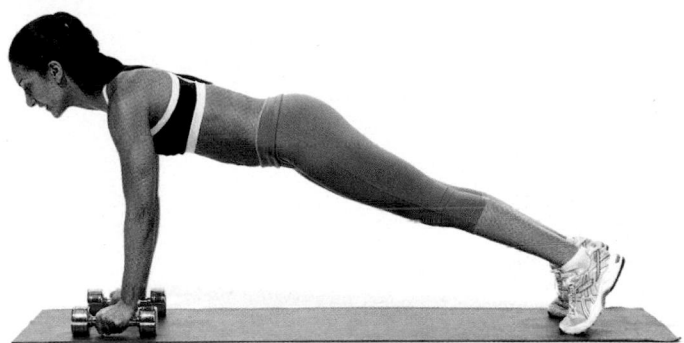

A

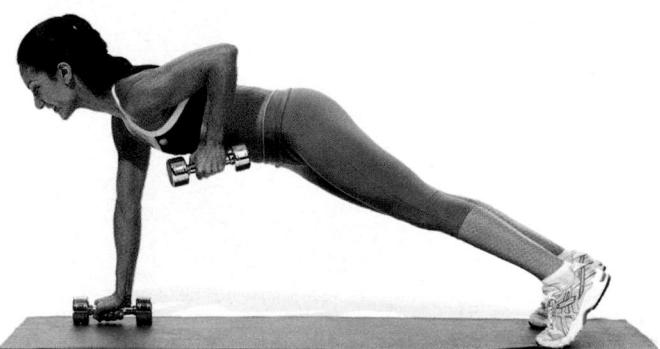

B

6 STABILITY BALL ROTATION

DO IT Get into plank position with your arms straight and slightly wider than your shoulders. Rest your shins on a stability ball, hip-width apart (**A**). Slowly roll the ball to the right, allowing your legs to move with the ball (**B**). Roll them as low on the ball as you can. Pause, then bring the ball back to start. Repeat to the left. Continue alternating until you've completed six reps on each side.

Tip: Don't just let the ball roll. Control its movement by contracting your abs.

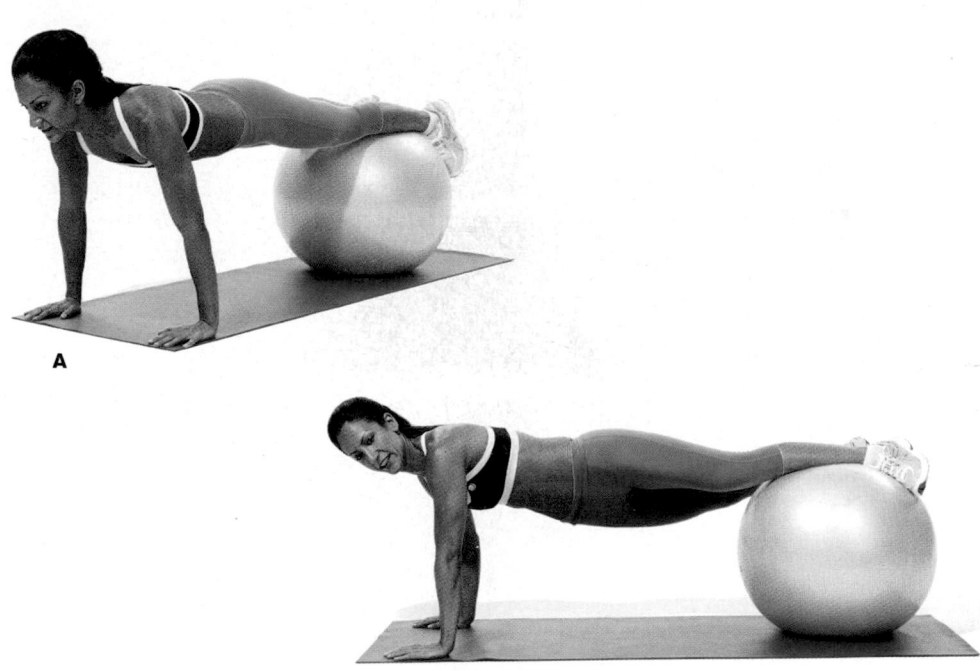

A

B

7 STABILITY BALL PASS-OFF

DO IT Grab a stability ball and lie on your back. Bend your knees slightly and raise your legs until they're directly above your hips. Hold the ball at arm's length behind your head (**A**). Crunch toward your legs, raise the ball in an arc over your head, and place it between your feet (**B**). With your torso raised, begin lowering your legs (**C**). When they're as close to the floor as possible without touching it, pause, then lift them back up and grab the ball. Lower your upper body back to the floor and repeat the sequence. Do 6 to 10 reps.

Tip: Keep your lower back glued to the floor to prevent strain.

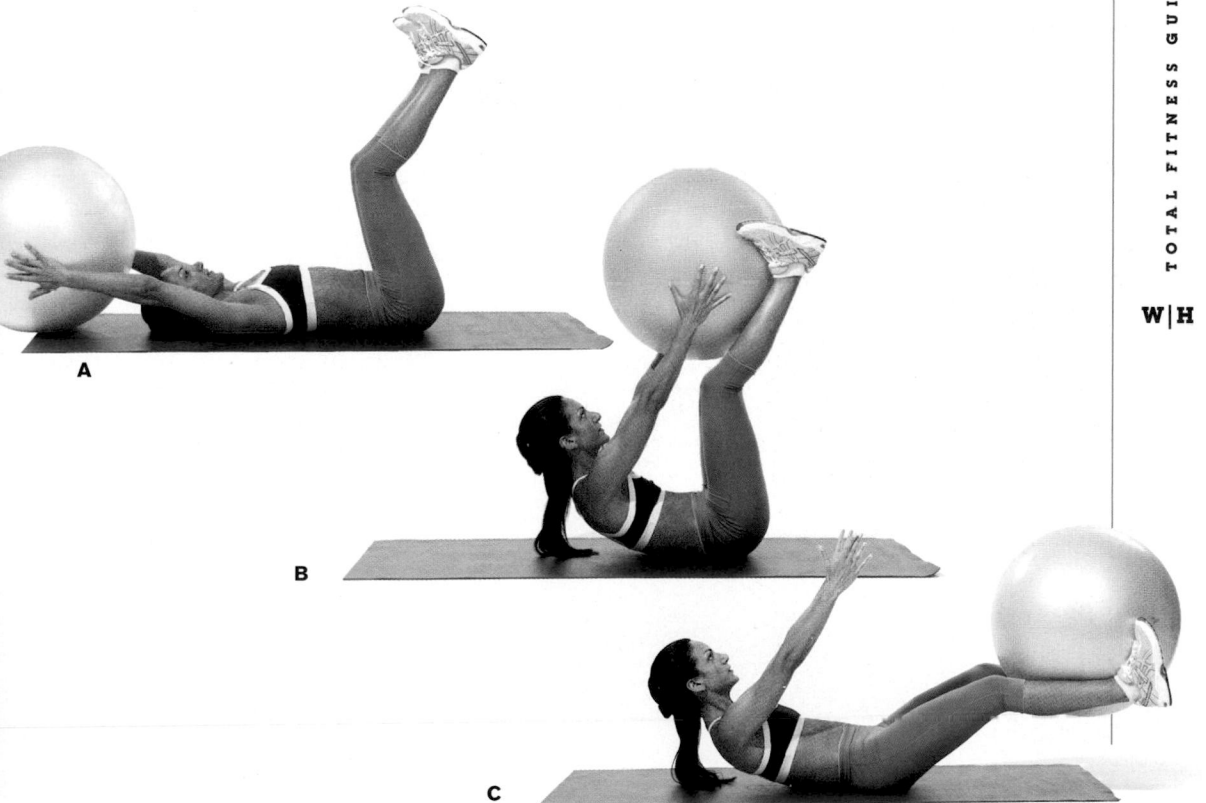

A

B

C

W|H

8 SAXON SIDE BEND

DO IT Grab a 2- to 5-pound dumbbell in each hand and raise them overhead. Straighten your arms and hold them shoulder-width apart, palms facing forward (**A**). Keeping your knees straight, lean as far to the right as possible without bending your elbows or bringing the dumbbells closer together (**B**). Once you've gone as far as possible maintaining perfect form (probably about 45 degrees), pause before bringing the weights back to start. Repeat to the left. Continue alternating until you've completed six reps on each side.

Tip: To avoid rotating your torso, focus on bringing your armpit toward your hip.

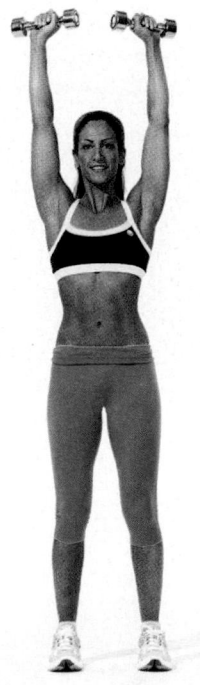

A

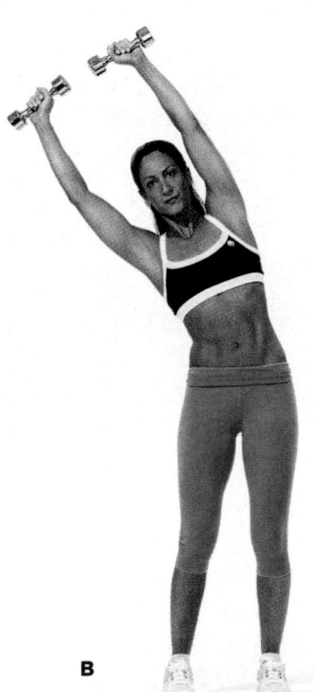

B

Stand and deliver

TAKE YOUR CORE WORKOUT FROM HORIZONTAL TO VERTICAL

Standing up to tone your abs isn't like fudging tax numbers or sneaking midnight lasagna. It's a legit way to work your entire core without yanking your neck or relying on your hip flexors, the way you might during on-your-back ab exercises. These four standing moves from Connecticut trainer Ellen Barrett will hone your balance and improve posture, while giving you straight-up great abs.

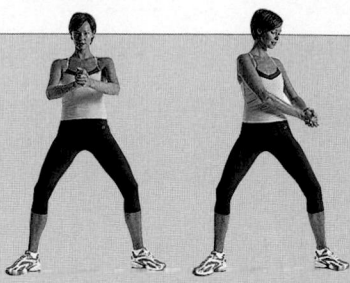

1 CANOE Stand with your feet 3 feet apart, knees slightly bent, and hands clasped. Keeping your hips still, bring your hands down to your left hip, "paddling" backward. Next, raise your hands up to chest level, and then paddle them to the right hip. Do 10 alternating reps for each side. If it's too easy, hold a 2- to 5-pound dumbbell in each hand.

2 KNEE CROSS CRUNCH Stand with your shoulders in line with your hips, and extend your right arm up and your left leg to the side, toes pointed. Next, lower your right elbow and raise your left knee, crunching them together on a diagonal line. Return to start and repeat for 10 nonalternating reps before switching sides.

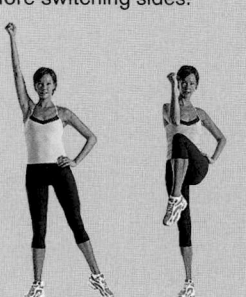

3 DOUBLE ARM REACH Stand with your feet 3 feet apart and hands clasped. Contract your abs and perform a plié, keeping your hands toward the floor. As you push up, raise your arms to the right. Next, lower your hands with another plié, and then lift them to the left. Alternate for a total of 20 reps. Too easy? Hold a 2- to 5-pound dumbbell in each hand.

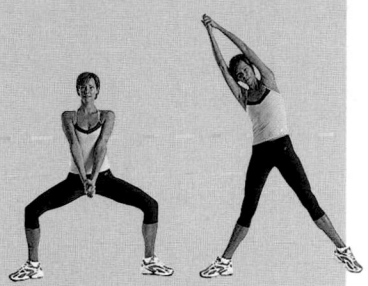

4 SIDE IMPRINT Stand with your shoulders in line with your hips and raise your right arm. Shift onto your left leg and rotate your right leg at the hip, turning your toes out. Crunch your right elbow and right knee together, pinching your waist. Return to start and do 10 nonalternating reps on each side.

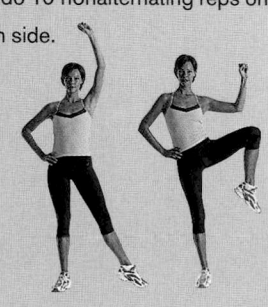

W|H

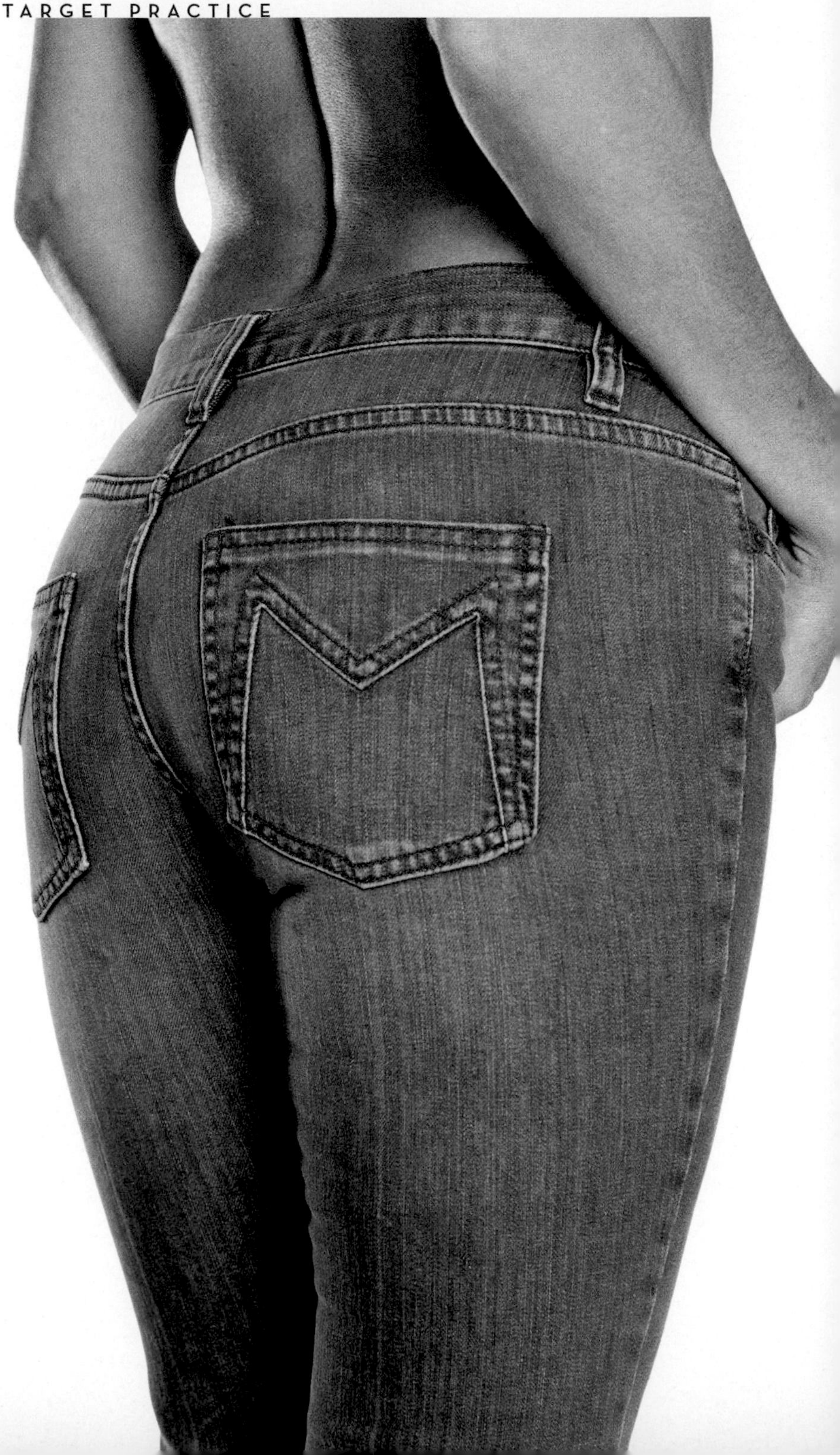

CHAPTER TWENTY-EIGHT

SITTING PRETTY

FOUR GREAT WAYS TO GET ONE BEAUTIFUL BUTT.

BY LARA ROSENBAUM

YOUR DARLING DERRIERE isn't the only thing that should be well-rounded: Your training plan should be, too. Which is why we asked a variety of fitness experts for their favorite glute-shaping moves. Do the exercises twice a week, and add 30 minutes of cardio three times each week to burn fat and make sure your back-porch swing remains a two-seater. (To target the muscles that surround your bum, try the B-Side Workout in Chapter 29.)

METHOD: **STRENGTH**

BOTTOM BENEFIT

"You need to build muscle in order to lose inches," says New York trainer Dolores Munoz, creator of *Trainer's Edge: Killer Butt* (VHS/DVD). Adding muscle will lift your glutes and make them rounder— not bigger. When you have more muscle, you'll burn more calories and fat; you might weigh more, but your body will look leaner.

THE MOVE: **SQUAT KICK**

STRENGTHENS GLUTES AND LEGS, AND THE HIGH REPS INCREASE YOUR HEART RATE, SO YOU'LL BURN EXTRA CALORIES AND FAT. Stand with feet slightly wider than hip-width and squat, bending your knees to 90 degrees, while keeping them behind your toes. Press up, and as you near the start position, kick with your right leg, keeping it straight and your right foot flexed. Step back and perform another squat, then kick with your left leg. Do three sets of 20 repetitions.

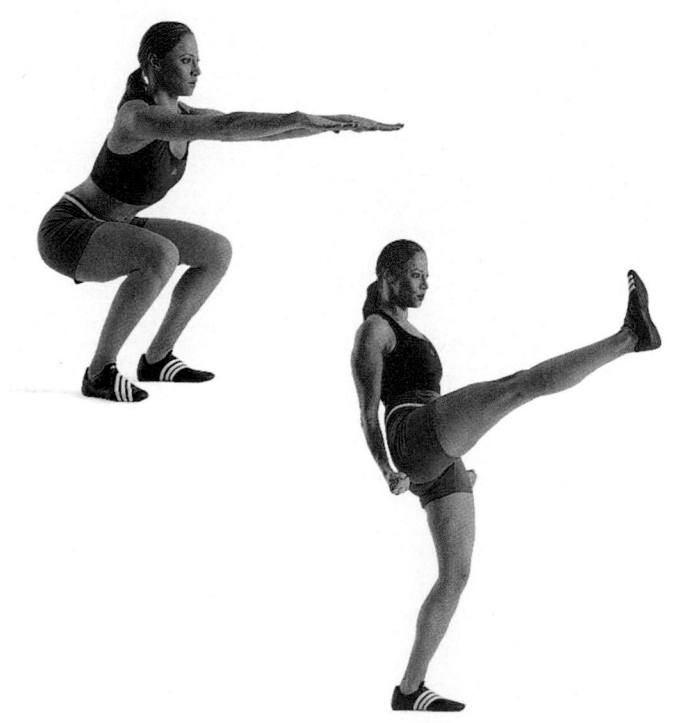

METHOD: **PILATES**

BOTTOM BENEFIT

"Pilates builds muscles, but it makes them long and lean," says Pilates instructor Lara Hudson, star of *10 Minute Solution: Pilates* (VHS/DVD). "When you contract your glutes, you're pulling the muscles in toward the bone. It keeps them looking tight and small."

THE MOVE: **GRASSHOPPER BEATS**

TONES AND TIGHTENS LEGS AND GLUTES— ESPECIALLY UPPER THIGHS, ERASING PANTY LINES.

Lie face down on the floor with your head resting gently on the backs of your hands. Pull your abs in toward your spine and raise your legs 3 inches off the floor (keep them straight; no bending at the knee). Rotate your hips so that your toes turn out, and quickly open and close your legs 6 to 8 inches, keeping them straight. Vigorously beat your heels together for two sets of 30 repetitions.

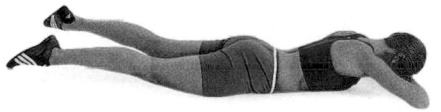

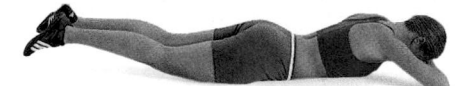

HOT (IN) PANTS

MEET THE WOMAN BEHIND THE BEST BUTT IN THE BIZ

Paige Adams-Geller has one perfect pair back there. Adams-Geller is known for filling out designer jeans brands like Earl and Seven, so we talked to her about the perks— and the work—that goes into being tops in the bottom business.

BLUE MOON

"This job makes you much more comfortable with your body. You can't be too precious, because at any moment, they're cutting the fabric off your body. 'Let's see how this looks.' And you're like, 'Hello? I'm naked here.' "

MAINLINE MAINTENANCE

"I avoid sodium and stay away from cheese, much as I love it. Water, protein, veggies, squats, and lunges— that's what works. And exercises with a Russian kettle bell: It hits every muscle in your body."

SEAT OF POWER

"I didn't buy pants for years. When I do go shopping, salespeople will say, 'It looks like these clothes were made for you.' And sometimes they were."

CELEBRITY CALLING

"Sheryl Crow would be great at this job. She's lean but with muscle tone; in good shape, but not too skinny."

METHOD: **PLYOMETRICS**

BOTTOM BENEFIT

According to a recent study published in the *Journal of Athletic Training*, plyometric jumps improve strength and corresponding jumps by 5.8 percent. What does this mean for you? More muscle and more fat loss. "Jumping stretches and then shortens your muscles, making them stronger and more explosive," says Nicole Chimera, an athletic trainer at West Chester University of Pennsylvania. Plyometrics may also help your muscles fire in a way that better protects your hips and knees from injury.

THE MOVE: **LATERAL BOUNDS**

TARGETS INNER AND OUTER THIGHS, HIPS, AND THE OUTER SIDES OF YOUR GLUTES, MAKING THE WHOLE PACKAGE LOOK SLIM.

Stand with your feet shoulder-width apart and knees and hips poised to jump. Push off with your left leg, jumping to the right, and land softly on the ball of your right foot (below left). Next, load and spring to the left, pushing off with your right leg. Do two sets of 10 jumps, giving maximum effort each time.

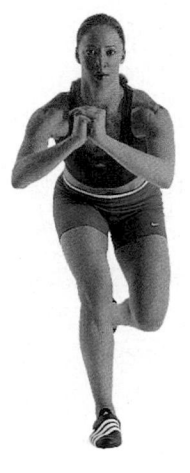
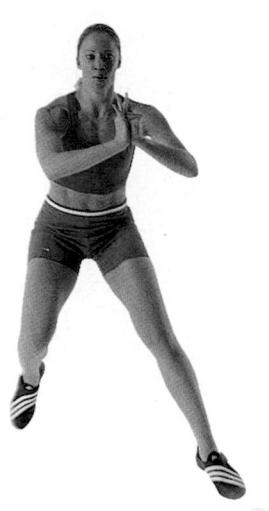

METHOD: **FLEXIBILITY**

BOTTOM BENEFIT

"You should always stretch when doing strength training to keep muscles balanced," says Tracy York, creator of *Shaping Up with Weights for Dummies* (VHS/DVD). Flexibility work won't necessarily tone your glutes, but it will keep the muscles long and improve your range of motion so that you can work muscles in their complete capacity. Stretching after a workout also allows your muscles to relax, making postworkout soreness less likely.

THE MOVE: **LYING GLUTE RELEASE**

STRETCHES AND RELAXES GLUTES
AND OUTER THIGHS.

Lie on your back with your knees bent and your feet flat on the floor. Next, place the outside of your right foot on your left thigh to form a triangle with your right leg. Gently pull your left leg toward you to stretch the right side of your buttocks. Hold for 30 seconds, release, and repeat on the other side.

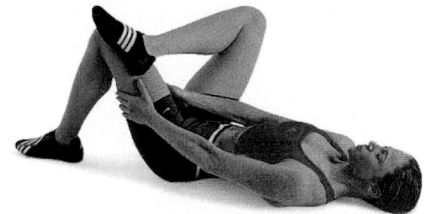
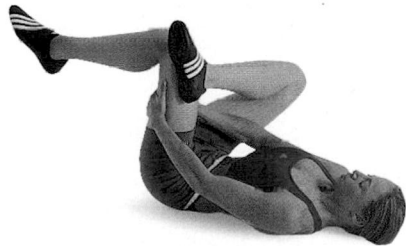

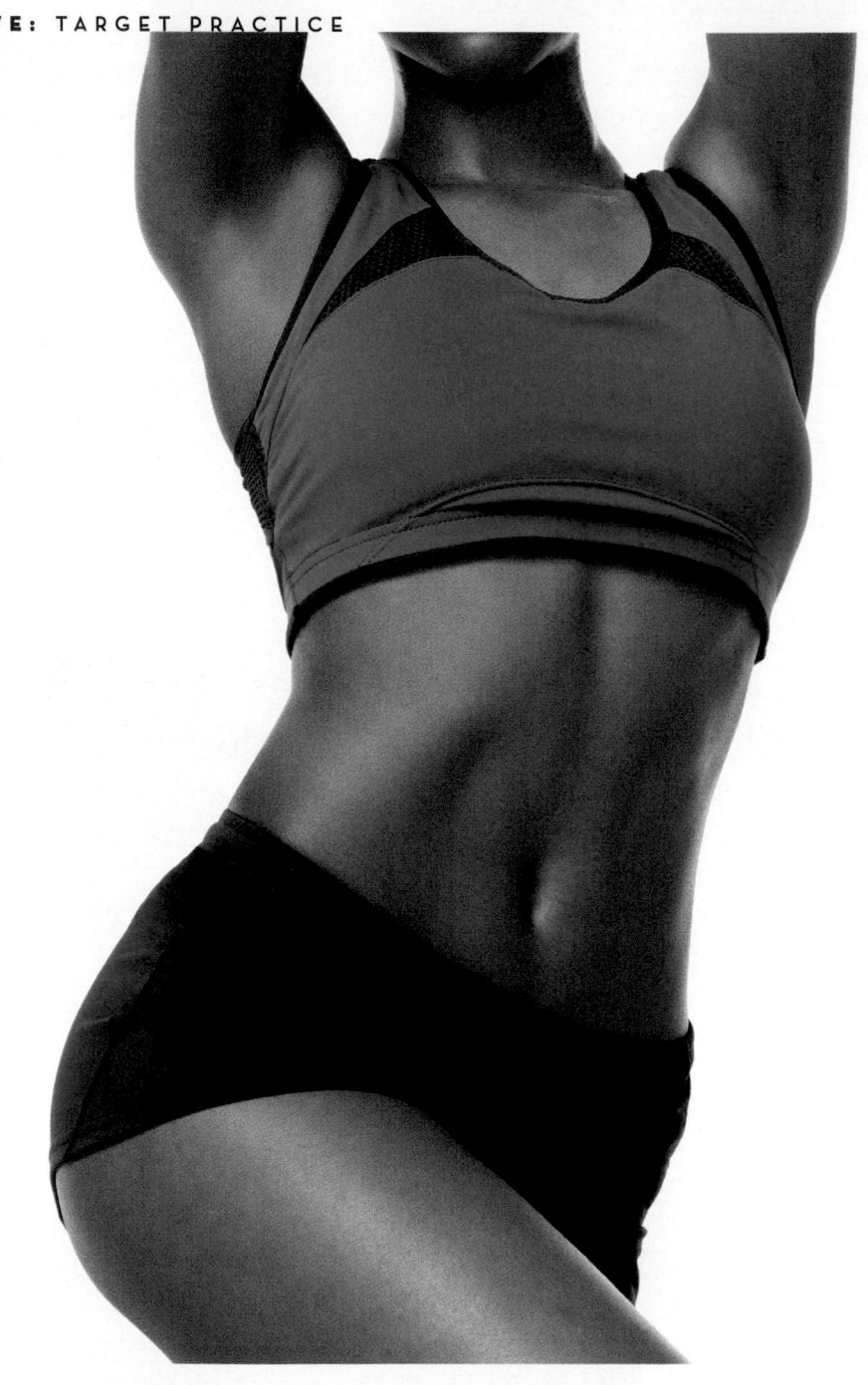

CHAPTER TWENTY-NINE

GUIDE TO
TO YOUR
B-SIDE

FOR A SCORCHING REAR VIEW, TARGET THE MUSCLES THAT SURROUND YOUR BUM.

BY MIKE MEJIA, C.S.C.S.

YOU WANT YOUR BUTT TO HAVE MORE perk than a sorority pledge on a latte bender, but no matter how many glute moves you do, your junk still jiggles. The key to a beauteous gluteus is a workout that targets your back, calves, and hamstrings. When this supporting cast is strong, your butt looks better and can work harder. Stick with our program and you'll start seeing results after just 10 workouts—at which point, invest in one of those dressing room–style mirrors. Admiring your own ass 24/7 can be a pain in the neck.

SUPPORT YOUR ASSETS

THE PLAN

Spend 2 to 4 weeks building the supporting muscles in your back, calves, glutes, and hams to stay injury free in Phase 2 (see page 299)— and get more bang for your butt.

Perform three sets of 12 to 15 reps, resting up to 60 seconds between sets, two or three nonconsecutive days a week.

WALKING SUPINE BRIDGE

WORKS GLUTES AND HAMSTRINGS

Lie on your back with your knees bent and feet flat on the floor. Lift your hips until your body forms a straight line from your knees to your shoulders (A). Slowly extend your left leg until it's in line with the rest of your body (B). Pause, then lower it and repeat with your right. That's 1 rep. Don't drop your hips until you've completed all reps.

Butt-kicker Press through your heels to maximize the involvement of your glutes and hamstrings.

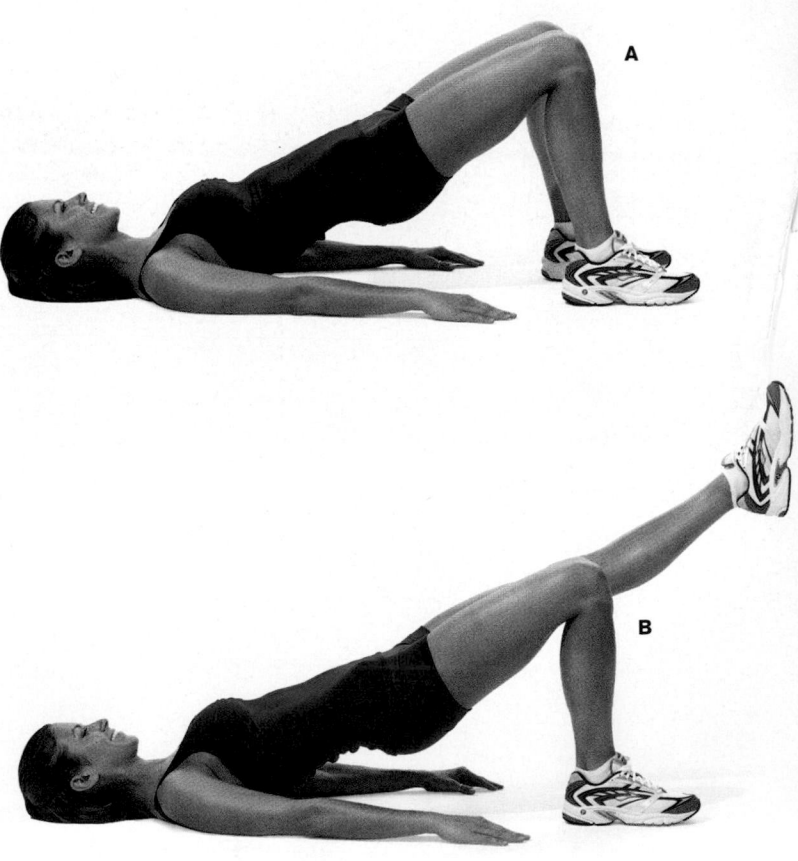

REVERSE HYPER-EXTENSION

WORKS ERECTOR SPINAE, GLUTEUS
MAXIMUS, AND HAMSTRINGS

Lie facedown on an exercise bench so your head,
chest, torso, and hips are on the bench but your legs
are mostly hanging off. Wrap your arms around the
bench and brace your abs (A). Lower your legs as far
as possible, then, keeping your legs straight and
together, lift them until they're just past parallel to the
floor (B). Pause, then lower and repeat.

Butt-kicker Place the entire bench on a step or
other stable platform to increase your range of
motion.

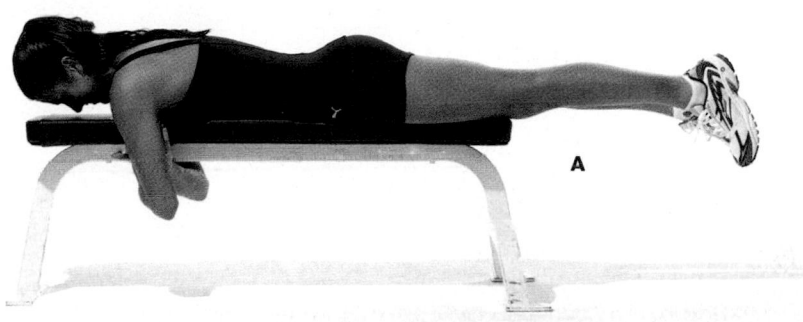

A

W|H

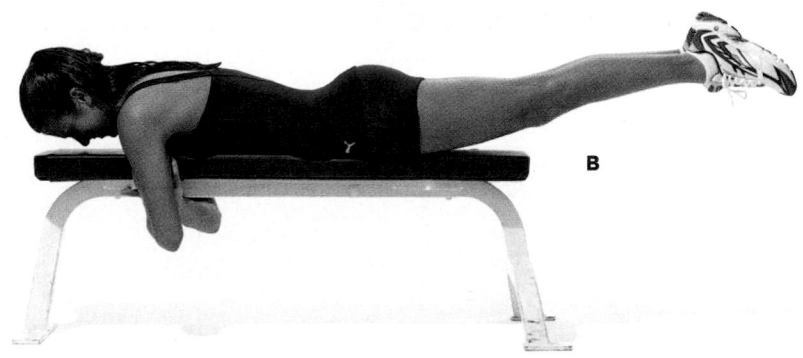

B

REVERSE WOODCHOP

WORKS CALVES, GLUTES (GLUTEUS MAXIMUS, MEDIUS, AND MINIMUS), AND HAMSTRINGS

Grab a 4- to 8-pound medicine ball and stand with your feet shoulder-width apart. Hold the ball with both hands outside your left hip, then perform a half squat (so legs lower 45 degrees) (A). Keeping your chest up and arms straight, press your feet into the floor and stand up as you "chop" the ball up and across your body until it's above your right shoulder (B). Pause, then lower the ball back to your left knee. Complete all reps before repeating on the other side. That's 1 set.

Butt-kicker Rather than using your arms, brace your core and push up with your legs as you drive the ball upward.

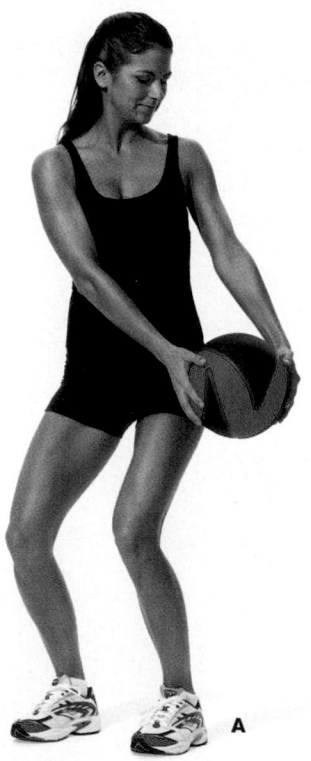

A

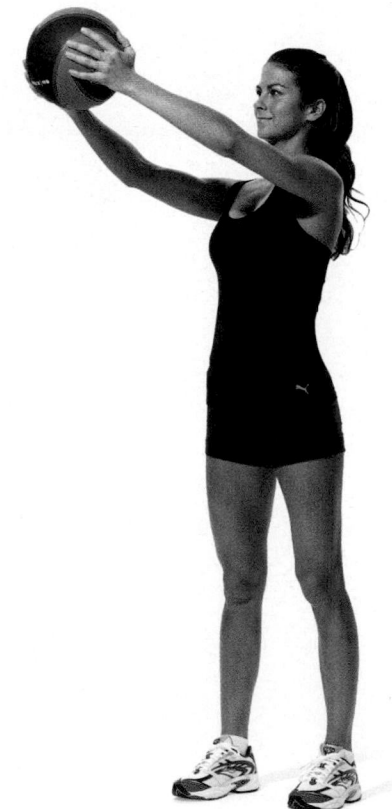

B

HYDRANT EXTENSION

WORKS GLUTES

Get on all fours with your knees directly beneath your hips and your hands under your shoulders. Keeping your knee bent, lift your left leg up and out to the side as high as possible (A). Next, extend your leg straight back so it's in line with your torso (B). Pause, then bring it back to start. Repeat with your right leg. That's 1 rep.

Butt-kicker Keep your lower back as still as possible throughout the exercise.

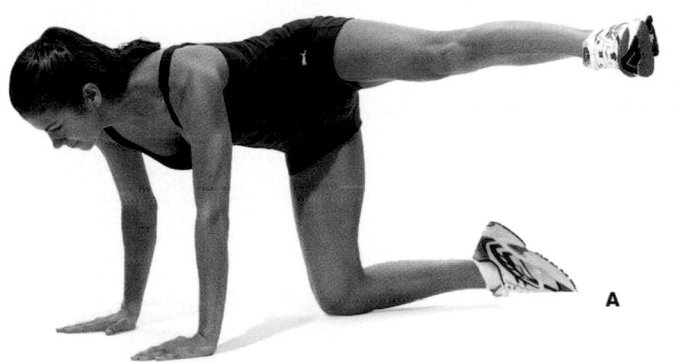

A

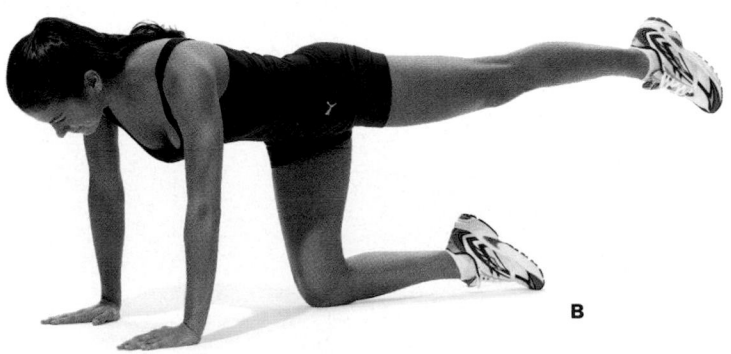

B

BIG MOMENTS IN BUTT HISTORY
2007 IS THE YEAR OF YOUR REAR

1346 The first recorded mooning: To mock King Edward III of England and his troops, Normandy soldiers drop trou—and take a few arrows in the ass.

1930 The invention of the Whoopee Cushion ushers in the age of flatulence humor.

1939 The thong debuts at the World's Fair. Sisqó (of "Thong Song" fame) won't be born for about another 40 years.

1969 On July 24, J.Lo's bum is born.

1987 Buns of Steel hits shelves to the delight of spandex-clad women with teased bangs everywhere.

1991 Prince flashes a pair of yellow ass-less chaps at the MTV Music Awards.

1992 Sir Mix-a-Lot releases "Baby Got Back."

2001 *South Park* airs an episode featuring a family with Torsonic Polarity Syndrome ("butts where their faces should be").

2006 A Maryland court rules that mooning counts as a legal form of expression backed by the First Amendment.

2008 May 2 will be No-Pants Day.

PHASE 2:
SCULPT A SUPERIOR POSTERIOR

THE PLAN

Phase 1 has prepped you to work more muscle safely so you can fry more fat and shape your butt as quickly as possible. For the next 4 weeks, 3 nonconsecutive days a week, alternate between Workout 1 and Workout 2 (you'll do one of the workouts twice each week). Do 3 sets of 10 to 12 reps of each exercise, resting up to 60 seconds between sets.

WORKOUT 1

1¼ BARBELL SQUAT
WORKS ERECTOR SPINAE, GLUTEUS MAXIMUS, HAMSTRINGS, AND QUADS

Place a barbell across your upper back and stand with your feet hip-width apart (A). Lower your hips until your thighs are parallel to the floor. Push back up a quarter of the way (B), then pause before going back down to parallel. Pause again, then return to start. That's 1 rep.

Butt-kicker Do this move first. It's a killer: If you wait until the end of your workout, you'll be too burnt.

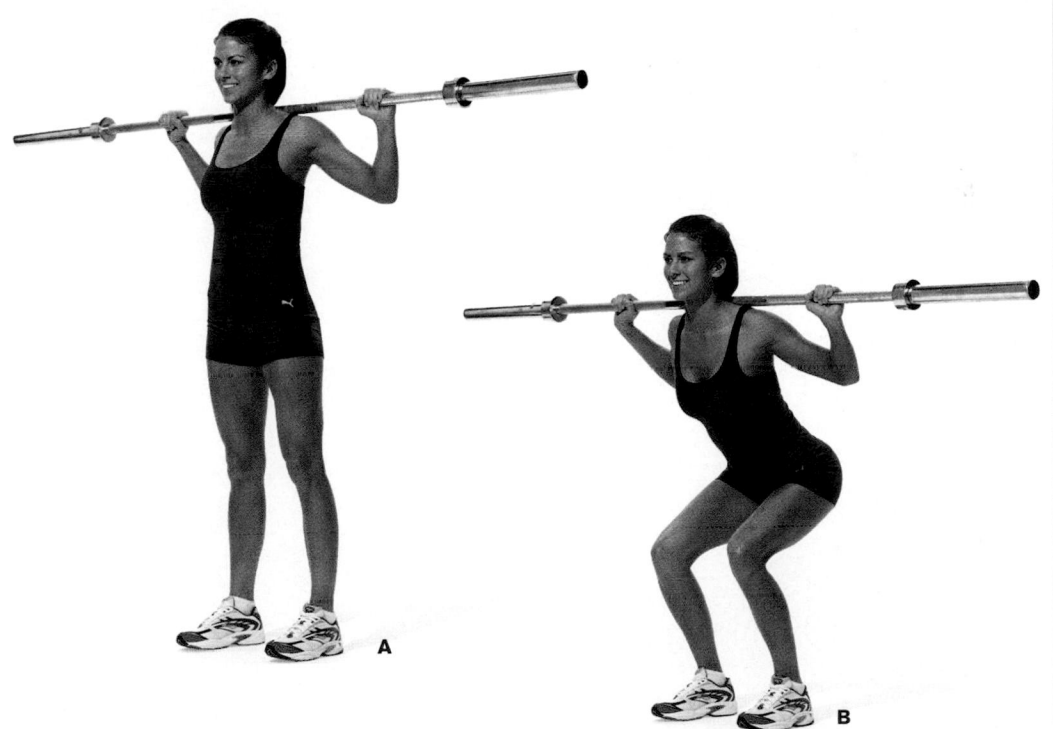

A

B

W|H

LUNGING STEPUP

WORKS GLUTEUS MAXIMUS,
HAMSTRINGS, AND QUADS

Grab a pair of 5- to 10-pound dumbbells and stand 2
to 3 feet from an exercise bench. Place your right foot
on the bench (**A**). Drive your right heel down and pull
your left leg up (**B**). Allow only your left toes to touch
the bench. Lower your left leg first and then your right.
Repeat, lunging up with your left leg. That's 1 rep.
Butt-kicker If you feel off balance, use 5-pounders
until you nail the form.

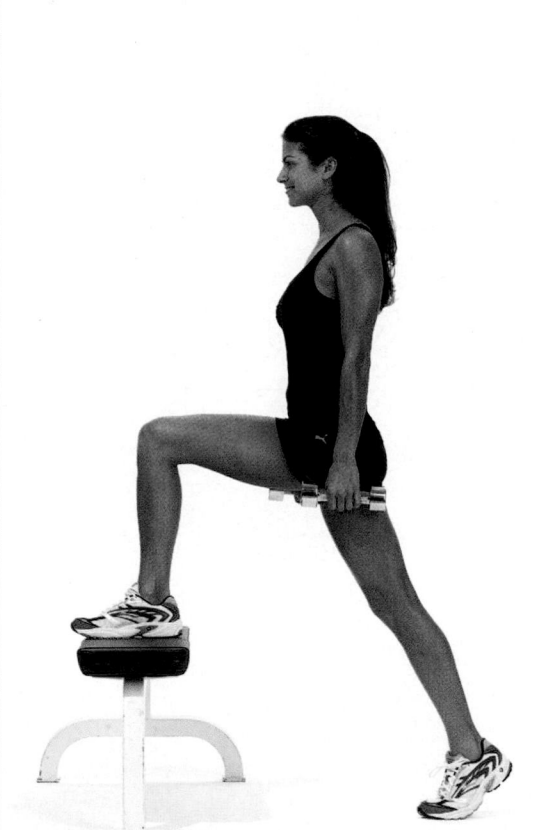

A

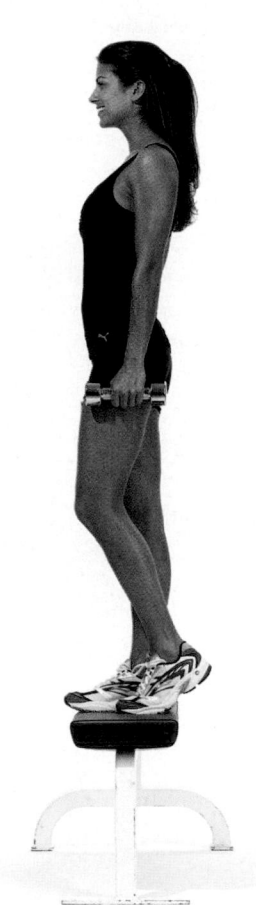

B

MODIFIED
GLUTE-HAM RAISE
WORKS CALVES, ERECTOR SPINAE, GLUTEUS MAXIMUS, AND HAMSTRINGS

Wrap a towel around the middle of a loaded barbell and place a mat under it. Kneel with your back to the bar and your ankles anchored beneath it (A). Slowly lower your torso (B). Use your arms to catch yourself when your legs give out (C). Return to start by pushing up with your arms and raising your torso until you're kneeling again.

Butt-kicker Finish the move with your hands beneath your shoulders, as if you're at the bottom of a pushup.

TOTAL FITNESS GUIDE 2008

W|H

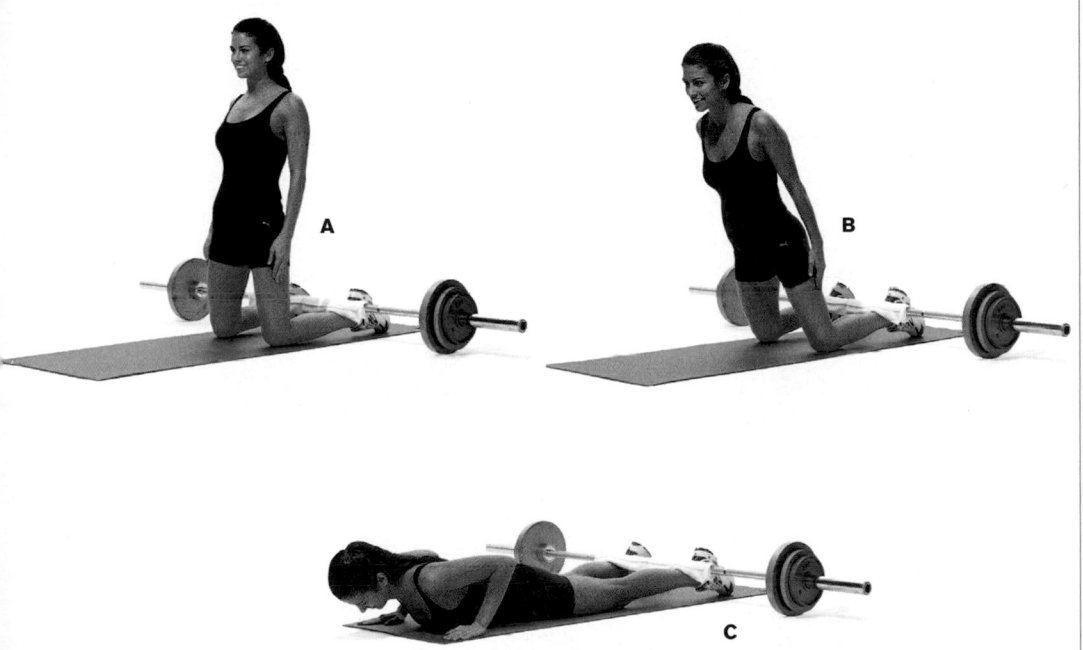

WORKOUT 2

ROMANIAN DEADLIFT
WORKS ERECTOR SPINAE, GLUTEUS
MAXIMUS, AND HAMSTRINGS

Grab a barbell with an overhand grip (add weight
plates once you can do all sets of all reps with perfect
form), hands shoulder-width apart, and stand with
your feet hip-width apart and knees slightly bent. Hold
the barbell with straight arms in front of your thighs
(**A**). Without rounding your back or changing the
bend in your knees, lean forward from your waist
while lowering the bar until your torso is parallel to the
floor (**B**). Pause, then rise to start.

Butt-kicker To work the glutes and hamstrings as
hard as possible, push your heels into the floor as you
stand.

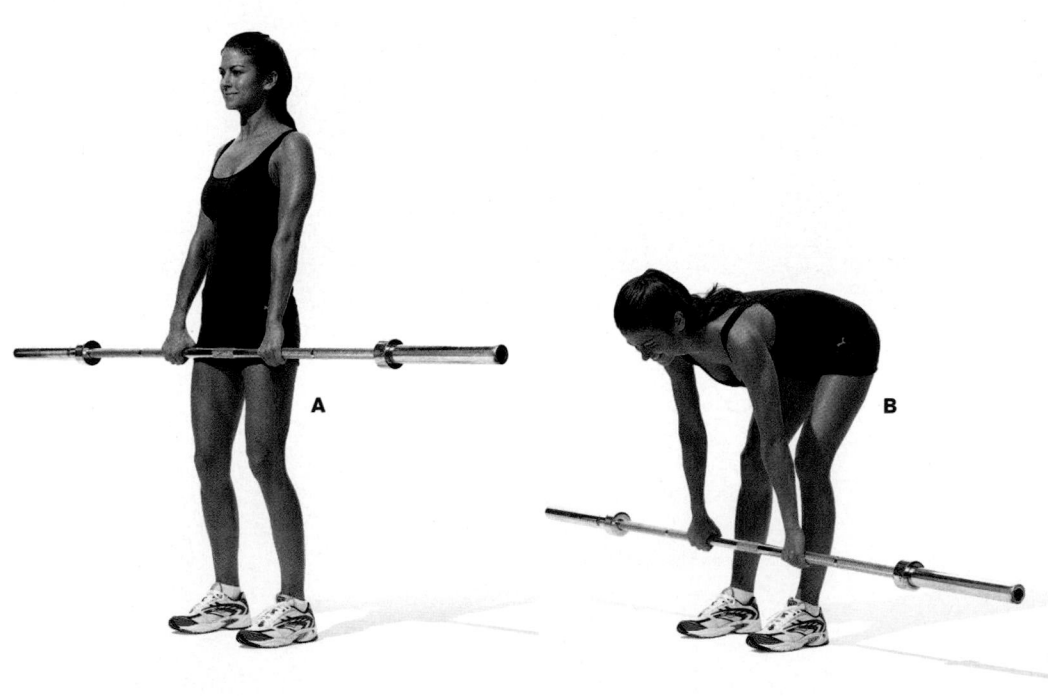

CABLE PULL-THROUGH

WORKS GLUTES, HAMSTRINGS,
AND QUADS

Stand about 2 feet from a pulley station set at a very
light weight (increase only once you've nailed the
form), with the cable on the setting closest to the
floor. With your back to the station, position your feet
shoulder-width apart, then bend from your hips as you
squat until your thighs are nearly parallel to the floor.
Reach back through your legs and grab the handle
(A). Keeping your head up, drive your heels into the
floor and straighten your legs (B) to standing. Pause,
then lower the weight and repeat.

Butt-kicker For a secure grip, use the rope or the
handle attachment (shown).

TOTAL FITNESS GUIDE 2008

W | H

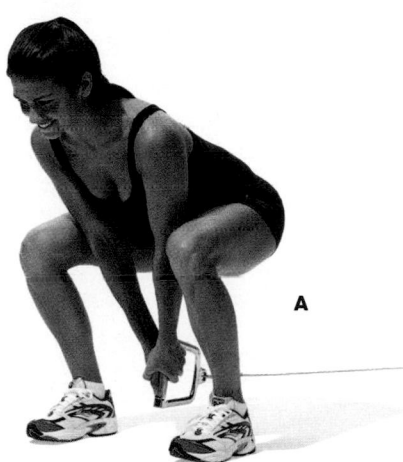

A

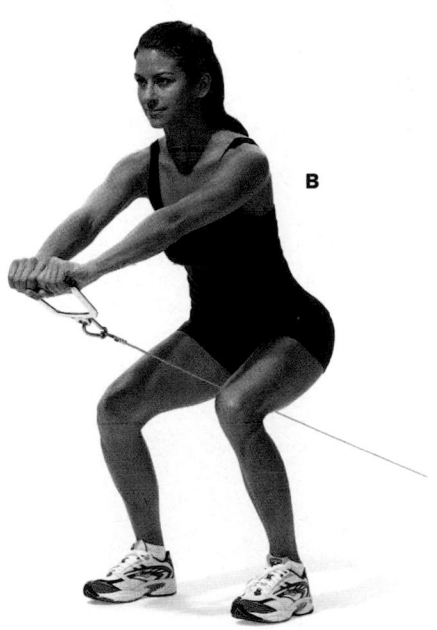

B

OFFSET SQUAT

WORKS GLUTES AND HAMSTRINGS

Grab a 5- to 8-pound dumbbell in your right hand, hold it at your right side, and lift your right foot so you're balancing on your left. Raise your right arm straight out in front of you until it's at shoulder level (A) and squat down until your thigh is as close to parallel to the floor as possible (B). Pause for a second and then push back up to start.

Butt-kicker Keep the dumbbell as far from your body as you can throughout the squat to work your glutes harder.

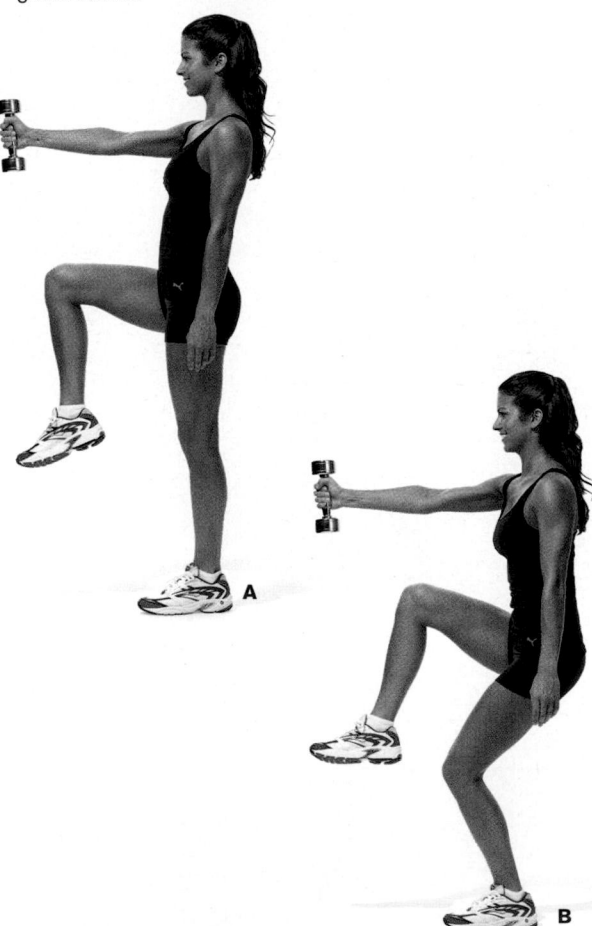

Your 4 weeks are up. Now what?

Create a butt-burning circuit. Do 10 to 12 reps of each exercise without resting in between. Once you've completed all six, rest for 60 seconds, then repeat.

RATE YOUR BUM

USE THIS FANNY FORMULA TO DETERMINE YOUR DERRIERE'S OVERALL APPEAL

BY YELENA MOROZ

From the "marginally scientific but totally entertaining" files: Last year, David Holmes, Ph.D., a leading psychologist in the U.K., devised this mathematical formula for defining the "perfect female ass." Dig out your calculator, kids, here it is.

Rear Rating =
[(S+C) x (B+F)/T]-V

S: Overall shape: Rate 1 to 5
1= Deflated beach ball;
5 = Volleyball

C: Cheek circularity: Rate 1 to 4
1 = Croissant; 4 = Grapefruit

B: Bounciness: Rate 1 to 5
1 = Jiggles like Jell-O;
5 = Rebounds like a rubber band

F: Firmness: Rate 1 to 4
 1 = Marshmallow;
4 = Bounce a quarter off it

T: Texture: Rate 4 to 1*
4 = Crater Island;
1 = Bambino-smooth

V: Vertical ratio: Rate 4 to 1*
4 = Upside-down heart;
1 = Right-side-up heart

*For T and V, 1 is best.

If you scored 80, or close to it, your buttocks are virtually perfect (à la Kylie Minogue, whose tush Holmes's focus groups deemed a perfect 80). If you scored below 40, get your butt in gear and re-test yourself after doing our workout for a month.

Booty Boosters

Three backside looks that make the most of your curves

IF YOU'RE SHOPPING FOR JEANS...
Look for snaps, flaps, and low-slung pockets because pockets that start below the midpoint of your bum are flattering whether you've got a bubble or a board, and buttons on the pockets draw the eye to the rear view we like to flaunt most.
Get it Paige Premium Denim Fairfax jeans, $189, paigepremiumdenim.com

IF YOU'RE SHOPPING FOR UNDIES...
Look for Stretchy hipster styles with a strong seam down the center because

Lycra and spandex blends lift and hold as seams separate, making uni-butt a nonissue.
Get it Warner's The End lace hipster, $9, bare necessities .com; Spanx Slim Cognito seamless midthigh bodysuit, $68, spanx.com

IF YOU'RE SHOPPING FOR A SKIRT...
Look for ruching, lacing, and bows near the waist, as well as a seam down the entire back of the skirt because upper-butt details pinpoint where your back ends and your rear begins, and the seam defines your sexy S shape. Add a 3-inch heel to force an arch in the back that naturally perks up your butt. Disclaimer: To protect your back, reserve the vixen heels for special occasions.
Get it Nanette Lepore lace-up skirt, $255, nanette lepore.com; Daryl K contoured short skirt, $260, shop bop.com; Cole Haan Carma Air peep-toe pumps, $275, colehaan.com

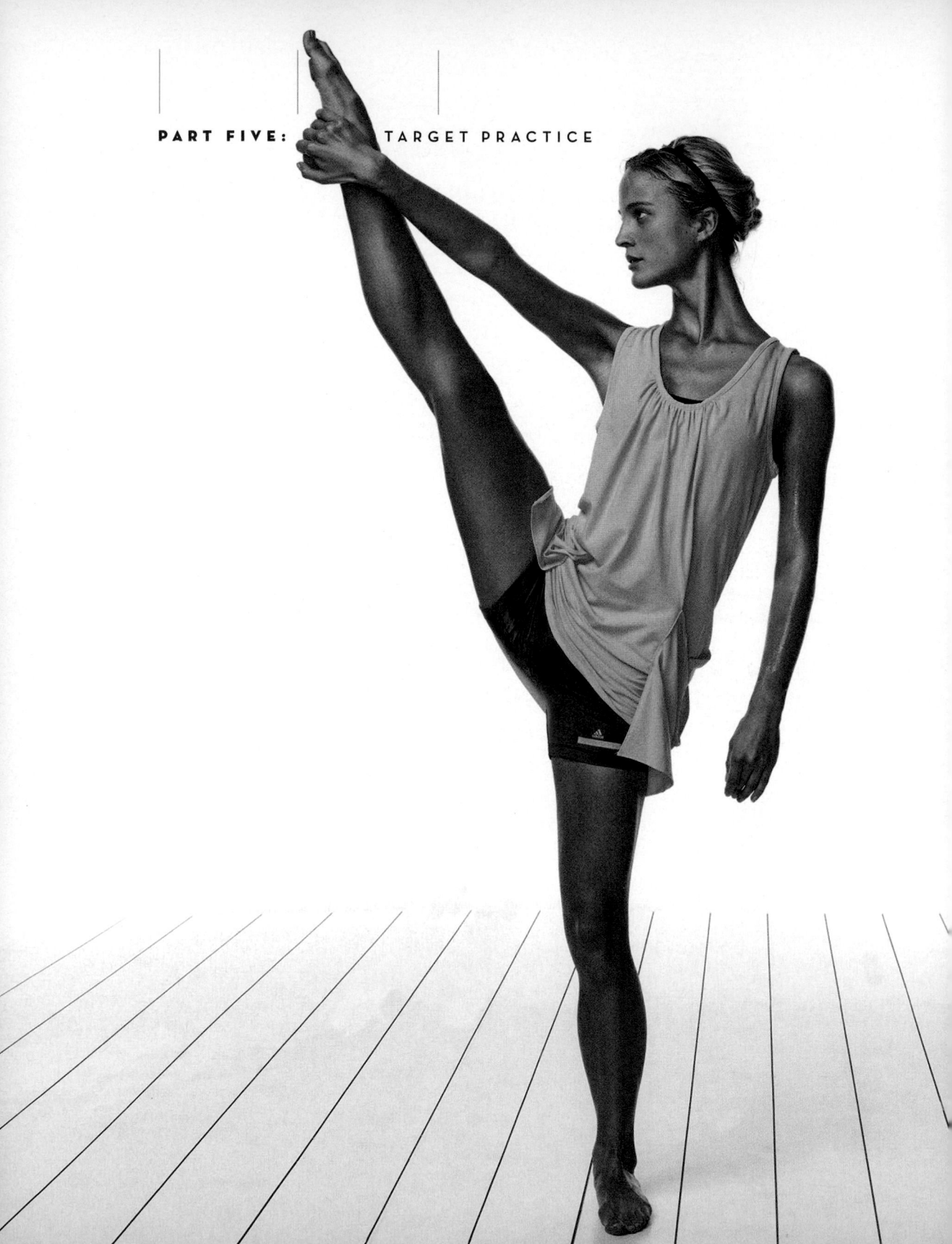

PART FIVE: TARGET PRACTICE

CHAPTER THIRTY

THE SECRET TO LEAN LEGS

THREE LEVELS OF MOVES THAT WILL SCULPT AND SHAPE YOUR LOWER BODY.

YOUR LEGS DO MORE than just get you up stairs and away from sharp-shooting paparazzi. They're also your body's main fat burners. Because the muscles in your legs are the biggest in your body, they're very effective in burning up calories (muscle burns calories because it takes a lot of energy to sustain that muscle). So adding a little muscle in your legs will not only help to tone them, it will also help you burn more fat all over. Here are some of the best leg-shapers there are—with three levels of variations, so you can keep challenging them as you get stronger and leaner.

LEVEL 1 MOVES

SQUAT

Starting position: Stand with your feet about shoulder-width apart, arms at your sides.

Movement: Keeping your back straight, lower yourself, bending from your knees and hips as though you're sitting down, as you inhale. Let your arms come out in front of you to help you balance. Stop just before your thighs are parallel to the floor. Hold for a second and then exhale as you slowly stand back up.

Technique: Don't let your knees move forward over your toes. Don't round your back.

BACK LUNGE (NO WEIGHTS)

Starting position: Stand with your feet together and place your hands on your hips.

Movement: Step your left foot back 2 to 3 feet. Inhale as you bend your right knee and lower your body straight down until your right knee is bent 90 degrees and your left knee nearly touches the floor. Your rear heel will come off the floor. Hold for a second and then exhale as you push yourself back up, bringing your left foot in. Finish all of your repetitions, then repeat the exercise stepping your right foot back.

Technique: Don't lean forward. Don't let your front knee move forward over your toes.

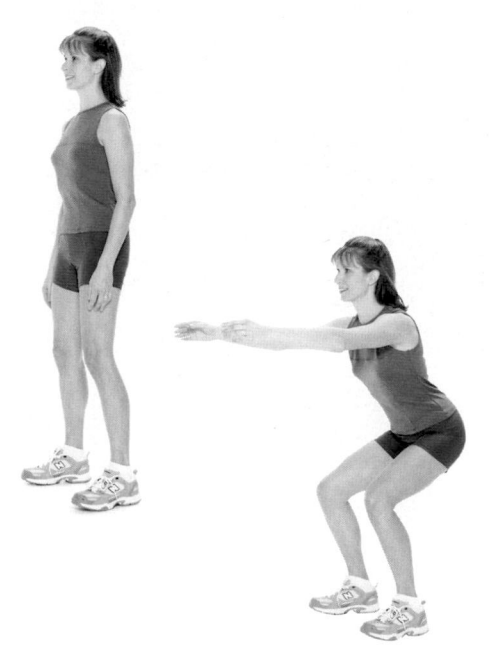

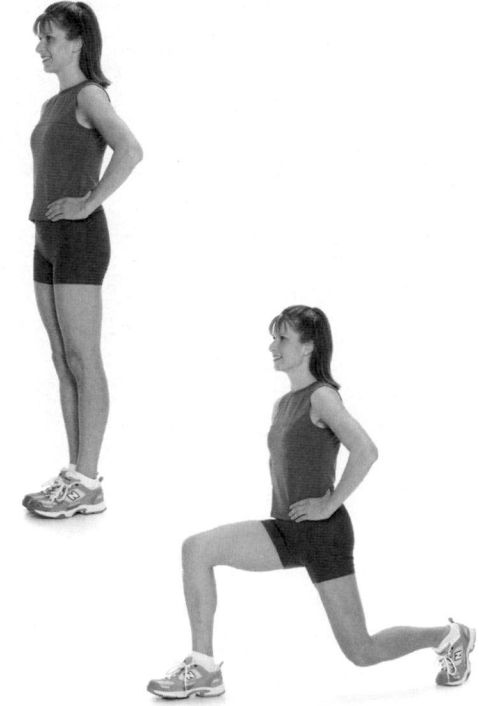

STEP SQUAT

Starting position: Stand with your feet together and your hands down at your sides.

Movement: Step your left foot out to the side 2 to 2½ feet. Keeping your back straight, lower yourself, bending from the knees and hips as though you're sitting down, as you inhale. Let your arms come out in front of you to help you balance. Stop just before your thighs are parallel to the floor. Hold for a second and then exhale as you push back up, bringing your left foot back in. Do five or six reps with your left foot and then do five or six reps stepping with your right foot.

Technique: Don't let your knees move forward over your toes. Don't round your back.

HEEL RAISE

Starting position: Stand with your feet together. Lightly hold on to a chair or wall with one hand if needed for balance.

Movement: Exhale as you slowly lift your heels off the floor, rolling up onto your toes. Hold for a second and then inhale as you slowly lower them.

Technique: Don't bend at the waist or lean forward, back, or to the side. Don't bend your legs.

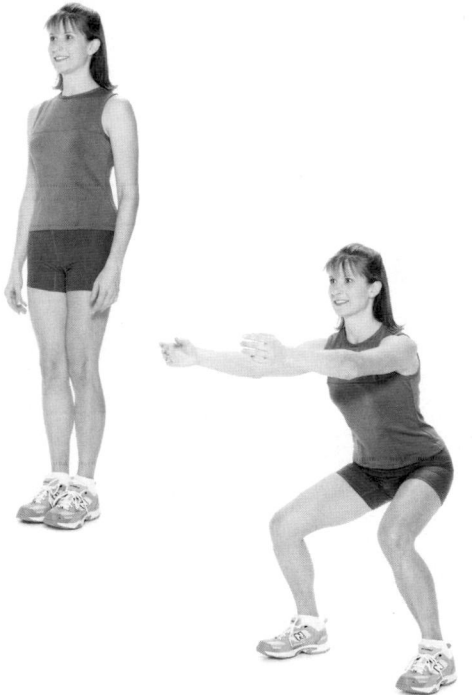

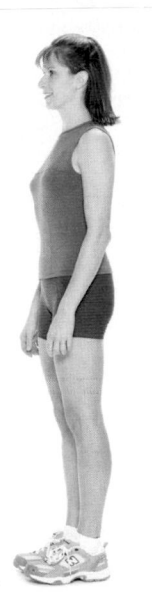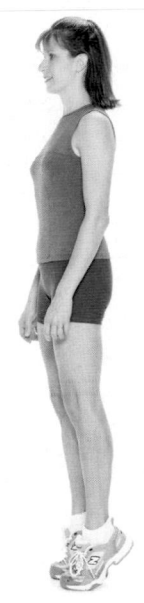

LEVEL 2 MOVES

PLIÉ SQUAT

Starting position: Stand with your feet wider than shoulder-width apart, toes pointing out. Hold a dumbbell with both hands down in front of you.

Movement: Keeping your back straight, lower yourself, bending from your knees, as you inhale. Stop just before your thighs are parallel to the floor. Hold for a second and then exhale as you slowly stand back up.

Technique: Don't let your knees move forward over your toes. Don't lean forward.

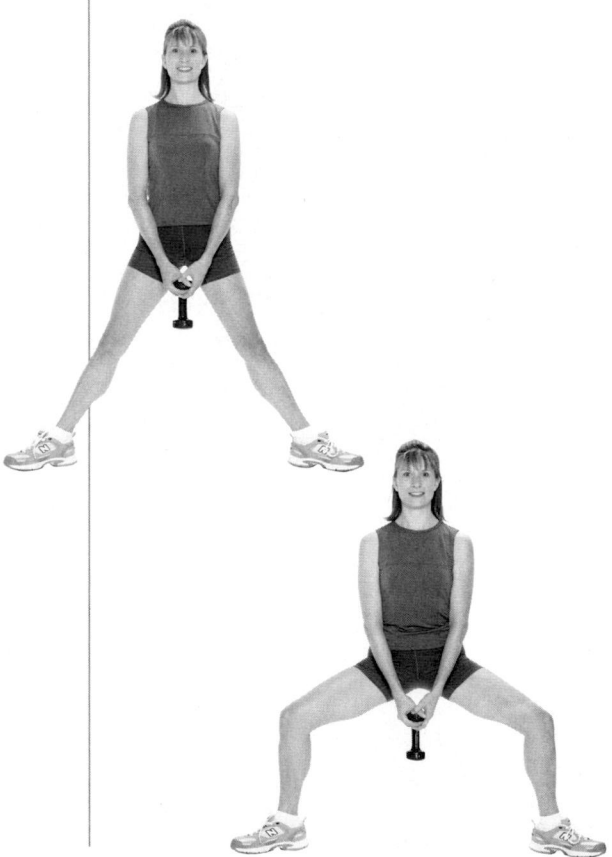

BACK LUNGE WITH KNEE LIFT

Starting position: Stand with your feet together. Hold a dumbbell in each hand, either at shoulder height or at your sides.

Movement: Step your left foot back 2 to 3 feet. Inhale as you bend your right knee and lower your body straight down until your right knee is bent 90 degrees and your left knee nearly touches the floor. Your rear heel will come off the floor. Hold for a second and then exhale as you push yourself back up. Lift your left knee up in front of you before bringing it back to the starting position. Finish all repetitions, then repeat stepping back with your right foot.

Technique: Don't lean forward. Don't let your front knee move forward over your toes.

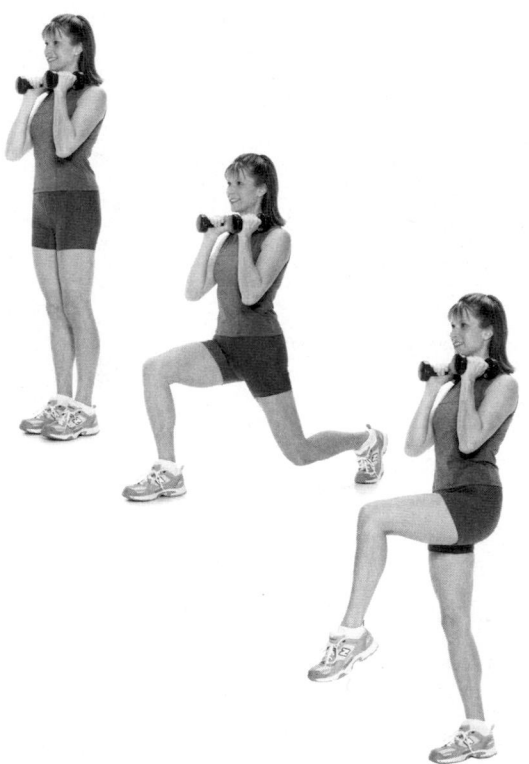

STEP SQUAT WITH KNEE LIFT

Starting position: Stand with your feet together. Hold a dumbbell in each hand, either at shoulder height or at your sides.

Movement: Step your left foot out to the side 2 to 2½ feet. Keeping your back straight, lower yourself, bending from the knees and hips as though you're sitting down, as you inhale. Stop just before your thighs are parallel to the floor. Hold for a second and then exhale as you push back up, lifting your right knee out in front of you before returning to the starting position. Do five or six reps with your right foot and then do five or six reps stepping with your left foot.

Technique: Don't let your knees move forward over your toes. Don't round your back.

SINGLE-HEEL RAISE

Starting position: Stand on one foot with the other resting on your calf. Lightly hold on to a chair or wall with one hand if needed for balance.

Movement: Exhale as you slowly lift your heel off the floor, rolling up onto your toes. Hold for a second and then inhale as you slowly lower it. Do the recommended number of reps and then switch feet.

Technique: Don't bend at the waist or lean forward, back, or to the side. Don't bend your supporting leg.

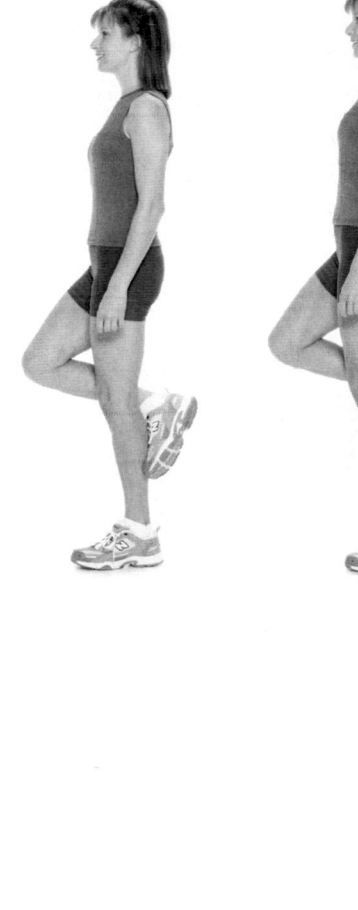

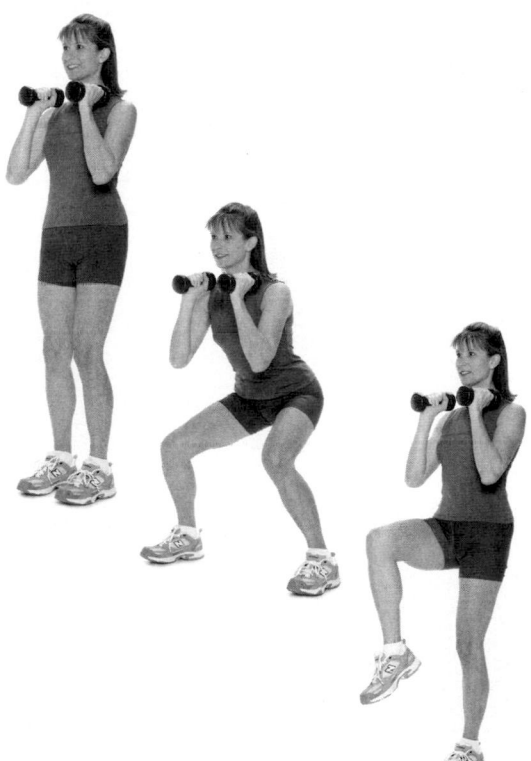

LEVEL 3 MOVES

ONE-LEG SQUAT

Starting position: Hold dumbbells in each hand at shoulder height or down at your sides. Shift your weight to your right foot and lift your left foot off the floor so that only your toes are lightly touching for balance.

Movement: As you inhale, bend your right knee and lean forward slightly from your hips, lowering yourself as if you were sitting in a chair. Go as low as is comfortable, but don't go past your right thigh being parallel to the floor. Hold for a second and then exhale as you slowly stand back up. Do the recommended number of reps and then switch legs.

Technique: Don't let your working knee come forward past your toes.

FRONT LUNGE WITH JUMP

Starting position: Stand with your feet together and your hands on your hips.

Movement: Step your right foot forward 2 to 3 feet. Inhale as you bend your right knee and lower your body straight down until your right knee is bent 90 degrees and your left knee nearly touches the floor. Your rear heel will come off the floor. Hold for a second and then exhale as you push off with your right foot and jump your feet together. Finish all of your repetitions, then repeat the exercise stepping forward with your left foot.

Technique: Don't lean forward. Don't let your front knee move forward over your toes.

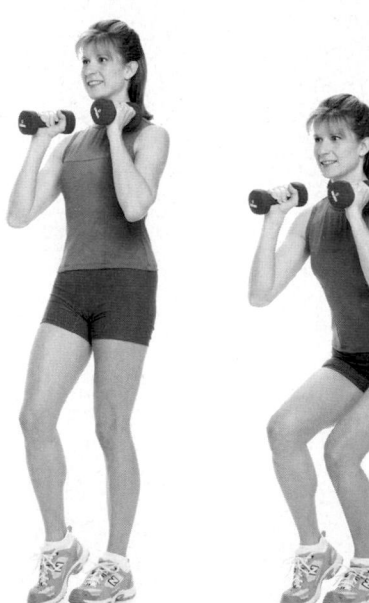

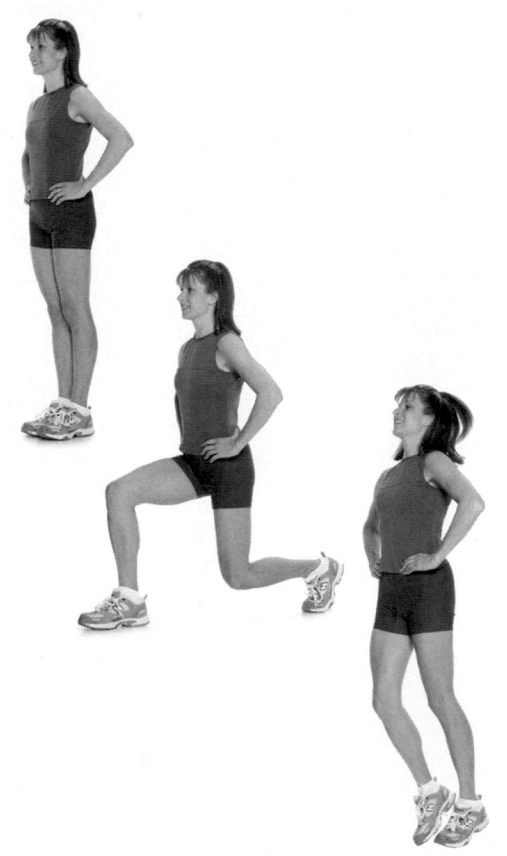

STEP SQUAT WITH JUMP

Starting position: Stand with your feet together and your hands down at your sides.

Movement: Step your left foot out to the side 2 to 2½ feet. Keeping your back straight, lowering yourself, bending from the knees and hips as though you're sitting down, as you inhale. Let your arms come out in front of you to help you balance. Stop just before your thighs are parallel to the floor. Hold for a second and then exhale as you jump and bring your left foot back in next to your right foot. Do five or six reps with your left foot and then do five or six reps stepping with your right foot.

Technique: Don't let your knees move forward over your toes. Don't round your back. Don't do this move while holding weights.

HEEL RAISE ON STEP

Starting position: Stand on the edge of a step so that your heels are hanging off. Lightly hold on to the railing, a chair, or a wall with one hand for balance.

Movement: Exhale as you slowly rise up onto your toes. Hold for a second, then inhale as you slowly lower, allowing your heels to drop below the edge of the step.

Technique: Don't bend at the waist or lean forward, back, or to the side.

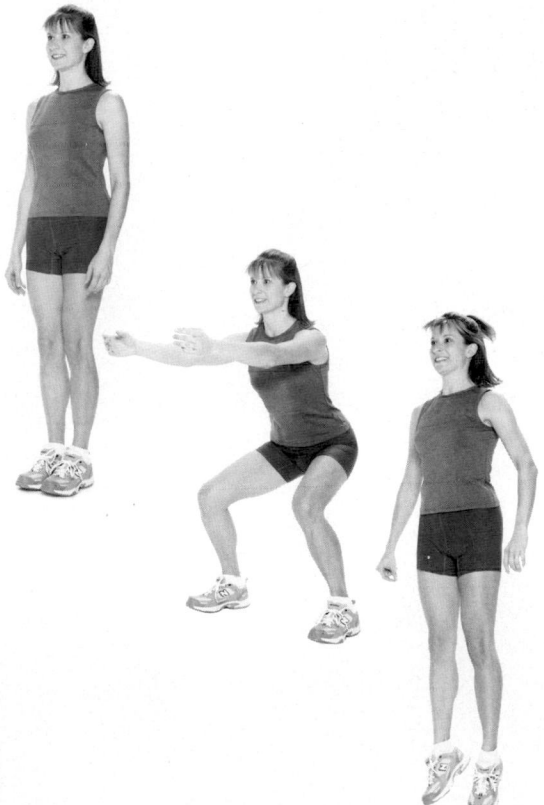
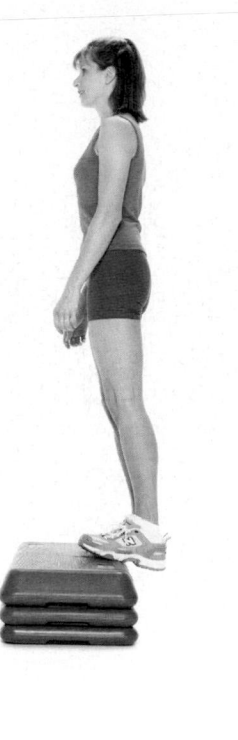
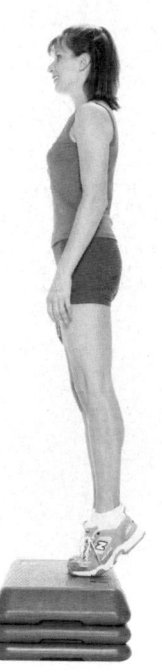

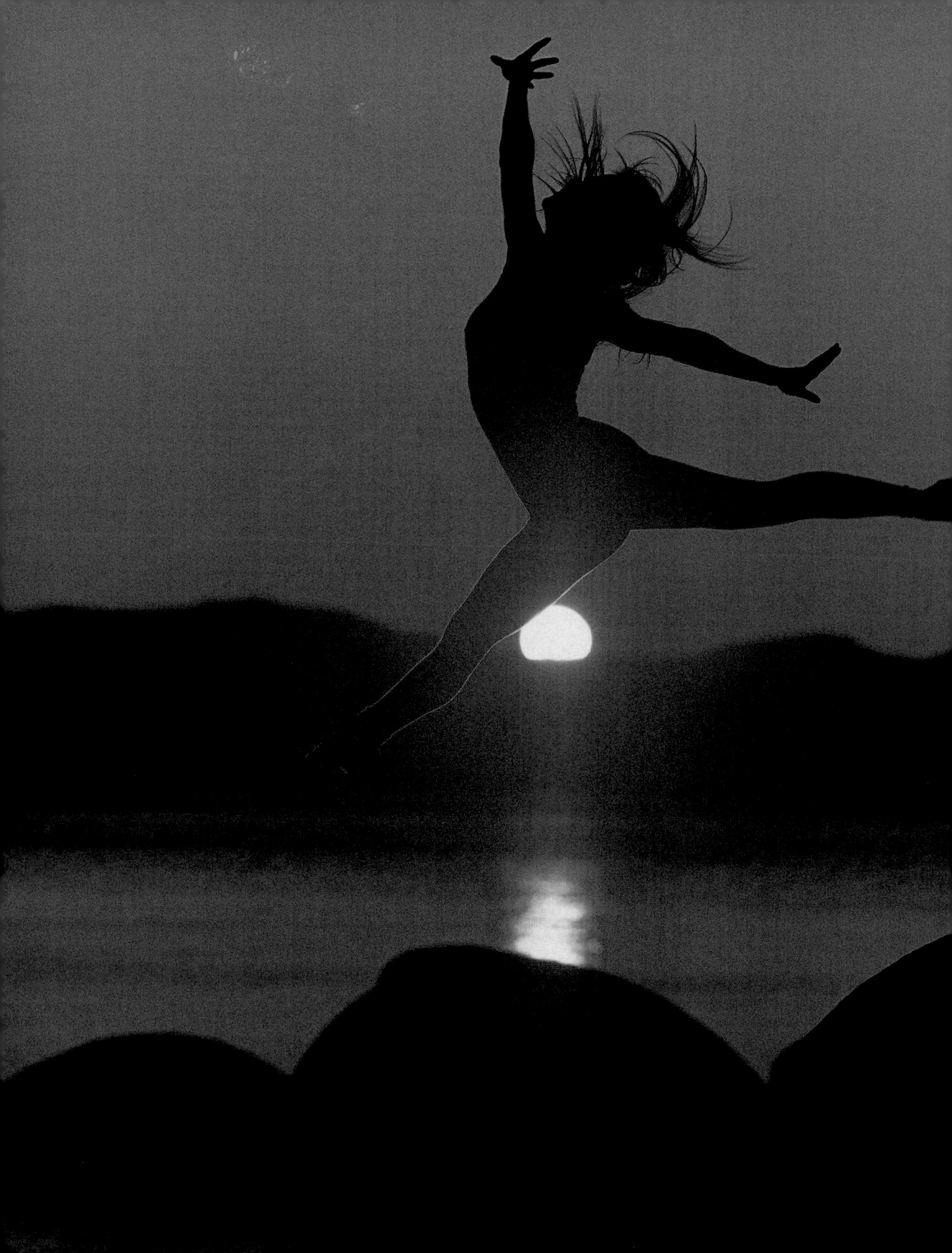

■ PART SIX

do everything right

You're on your way to a slammin' body. Now it's time to up your game a few notches by avoiding common pitfalls and perfecting your workout. Use these fitness finesses and fix-its for long-lasting success.

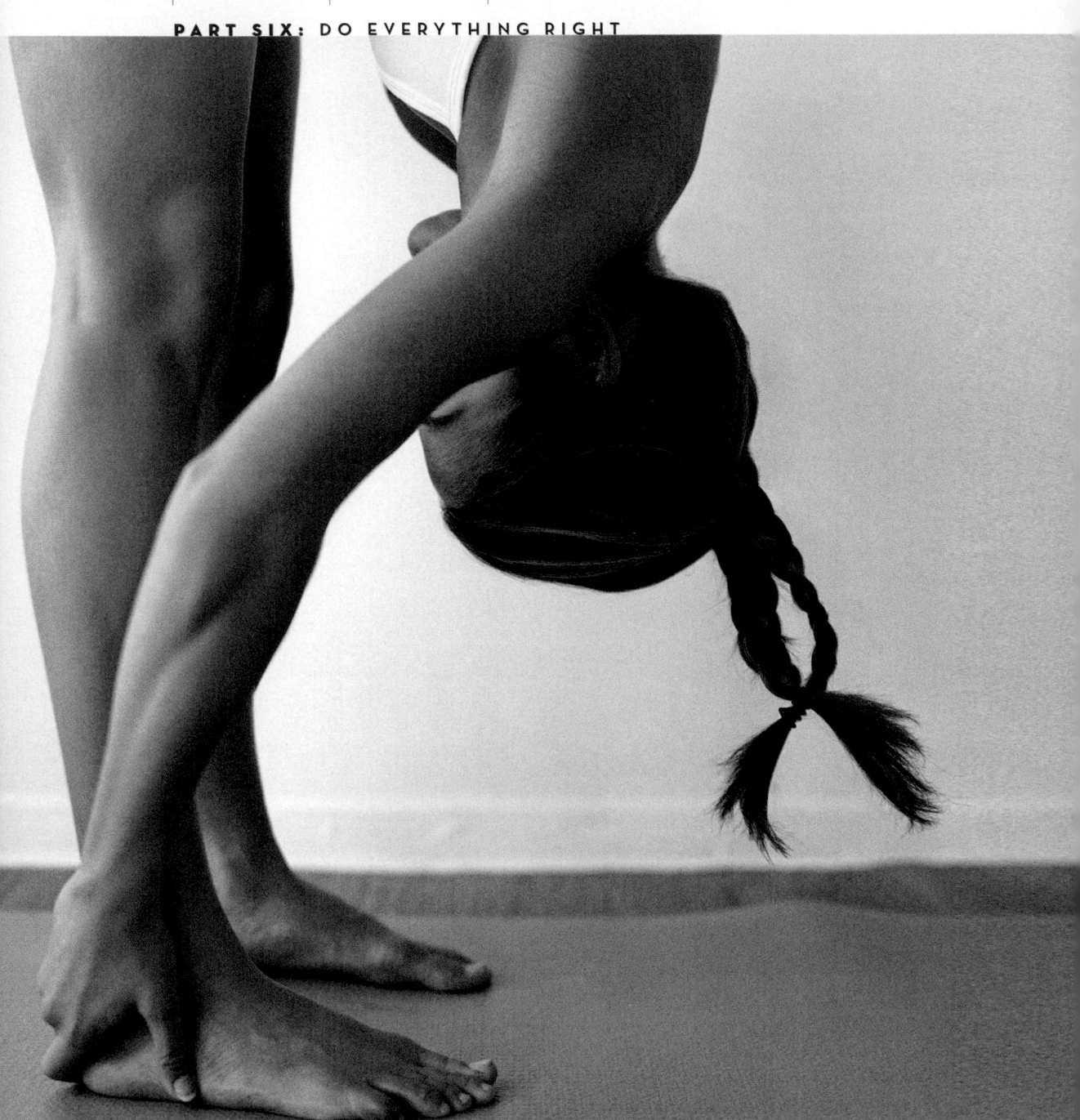

CHAPTER THIRTY-ONE

NO PROPS?
NO PROB

THE CHEAPEST, MOST CONVENIENT WORKOUT ON THE PLANET WILL GET YOU JAW-DROPPING RESULTS.

BY MIKE MEJIA, C.S.C.S.

TOTAL FITNESS GUIDE 2008

W|H

YOUR EQUIPMENT LIST FOR THIS WORKOUT: (1) 10 square feet of floor space, (2) you.

No stretchy bands, balls, or dumbbells (even a mat is optional). No state-of-the-art machinery to wait in line for at the gym. What's the point? Aside from leaving you with extra cash for Labor Day sales, this routine can be done anywhere, anytime, and in just 15 minutes. Most important, it can lead to superior results. While machines and props isolate and strengthen individual muscles, they don't build overall functional strength. "Hoisting your own body weight distributes the exercise load over multiple muscle systems, providing strength and tone without bulk," says Juan Carlos Santana, C.S.C.S., CEO, of the Institute of Human Performance in Boca Raton, Florida.

This total-body workout, unrestricted by fancy equipment, is designed to do just that. Aim for 2 or 3 sets of 8 to 12 reps of each exercise, resting 30 to 60 seconds between moves. Do the routine 2 or 3 nonconsecutive days a week—and after 4 weeks, change the "you" on your list to "your scorching body."

SIDE BRIDGE WITH ABDUCTION
WORKS CORE AND GLUTEUS MEDIUS

Lie on your left side with your elbow directly beneath your shoulder and legs stacked. Brace your abs and lift your hips off the floor until you're balancing on your forearm and feet and your body forms a diagonal line (A). Lift your right leg at least 6 inches (B). Lower and repeat. Complete all reps, then repeat on your right side. That's 1 set.

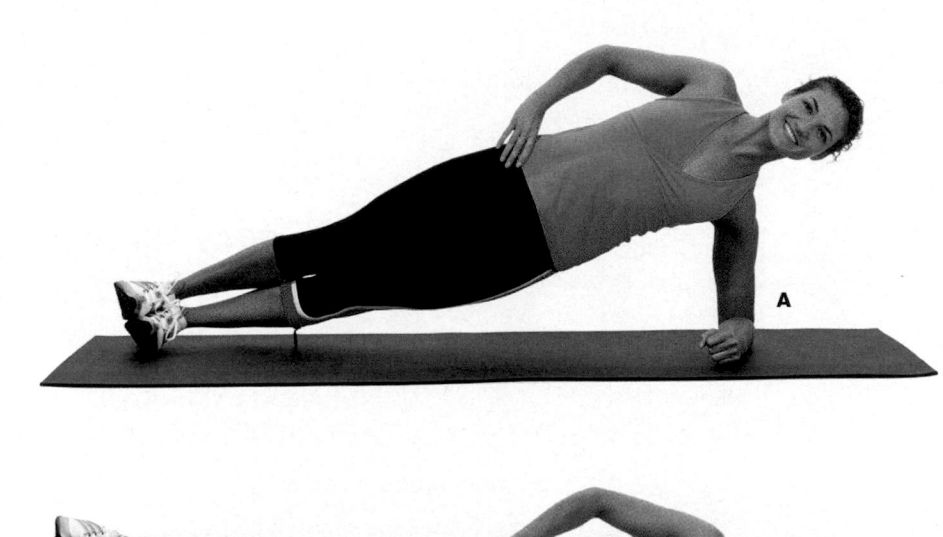

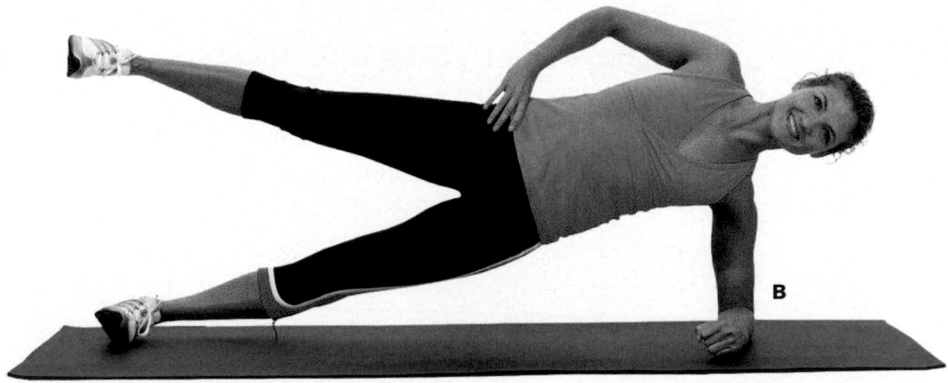

WRAPAROUND ANKLE TOUCH

WORKS CORE, GLUTES, HAMSTRINGS, AND QUADS

Stand with your legs together and bend your right knee 90 degrees so you're balancing on your left leg (**A**). As you squat, reach your right arm across your body and try to touch the outside of your left foot with your fingertips (**B**). Keep your back as straight as possible while reaching. Press back up to start. Complete all reps, then repeat on your right leg. That's 1 set.

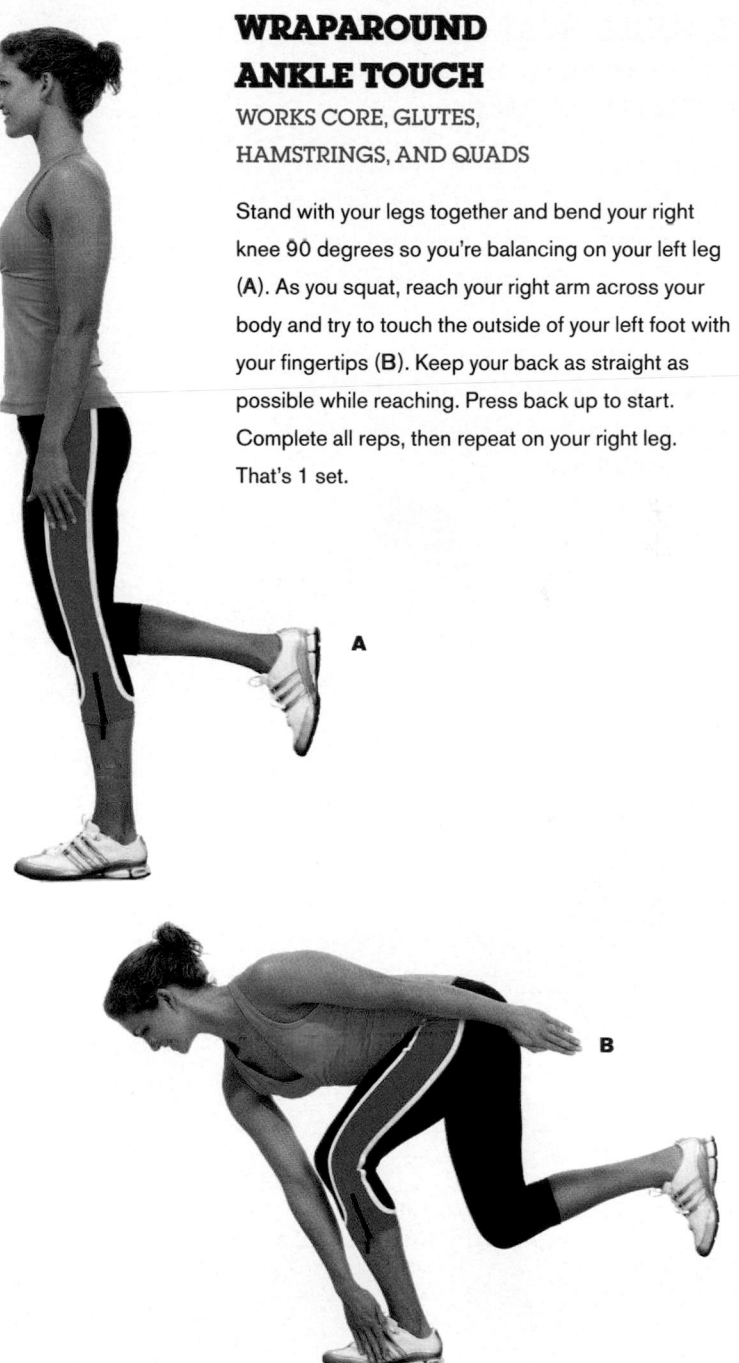

A

B

W|H

DOUBLE-STOP PUSHUP

Assume a pushup position with your hands slightly
wider than your shoulders and your back straight (**A**).
Keeping your neck in line with your spine, lower
yourself halfway and hold for 1 second (**B**). Continue
lowering until your chest is only a couple of inches
from the floor (**C**). Pause, then push back up to the
halfway point and pause again before finally pressing
back up to start. Too hard? Do the move with your
knees on the floor.

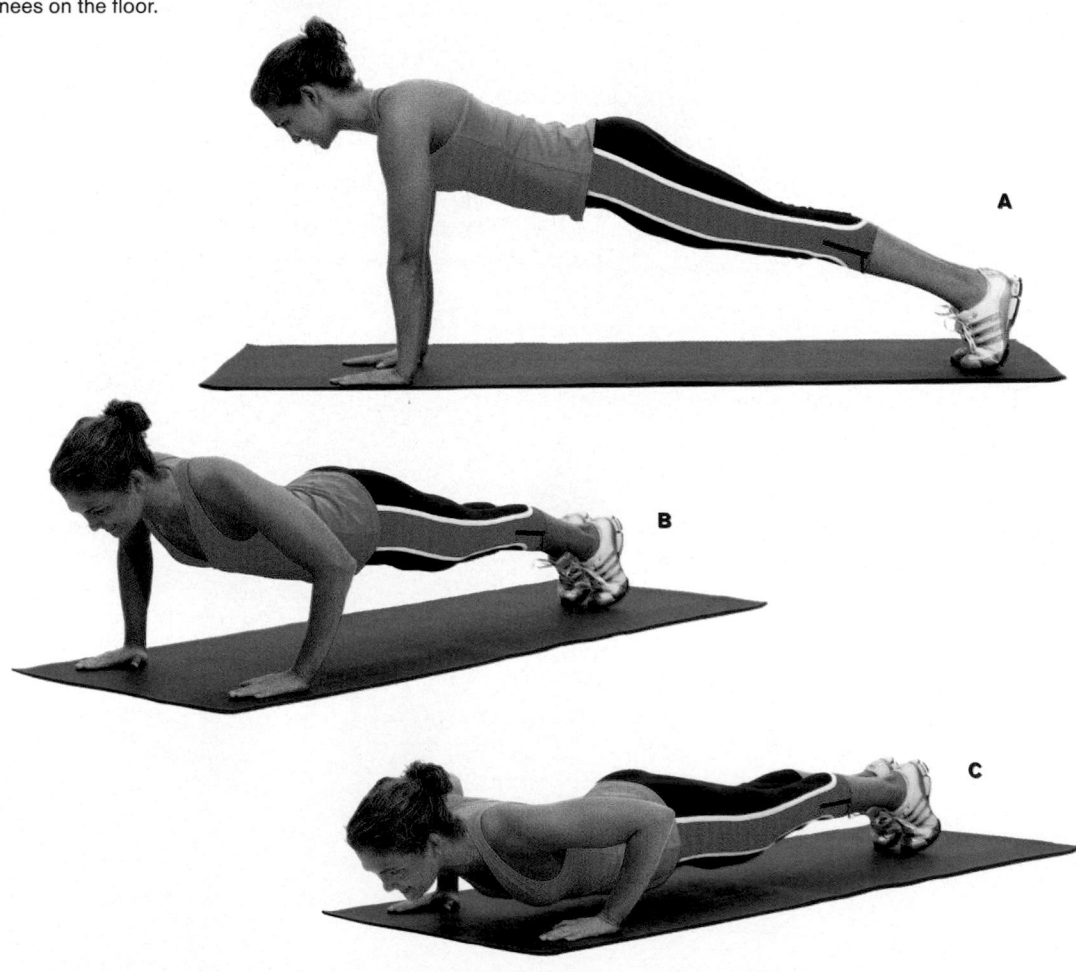

PUSHUP POSITION BIRD DOG

WORKS CORE, GLUTES, AND
LOWER AND UPPER BACK

Assume a pushup position with
your hands slightly wider than
your shoulders and your back
straight (**A**). Brace your abs as
you extend your right arm and
left leg (**B**). Lower them both—
but not your torso—and repeat,
lifting your left arm and right leg.
Continue alternating until you've
completed 8 to 12 reps on each
side. That's 1 set.

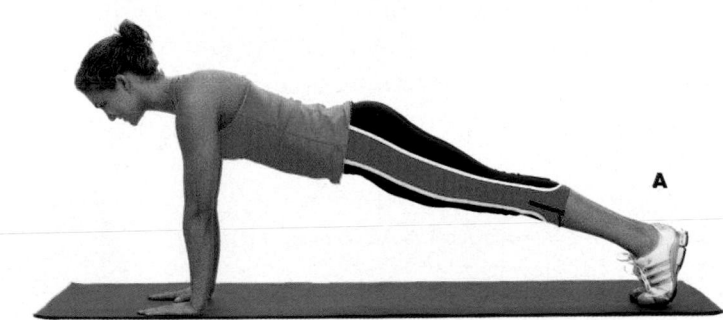

A

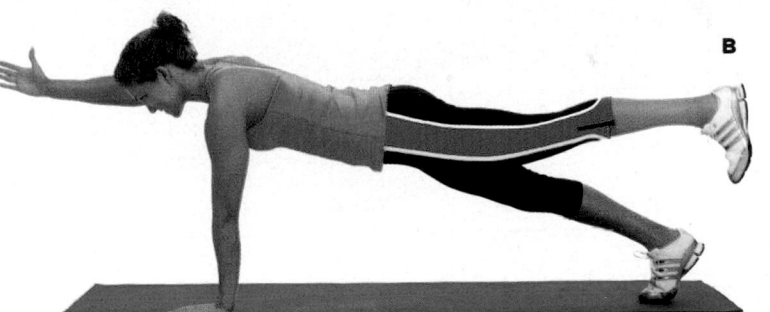

B

W|H

ROCK YOUR BODY
HOW TO AMP UP THE CHALLENGE WITHOUT ADDING PROPS (OR GOING ON AN ALL-PIZZA DIET)

S-L-O-W down Tapping the brakes forces your muscles to contract longer, so they work harder. Try taking 3 seconds to do the lowering and lifting portions of each rep.

Hold the line When you get to the most difficult part of the move (say, when your legs are hovering above the floor in the windshield wiper on page 322), stop completely for 1 second.

Go blind Close your eyes throughout the movement. Seriously, it's really tough. This forces your brain and muscles to work harder to communicate with each other, since usually your eyes are a main source of sensory feedback. The upshot: increased coordination.

WINDSHIELD WIPER
WORKS CORE

Lie on your back with your legs together and arms extended at shoulder level, palms flat on the floor. Bend your knees and lift your legs until your thighs are above your hips (**A**). Press your palms into the floor and lower your legs to the left. Go as far as possible while keeping your right shoulder glued to the floor (**B**), then bring your legs back to center. Next, lower them to the right. Alternate until you've completed 8 to 12 reps on each side.

SUPINE ROW

WORKS MIDDLE AND UPPER BACK

Lie on your back with your knees bent, feet flat on the floor, and arms at your sides with elbows bent 90 degrees (**A**). Pinch your shoulder blades together as you dig your elbows into the mat and lift your head and torso a few inches off the floor (**B**). Lower and repeat.

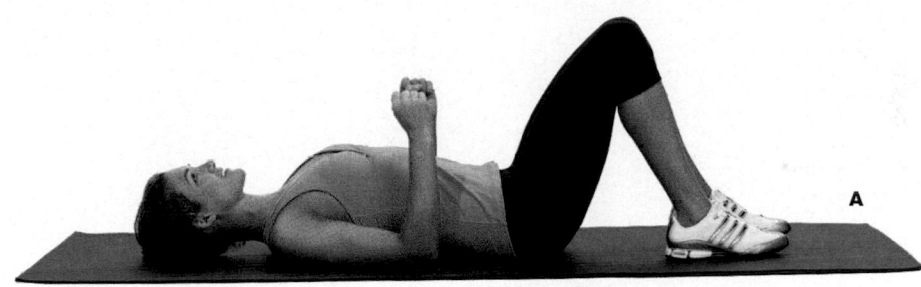

A

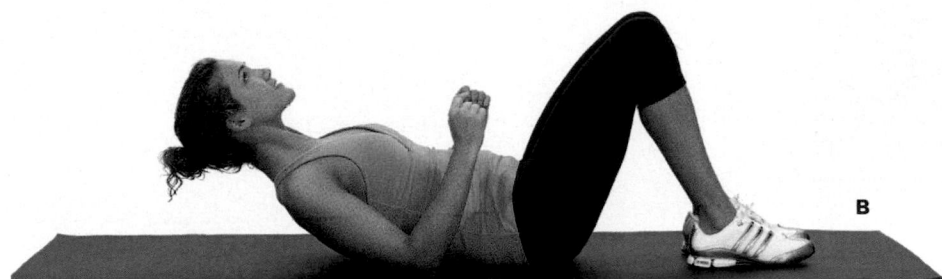

B

TOTAL FITNESS GUIDE 2008

W|H

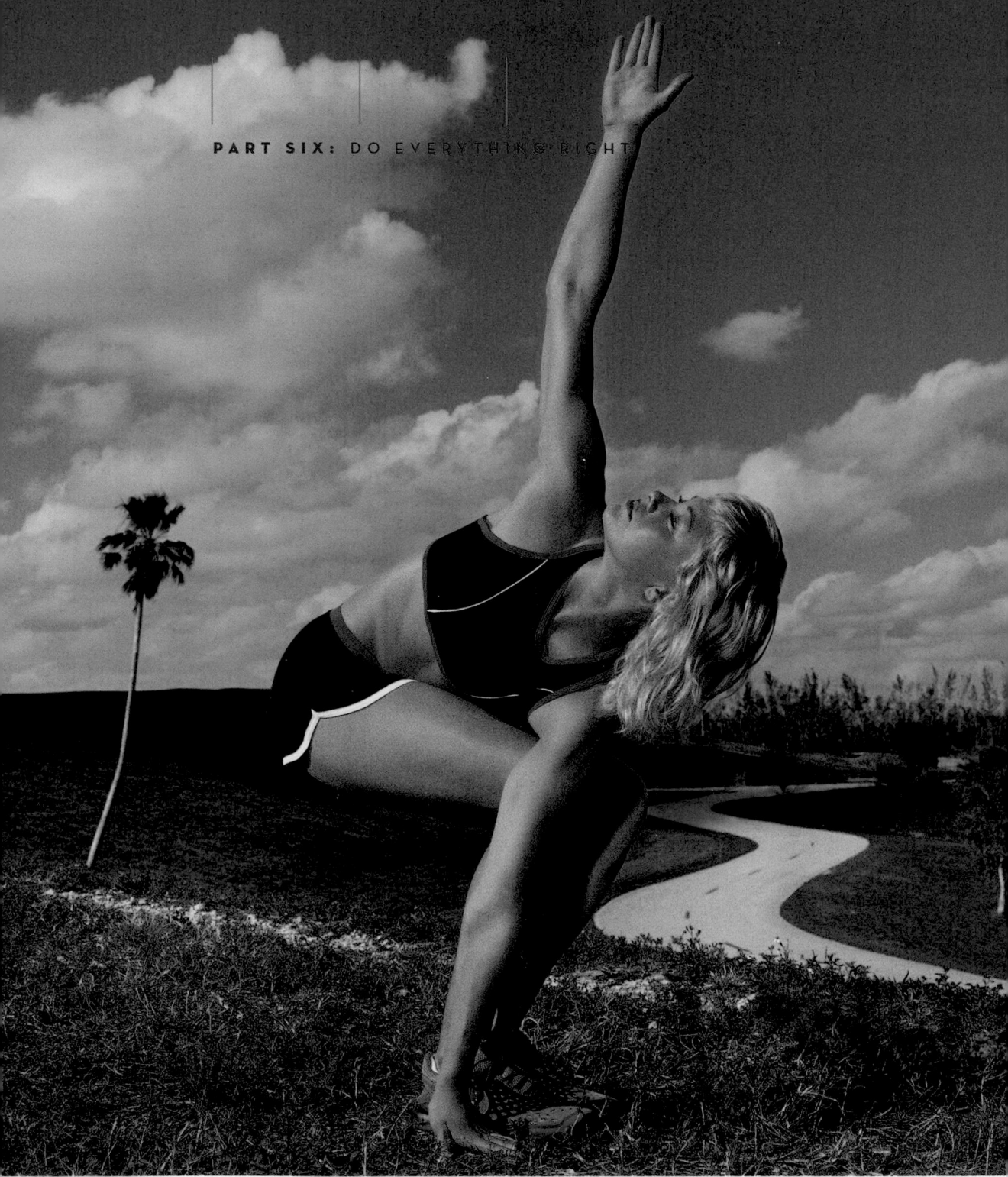

CHAPTER THIRTY-TWO

STRETCH YOURSELF

USE YOGA TO BULLETPROOF YOUR BODY– AND GO LONGER AND STRONGER THAN EVER.

BY PAIGE GREENFIELD

IF YOU'RE IN A ONE-ON-ONE LOVE AFFAIR with your sport, do yourself a favor: Get out, play the field—and start fooling around with yoga. Sure, running, biking, hiking, swimming, and weight lifting are far superior to yoga when it comes to calorie busting. But you're constantly using the same muscles, leaving some exhausted and others neglected entirely. The result: overworked muscles that feel the way you do after a bad day at the office (tight and ready to pop) and underworked ones in a three-martini-lunch stupor.

Yoga, on the other hand, stretches and strengthens every muscle group. You don't have to trade in your running shoes for a 100-degree Bikram room—but you'll see tremendous results if you supplement your workout with just 15 minutes of yoga during your warmup or cooldown. After all, yoga doesn't just correct imbalances; all that stretching and breathing also boosts oxygen flow to your muscles, letting you run longer, pedal faster, and play harder. These 15 moves will maximize your performance—and keep you out of the orthopedist's office.

Swimming

Swimming is great for keeping your joints well oiled, but mat work can take you beyond your perceived limits of joint motion and power, according to Corinne Friesen, a certified yoga instructor and the author of *Hurry Up–Relax!* Experts estimate that regular yoga sessions (at least four a week) can also increase your oxygen intake by 200 to 300 percent. That means less fatigue and cramping because extra oxygen brings more power to every stroke. Do each pose three times–alternating spider, butterfly, then bow–before swimming. The first round is a warmup, the second finds your limit, and by the third you'll be able to stretch beyond that limit.

SPIDER

STRENGTHENS ABS AND UPPER BODY; STRETCHES HAMSTRINGS, HIPS, INNER THIGHS, AND LOWER BACK

Lie on your back with arms by your sides. Bring your right knee up toward your chest. Keeping your right arm on the inside of your leg, reach out and grab your toes (**A**). With every exhale, tug your foot toward your shoulder. After a few breaths, straighten your knee (**B**). Lift your chest toward your knee and hold for three to five breaths. Lower your leg to the floor. Repeat on the opposite side.

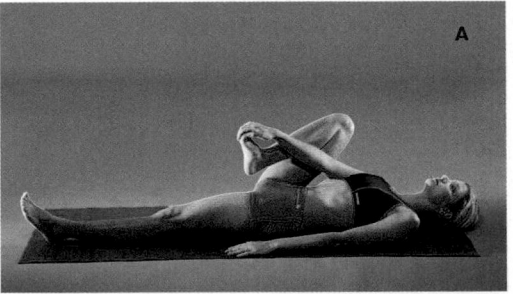

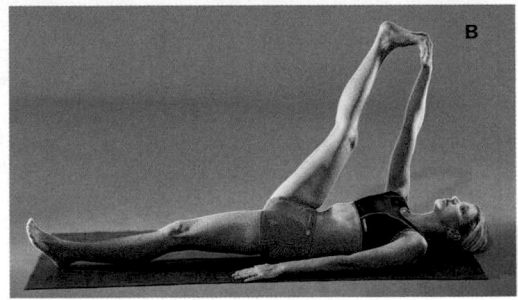

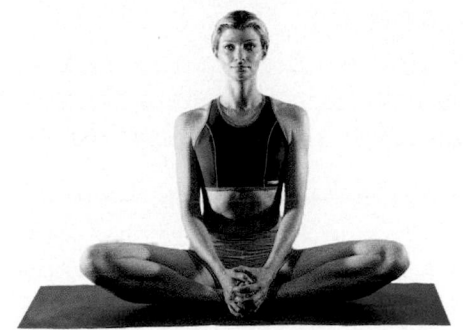

BUTTERFLY

STRENGTHENS ABS, ANKLES, BACK, BICEPS, AND KNEES; STRETCHES INNER THIGHS

Sit with the soles of your feet together. Cup your feet in your interlaced fingers. Take three to five breaths as you feel your muscles stretching. Press the soles of your feet together and lower your knees to the floor until you feel a good stretch. Hold for three to five slow breaths.

BOW

STRENGTHENS BACK, BICEPS, AND QUADS; STRETCHES CHEST, QUADS, AND SPINE; IMPROVES SHOULDER ROTATION

Lie facedown on the floor. Bend your knees and bring your feet toward your butt, keeping your thighs on the ground. Grab the tops of your feet and lift your thighs off the floor. Now bring your chest off the floor. Feel the opposing forces and pull a little more with each inhale. If you're up for it, rock back and forth from your chest to your thighs 2 to 10 times (or hold for three to five breaths if you're not into rocking).

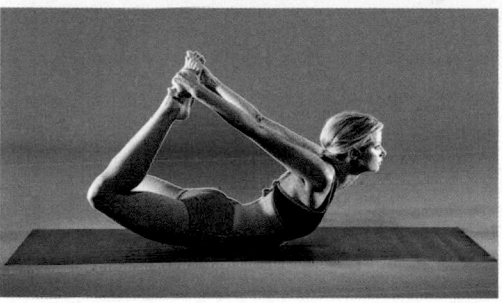

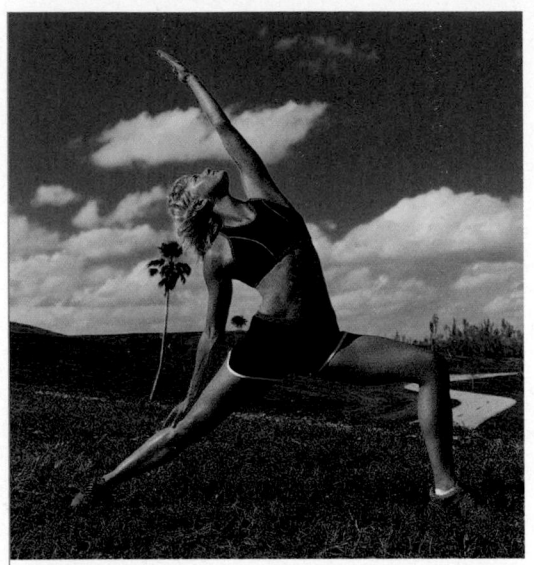

Lifting

Weight lifting can leave your muscles tired, sore, and tauter than a circus tightrope. "Lifting reduces range of motion as a result of bulking and tightening of the muscles," says Lynn Burgess, a certified yoga instructor and the founder of the Yoga from the Heart studio in Sarasota, Florida. Over time this limits gains because muscles need to contract to build strength, but they can't contract properly when they're tight. Luckily, a 2004 study by Springfield College in Massachusetts found that doing 5 minutes of yoga after lifting speeds recovery. Do each of these moves once before your workout and again when you're done.

WARRIOR I

STRENGTHENS ARMS, BACK, LEGS, AND SHOULDERS; STRETCHES ANKLES, CALVES, CHEST, LOWER BACK, AND SHOULDERS

Extend your arms out to the sides, level with your shoulders with palms down, your feet about 4 feet apart. Turn your left foot slightly in and your right foot out 90 degrees. Turn your palms to face the ceiling and bring your arms toward each other until they're parallel, fingers pointing up. Rotate your pelvis and chest to the right so they are facing in the same direction as your right toe. Bend your right knee to 90 degrees. Concentrate on stretching the back leg and lengthening the spine as you reach up. Stay here for 15 to 30 seconds before repeating on the left side.

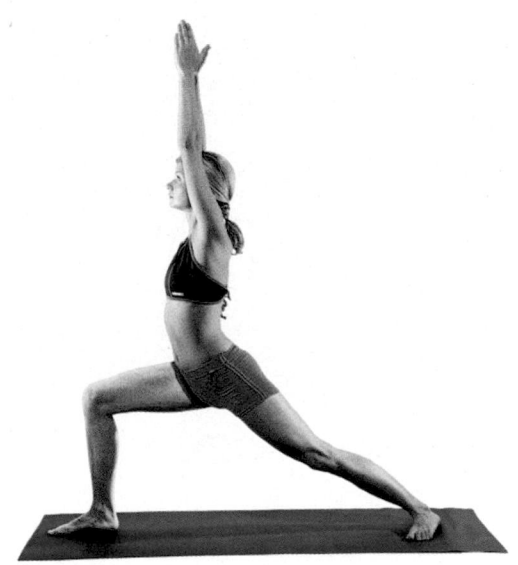

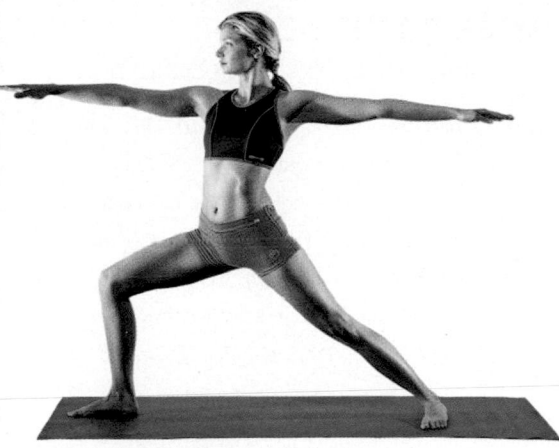

WARRIOR II

STRENGTHENS ABS, ANKLES, AND LEGS;
STRETCHES CHEST, GROIN, AND SHOULDERS

Extend your arms out to the sides, level with your
shoulders with palms down, your feet about 4 feet
apart. Turn your left foot slightly in and your right foot
out 90 degrees. Keep your hips facing forward.
Inhale, then bend your right knee. Try to get your right
thigh parallel to the floor. Turn your head to the right
as you look over your right fingers. Hold for 15 to 30
seconds. To release, straighten your right leg, turn
your feet so they're facing forward, and repeat on the
opposite side.

MODIFIED EAGLE STRETCH

STRENGTHENS JAW AND NECK; STRETCHES
SHOULDERS AND UPPER BACK

Wrap your arms around your torso, left arm under
right, hugging yourself. Keeping your arms close to
your body, bring your hands up, your right elbow
resting in your left in front of your chest, with your
palms touching each other. Relax your jaw and
shoulder blades. Hold for 10 seconds, breathing
evenly. Release and repeat with your right arm under
your left. To make it harder, cross your right leg over
your left and place your right foot behind your left
calf. Squat slightly.

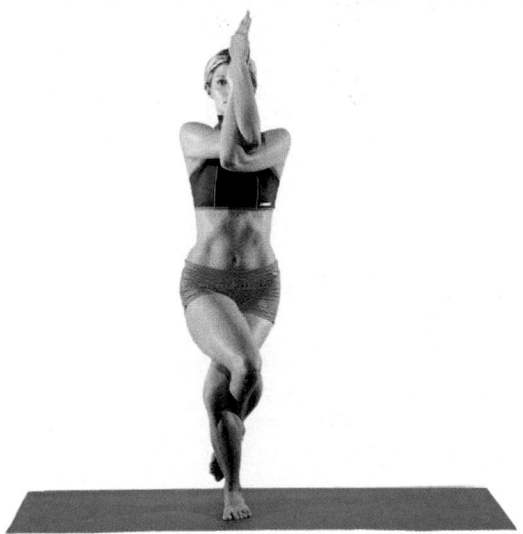

Running

During a 3.5-mile run, your feet pound the pavement more than 6,000 times at a force that's three to five times your body weight. If you don't stretch, the muscles from your Achilles tendon through your legs, hips, and back become tighter and shorter, says Beryl Bender Birch, author of *Power Yoga* and former wellness director of the New York Road Runners Club. To ease your taut muscles, perform these moves after every run, long or short. Each one strengthens your entire body while giving key areas of your lower body a much-needed stretch. Do one rep on each side.

KNEE TO CHEST
STRETCHES GLUTES AND HIP FLEXORS

Stand up straight with your feet together. Grab your left knee with both hands just below the kneecap. (Hold behind your knee if you have any injuries.) Use your biceps to pull your knee into your chest. Resist the urge to lean back, and keep your rib cage lifted and shoulders down. Take five slow breaths. Repeat, this time hugging your right leg.

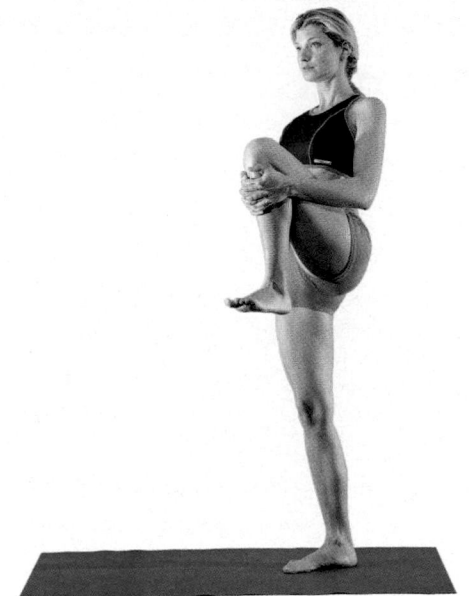

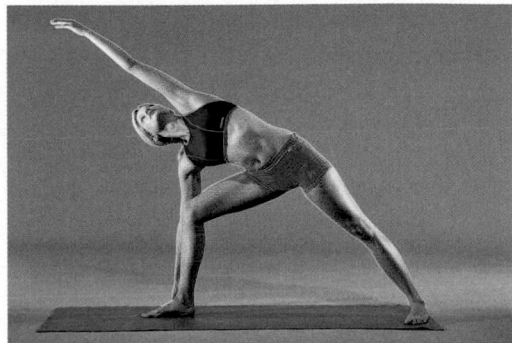

EXTENDED SIDE ANGLE

STRENGTHENS ARMS AND QUADS;
STRETCHES BACK, GROIN, AND HAMSTRINGS

With feet about 4 feet apart, turn your right foot out 90 degrees and your left foot in slightly. Extend your arms, level with shoulders and palms down. Bend your right knee until it's aligned over your ankle. Place your right hand outside your right foot. (Can't reach the floor? Place it on the inside of your foot instead.) Reach your left arm over your ear and turn your chin toward your left armpit. Look up and take five slow breaths. Switch sides.

EXTENDED TRIANGLE

STRENGTHENS HIP FLEXORS AND QUADS;
STRETCHES HAMSTRINGS AND HIP FLEXORS;
IMPROVES STABILITY

Stand with your feet about 4 feet apart, right foot turned out 90 degrees and left foot in slightly. Extend your arms out to the sides at shoulder height, palms down. Bend over to the right (from the hip) keeping your arms in line with your shoulders. Grab your right ankle with your right hand (place your right hand on your thigh or shin if you can't reach). Stretch your left hand toward the ceiling and look up at your thumb, putting minimal pressure on your right hand. Hold for five slow breaths. Switch sides.

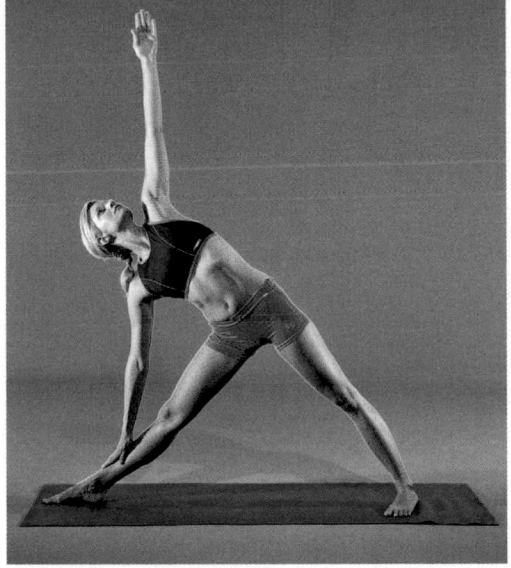

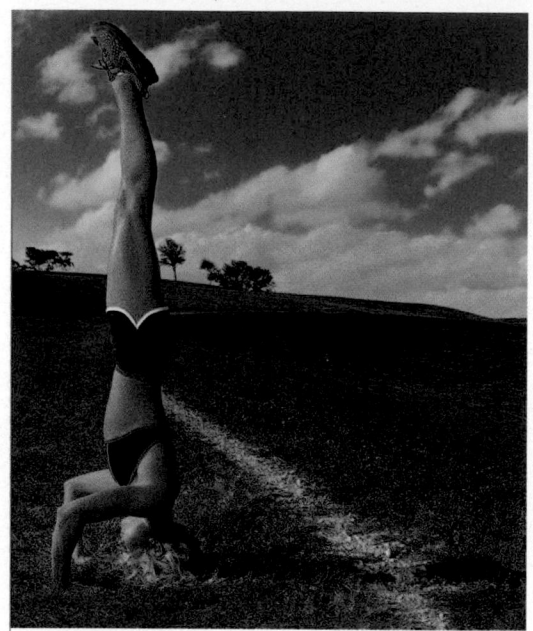

Hiking

Hauling a pack the size of a Volkswagen (and your fair share of the peanut M&Ms) over rock- and root-strewn terrain puts a lot of strain on your body, says Erin Widman, author of *Sleeping Bag Yoga*. Yoga stretches muscles and tissues– like your shoulders and Achilles tendons–that compress under this weight. And it strengthens the muscles in your back and legs to power you uphill and control your descent. Plus, breathing like a yogi boosts endurance, so you need fewer catch-your-breath breaks and can summit that super-technical trail. Use these moves to prep your body for the climb, then finish with them to get all your pieces back where they belong.

FIERCE

STRENGTHENS WHOLE BODY; STRETCHES ACHILLES TENDONS AND CALVES; INCREASES FOOT CIRCULATION

Stand with your feet parallel, hip-distance apart, and your hands on your hips. Exhale and bend your knees as if sitting back into a chair. Tuck your tailbone in to help bring the torso upright. Lift your chest and extend your arms in line with your ears, palms facing each other. Hold for 5 to 10 slow breaths.

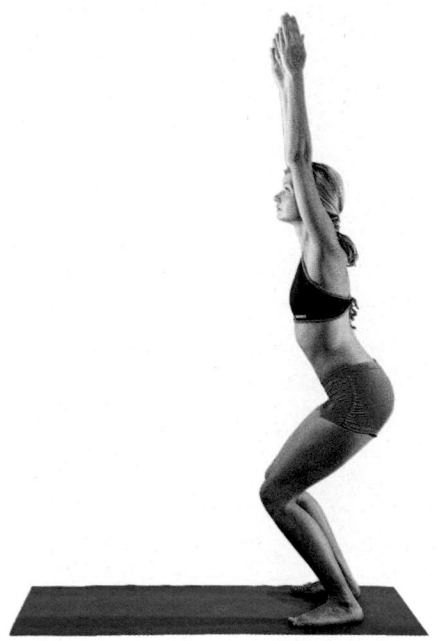

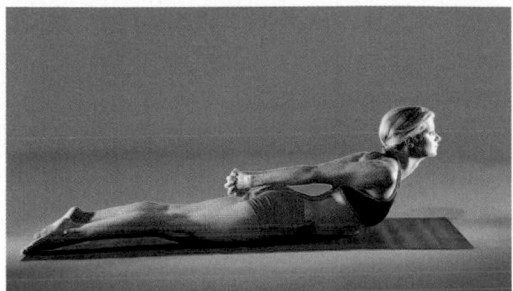

LOCUST
STRENGTHENS UPPER BACK; STRETCHES
CHEST AND SHOULDERS

Lie on your belly with your toes pointing straight back behind you. Press the tops of your feet, including your toenails, strongly into the floor. Interlace your hands behind you and rest them on your butt, elbows slightly bent. Push your tailbone toward the floor to stabilize your lower back; inhale and raise your chest forward and up toward the ceiling. Keep your feet pressing into the floor for stability. Hold for 5 to 10 slow breaths.

ONE-LEGGED KING PIGEON
STRENGTHENS LEGS; STRETCHES CHEST, HIP
JOINTS, SHOULDERS, AND THIGHS

Start on all fours. Slide your left knee forward to the back of your left wrist and your left foot toward your right hand. Slowly slide your right leg back, straightening your knee and placing the front of your thigh on the floor. Turn your pelvis to face toward the front. Press the top of your front foot into the floor and bend the back knee. Reach back with your right hand and hold the top of your back foot. Press your foot into your hand and your back knee into the floor; bend your elbow toward the ceiling. Hold for 5 to 10 breaths. Switch sides. Never force this pose.
To make it easier: Don't lift your back leg.

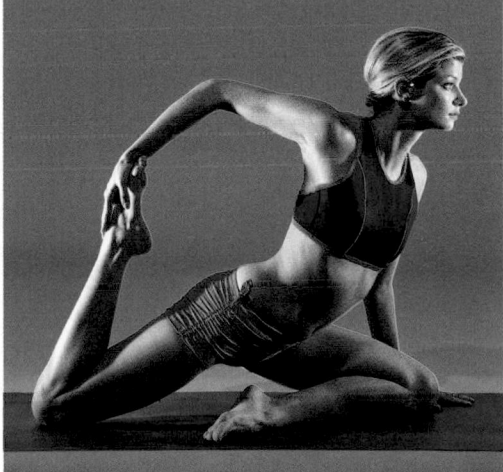

Cycling

There's nothing natural about the Cro-Magnon hunch on a bike. Preride, these yoga poses counteract that bent-over posture and prevent injury by stretching your back and overworked leg muscles, says Prisca Boris, a certified yoga instructor who teaches athletes in Vail, Colorado. Practicing for at least 10 minutes right after your ride will increase overall circulation to help you recover faster. Do one rep on each side.

FORWARD BEND HANG
STRETCHES GLUTES, HAMSTRINGS, AND LOWER AND UPPER BACK

Stand with your feet parallel about shoulder-distance apart. Slide your hands down the front of your legs and grab them above or below your knees. Lift your sit bones and lean forward from your hips, keeping your thighs contracted and your back straight. Hold for five breaths. Next, slide your hands down and grab your ankles, keeping your tailbone pointing up (A). Pause here for three breaths. Staying bent over, hold your left elbow in your right hand and your right elbow in your left hand in front of your face (B). Relax your torso so you're hanging. Take five slow breaths.

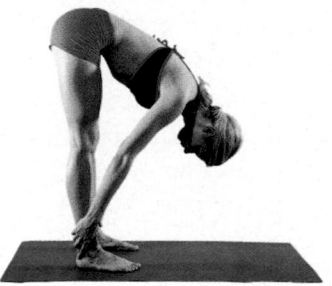

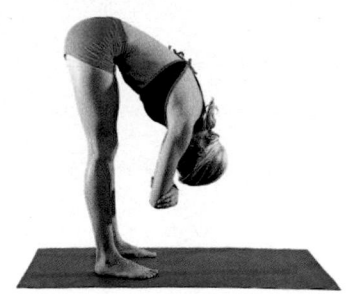

ONE-LEG CROSSOVER

STRETCHES GROIN, INNER THIGHS, KNEES, AND LOWER BACK

Lie on your back and cross your left ankle over your right thigh. Lift your right foot off the floor, bend your right knee, and bring your right thigh close to your chest. Thread your left arm in the space between your legs and bring your right arm around the outside of your right leg. Interlace your fingers underneath your right knee. Use your left elbow to press your left knee away from your chest. Take five slow breaths. Repeat on the other side. To make it harder: Lift your head, neck, and shoulders a few inches off the ground toward your right knee to challenge your core.

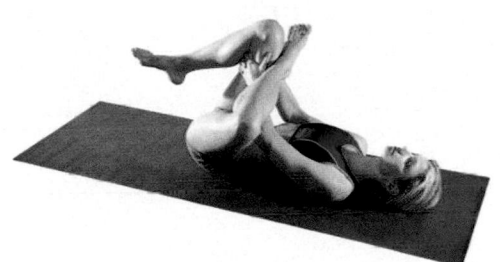

SPINAL TWIST

STRENGTHENS AND STRETCHES GLUTES, SHOULDERS, AND SPINE

Lie on your back and place the bottom of your right foot on top of your left thigh. Place your left hand on your right knee and lower it across your body to the left until it touches the floor. Twist your upper body to the right, extending your right arm out to the side at shoulder level. Turn your head so you're looking at your right hand. Take five slow breaths. Repeat on the other side.

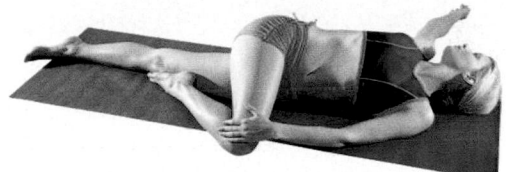

WHERE DO YOU STAND?

Whether you're Wonder Woman, Olive Oyl, or Dame Edna, the way you're standing usually falls into one of three categories. And when you identify and work with it, you can dramatically reduce injuries, especially knee and back pain, says Heidi Gremaud, a human kinetics specialist in Vancouver, Canada. Here's how to find your type.

THE TEST

Lie face up on the floor with your legs extended. Try to slide your hand underneath your back. If it slips easily to the other side, you're probably lordotic. If your hand is squished, you probably have a flat back. If the back of your knees and calves touch the floor, you probably have a sway back. (Since most Web sites with posture information come from private practitioners, visit a spine specialist for a more complete analysis, including a digital map of your posture and customized exercises for about $150.)

THE FIXES

If you're LORDOTIC

THINK JENNIFER LOPEZ.

You probably have a large arch in your lower back, a round butt, and a stomach that pops out a little bit. You also often walk on your toes.

TIPS

» Lordotics tend to slump. Think of zipping up the front of your jacket to help lift your chest and then zipping down the back to help you sit taller.

» When you're wearing high heels, pull your belly button in toward your spine, which will help you avoid back pain (and make you look even better in that dress).

If you have A FLAT BACK

THINK GWYNETH PALTROW.

You have almost no arch in your lower back, you've got a flat butt, and when you stand, you generally check out the floor. You also tend to stand with your weight on your heels.

TIPS

» Think about lifting your chest and arching your back, to help alleviate the upper neck pain and headaches many flat-backed people suffer.

» When you're walking or standing, remind yourself to look ahead—and we don't mean two steps in front of your feet.

If you have A SWAY BACK

THINK PARIS HILTON.

Your pelvis is thrust forward, your shoulders are rounded, and you tend to hyperextend your knees.

TIPS

» Make "soft knees" your mantra, keeping them unlocked and slightly bent and relaxed when walking or standing, to reduce overstretching your ligaments for fewer knee and lower-back problems.

» Rock gently from your heels to your toes while standing to keep from hyperextending your knees.

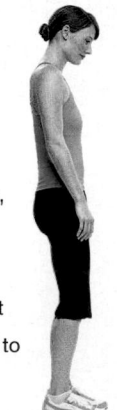

STRENGTH TRAINING
Seated Stability Ball Row

Posture payback

It strengthens your upper back and shoulders to keep them from rounding forward. "This can improve your breathing and increase energy," Dr. DeMann says.

How to do it

Sit on a stability ball with your knees bent, feet flat on the floor, and your neck in line with your back. Grip a 5-pound dumbbell in each hand with your palms facing each other and your elbows bent at 90-degree angles. Row the weights to your sides, squeezing your shoulder blades together. Do three sets of 10.

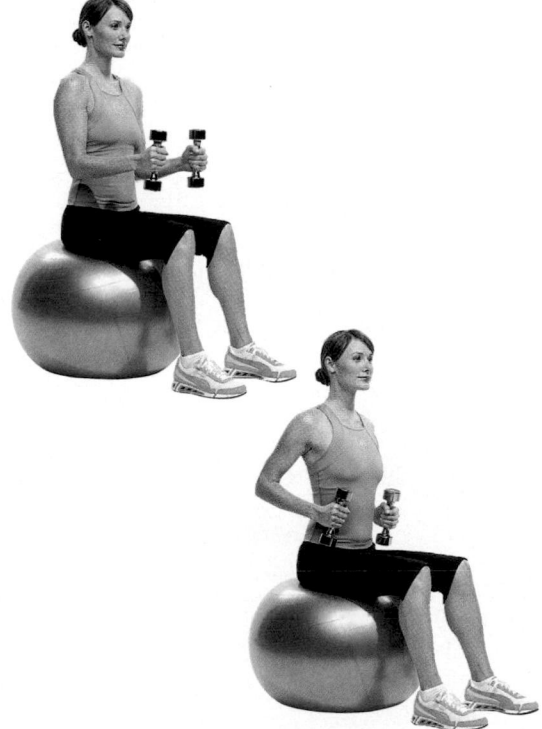

ALEXANDER TECHNIQUE
Spinal Stretch

Posture payback

It will help elongate your spine. "Your head weighs the same as a small TV set," says Richard Brennan, author of five books on the Alexander Technique, which is a gentle, dance-inspired method known for enhancing posture. By relieving your spine of that compression, he says, you can stand half an inch taller.

How to do it

Lie on a mat with your knees bent and your feet flat on the floor. Support your head with a small pillow and, with your eyes open, let your body sink into the mat as you focus on lengthening your spine. Think of your pelvis releasing away from your head. Allow yourself to breathe deeply and continue for 20 minutes. "You won't notice much at first, but after a few weeks, you'll have better posture," Brennan says. But don't confuse this exercise with sleep. "It's different because you're lying still, consciously releasing your spine. And bending your knees especially relieves spinal pressure," says Mischul Brownstone, a bodywork specialist in Charlotte, Vermont.

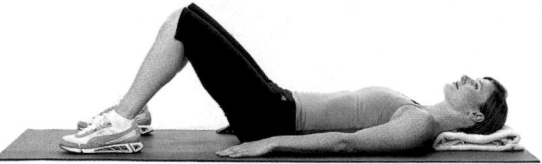

W|H

Stomach Massage

Posture payback

This move stretches your back, strengthens your abs and legs, and aids circulation and digestion. "Good posture comes from a strong core, and Pilates strengthens the powerhouse," says Brooke Siler, author of *Your Ultimate Pilates Body Challenge*.

How to do it

Balance on your tailbone with knees bent shoulder-width apart and toes resting lightly on the mat. Reach forward with both arms and lift your spine up, imagining you're on a balance beam. Next, stretch your legs out and twist your upper body to follow the reach of one arm behind you. Keep your arms straight and think of chopping a tree behind you. Inhale as you reverse the twist, pulling your knees back toward your chest and lightly touching the mat with your toes. Repeat on the other side and do three to five sets, alternating sides with each rep.

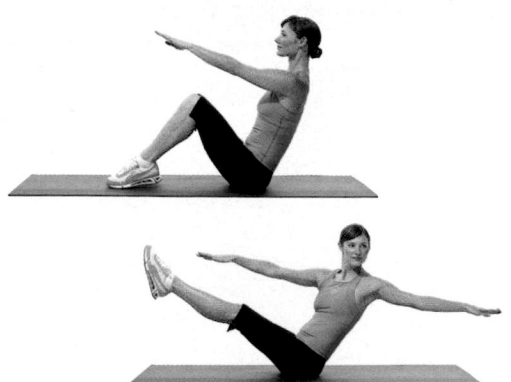

Bosu Angels and Overhead Lift

Posture payback

It stretches and opens your chest muscles, pulls the shoulder blades down, and elongates the neck. "Your head will look lifted like that of a dancer," says Julie O'Connell, the physiotherapist for Chicago's Joffrey Ballet.

How to do it

Lie face up on a Bosu with your bra strap hitting the center of the Bosu, your knees bent and your abs engaged. Next, sweep your arms outward and upward, as if you're making a snow angel. Hold this stretch for 30 to 40 seconds. To deepen the stretch, grip each end of a hand towel and hold it overhead for 30 to 40 seconds.

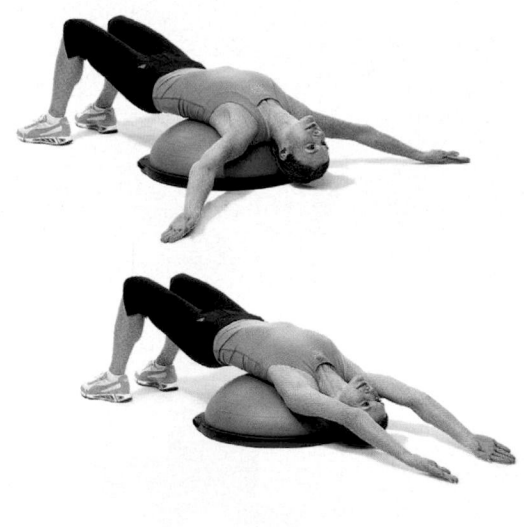

YOGA
Prayer Pose

Posture payback

It stretches your spine, arms, shoulders, glutes, and hamstrings and helps straighten your spine and neck. "Slightly tilting your head back and folding your neck is common, but it's like crimping a garden hose—we can only guess what that's doing to your brain," says Jean Couch, owner of the Balance Center in Palo Alto, California. Couch also uses this move to correct the American habit of pushing the pelvis forward. (African women, according to a study in the science journal *Nature*, can carry 20 percent of their body weight on their heads—without expending a single extra calorie—because of their proper pelvis alignment.)

How to do it

Begin on all fours, with your knees and feet about a foot apart. Tip your butt bones up and move your torso back so that your hipbones rest on your thighs. Then walk your hands out, keeping your palms flat, until your forehead rests on the floor. Let your spine lengthen and your pelvis continue to rise up behind you.

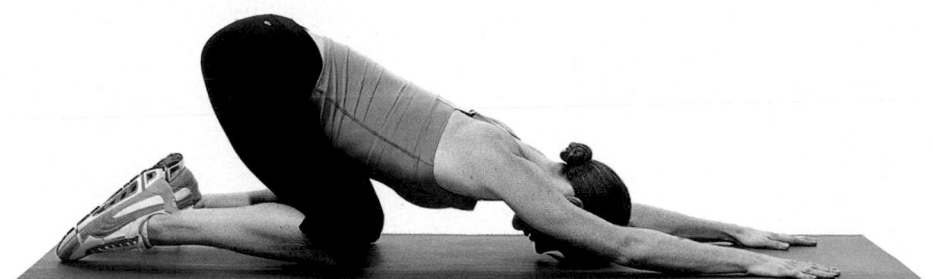

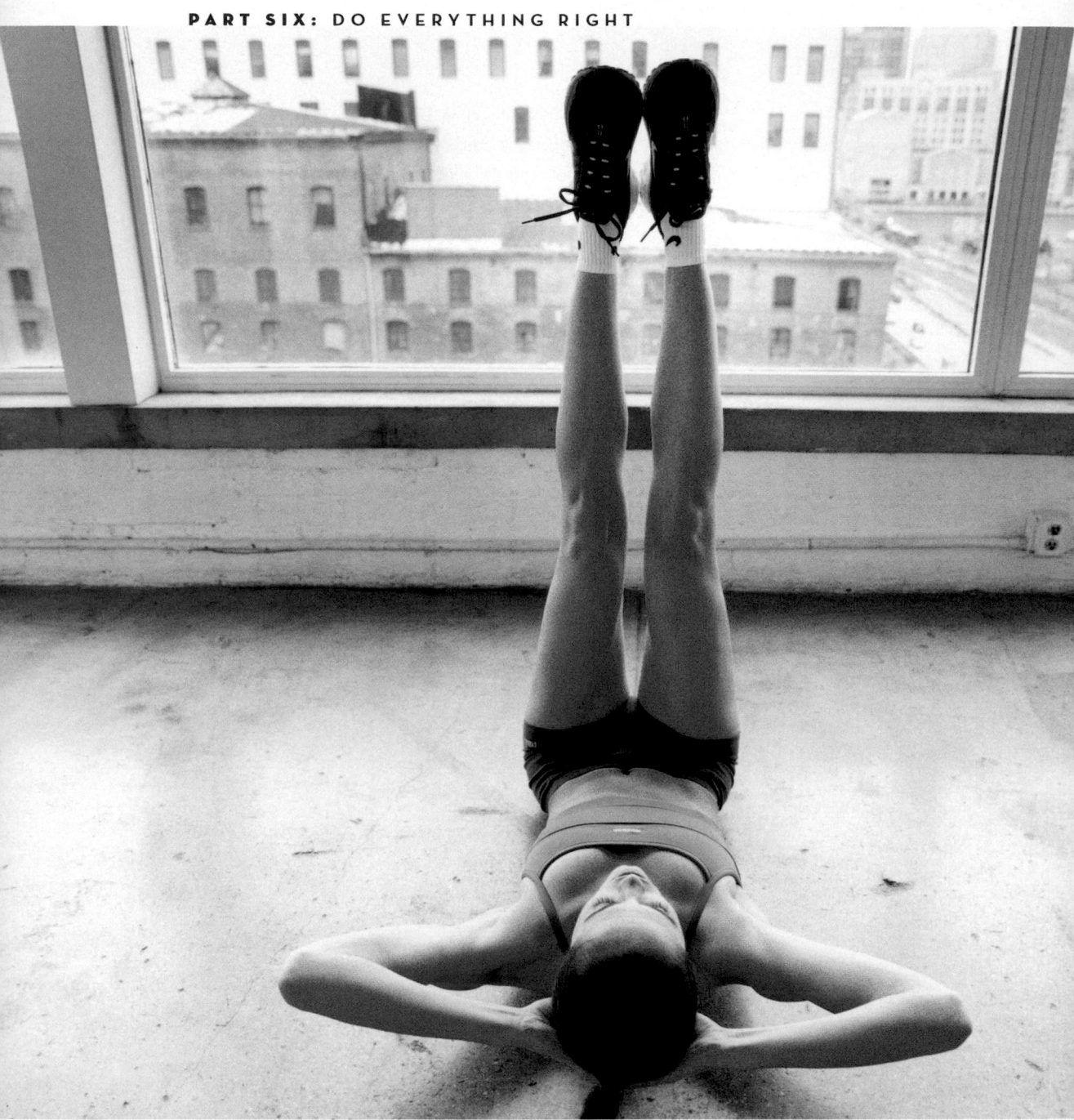

CHAPTER THIRTY-FOUR

FIX YOUR FITNESS MISTAKES

FROM THE WRONG FORM TO THE WRONG ENERGY BAR, SIMPLE MISTAKES CAN WIPE OUT YOUR BEST SWEAT SESSION. HERE'S HOW TO DETECT THEM AND CORRECT THEM.

BY ALEXA JOY SHERMAN

WE'VE ALL SEEN PEOPLE make mistakes at the gym (see-through white shorts come to mind). But the gym is a little like Spring Break—pretty much anything goes. Some people run fast, some slow. Some people do 15 reps, some do 8. Some go with the iPod, some request a Bee Gees mix during spinning class. The thinking: As long as we're doing some kind of exercise, it's got to be good. But the fact is that the gym is a place where you can make mistakes—the kind that can lead to injury, stop any progress you've made, or derail all of your exercise and bodily goals. No, these workout blunders won't draw stares the way a leather

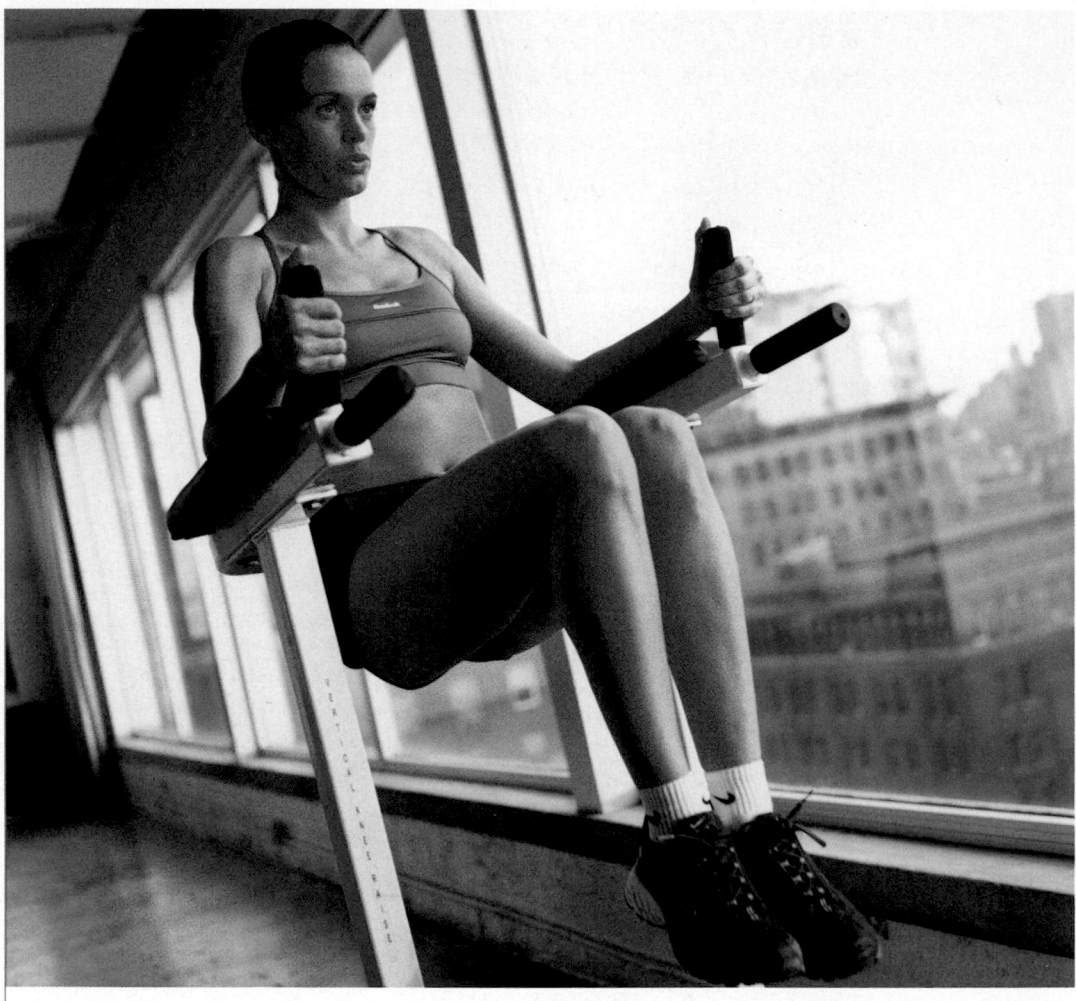

sports bra would, but they're the ones even more worthy of correction.

FITNESS FLAW:
Getting married to the machines.

Sure, weight machines are the lowest-maintenance pieces of workout equipment since the jump rope. That's because using machines means there's no searching for dumbbells or fighting for a free bench with the no-neck crowd. But don't rely solely on the easy-made equipment, because typically you can work more muscles and build greater practical strength with free weights or even no weights, says Jay Dawes, instructor of kinesiology and health studies at the University of Central Oklahoma. For example, although a leg curl will strengthen your hamstrings, it isn't exactly a move you'll make in life. A lunge-and-press (see below), on the other hand, strengthens your quadriceps, hamstrings, buttocks, calves, upper back, and shoulders—and also builds the balance and coordination used in daily activities like bending down, lifting kids, and playing sports.

The Fix: To get the most benefit from each workout, try to perform a mix of all kinds of exercises—ones using machines, body weight, free weights, and dumbbells, says Cedric X. Bryant, Ph.D., chief exercise physiologist and vice president of educational services for the American Council on Exercise. Dawes suggests including two to three sets of a move like the lunge-and-press several times a week. To do it, hold a dumbbell in each hand at shoulder height with your arms bent close to sides and palms in. Keep your feet hip-width apart with one foot about a stride ahead of the other and your back heel lifted. With your abs contracted, bend your knees so the front knee aligns with your front ankle and the back knee points toward the ground. At the same time, straighten your arms to press the dumbbells overhead. Straighten your legs and lower the dumbbells to the starting position, and repeat for 12 to 15 repetitions.

FITNESS FLAW:

Speeding through your workouts to raise your heart rate.

Moving quickly through your sets may help you make it back in time for *Grey's*, but it could also be sign you're misusing momentum, executing the

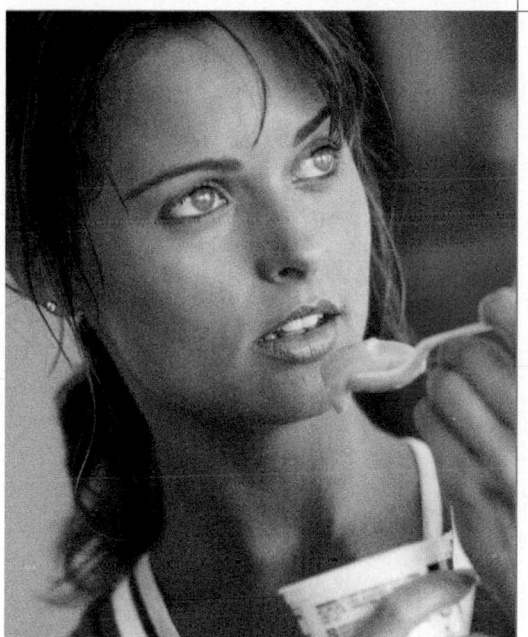

GYM CANDY
DON'T LET A BAD SNACK WIPE OUT A GOOD SWEAT

The right kind of snack can help your body prepare for a workout and recover from one faster. The wrong kind can erase that 45 minutes of hard work you just put in. So skip the sugar-loaded fixes that promise an energy *boost* but mostly just deliver empty calories, says Susan M. Kleiner, Ph.D., a sports nutritionist in Washington, D.C., and author of *Power Eating*. If you grab an energy bar, choose one that goes easy on the sugar and has the right mix of protein, carbohydrates, and unsaturated fat. An apple with some peanut butter or a cup of low-fat yogurt is also a good option, Dr. Kleiner says. The ideal workout snack for a woman should be no more than 200 calories with at least 10 grams of protein, 20 g of carbs, and 2 g of unsaturated fat, she says.

temptation: lunges. Speeding through them increases the risk of pulled muscles or joint strains and sprains.

The Fix: With any strength move, go at a slow, controlled pace in the lifting and lowering phases (2 seconds up, 2 seconds down). "There should be no point at which you pick up speed," says California trainer Jay Blahnik, author of *Full-Body Flexibility*. With crunches, hold dumbbells or a medicine ball on your chest to slow you down. For lunges, hold a dumbbell in each hand as you perform your reps or try doing them with your front foot on a Bosu balance trainer. (If you want to raise your heart rate during circuit training, decrease the time of rest between exercises rather than rushing through the exercise.)

FITNESS FLAW:
Using the same setting he just did.

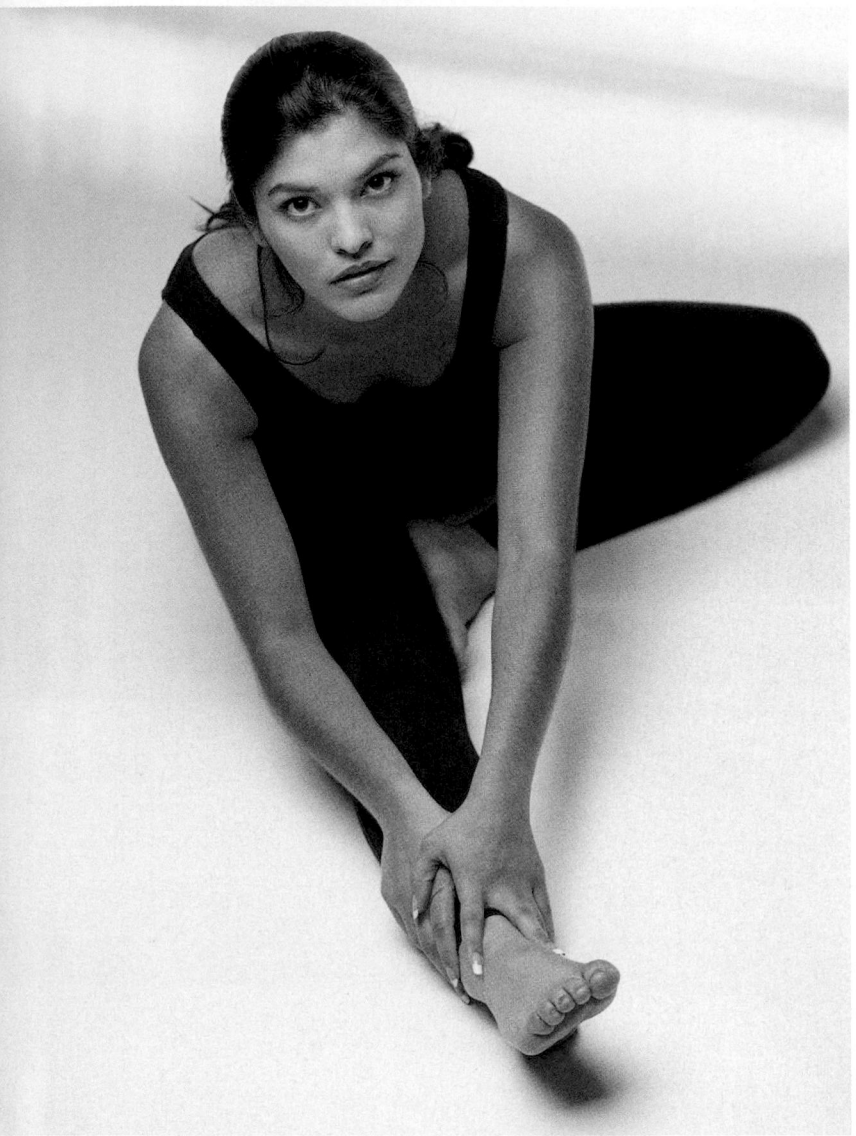

exercise incorrectly, or using too much or too little weight. Many women tend to use momentum with crunches, potentially straining the neck, says Janet Huehls, clinical exercise physiologist for the weight center at the University of Massachusetts Memorial Medical Center. Another momentum

You wouldn't drive without adjusting the seat and mirrors, so don't do sets on exercise machines in somebody else's seat settings. "On the leg extension, if the knees are out too far in front of the feet, you put more sheer force on the knee, which can cause ACL strains," Dawes says. You can also strain your shoulder if your arms are positioned too far back on the chest-press machine.

The Fix: A certified trainer can show you the correct settings for your size, but you can also do it by feel. In general, the rule is: "You should be able to go through the full range of motion and maintain good posture with back and feet well-supported," Dr. Bryant says. With the leg extension, make sure your thighs are in the center and the backs of your knees just about touch the front of the seat. With any upright machine, put your head, back, and hips in contact with the back pads.

FITNESS FLAW:
Making stretching the first thing you do at the gym.

For years people thought preworkout stretching was essential to prevent injury. But cold muscles are like uncooked noodles; they need to be heated up before they can move freely. "We now suggest you don't stretch before you work out because it doesn't appear to reduce the risk of injury. It may even lead to injury and compromise performance," Blahnik says.

The Fix: To warm up before a workout, skip stretching and do 5 to 10 minutes of cardio or a lighter, easier version of whatever movements you do in the workout itself. But don't ignore stretching completely, because muscle flexibility will relieve overall tightness and reduce injury over the long term. You can focus on traditionally tight areas like your hamstrings, but don't ignore the most neglected muscles: your back, neck, and feet (common areas of tightness for women who

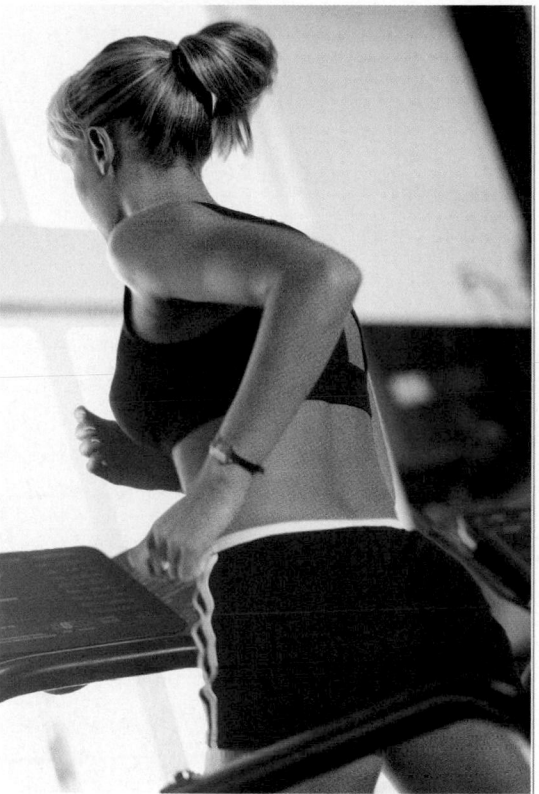

W|H

sit at desks or wear heels). To prevent neck strain, for example, do this full-motion stretch 10 to 12 times on each side using slow, controlled, fluid movements: Stand with your feet shoulder-width apart and, keeping your chin up, turn your head as far to one side as possible, then turn back to the opposite side, and repeat.

FITNESS FLAW:
Using 2 for the price of 1.

It's not a mistake per se to do leg extensions and biceps curls with both legs or arms at once. But it can lead to

THE MACHINE MISTAKE

THE PROBLEM WITH THE CALORIE-COUNTERS ON CARDIOVASCULAR EQUIPMENT

Many of us watch calories the way some people watch stock prices—every little bit counts. But it's a mistake to trust cardio machines for a perfect recording. "The calorie burn on cardio machines is more accurate than it used to be. If it asks you to enter your weight, there's always going to be an error, because they make several assumptions," says exercise physiologist Cedric X. Bryant, Ph.D.

First, weight-bearing machines like stairclimbers, elliptical trainers, and treadmills assume you're not leaning on the handrails, but research shows people off-load their weight on these machines by as much as 20 percent. "So if the machine says you're burning 300 calories, you're probably only burning about 240," Dr. Bryant says.

Machines also assume your exercise efficiency is average. Some people are more efficient in the way they stride or step. In one of your body's great injustices, you burn fewer calories by using better form. That means a machine could also be overestimating your caloric total. "There's no way to make that determination for individuals based upon the input that they provide on cardio equipment," Dr. Bryant says.

Finally, people with more body fat and less muscle mass will burn considerably fewer calories than those who have more muscle and less fat. For instance, a 140-pound woman with 20 percent body fat will burn calories more effectively than the same woman with 25 percent body fat. The only reliable way to figure out how many calories you burn is via metabolic testing. (Some gyms, such as Bally Total Fitness, offer this using devices like the BodyGem, which measures your metabolism in a breath test.) Short of that, experts say you should decrease the estimated number of calories burned by 30 percent to get a more accurate reading.

lopsided strength gains. "We're asymmetrical by nature with one dominant side," Dawes says. "So [when working both legs] your stronger side will dominate and help you through those sticking points. Then you get more development on one side, setting you up for imbalances and injury."

The Fix: Do some unilateral exercises within each total-body workout to correct imbalances, using machines that let you work the arms or legs separately, or doing free-weight exercises so you have that option. "Start an exercise with the non-dominant side and do as many reps as you can, then do the dominant side," Dawes says. "If, say, you do three more reps with the dominant side, go back and do those last three with the nondominant side to try to reduce that deficit."

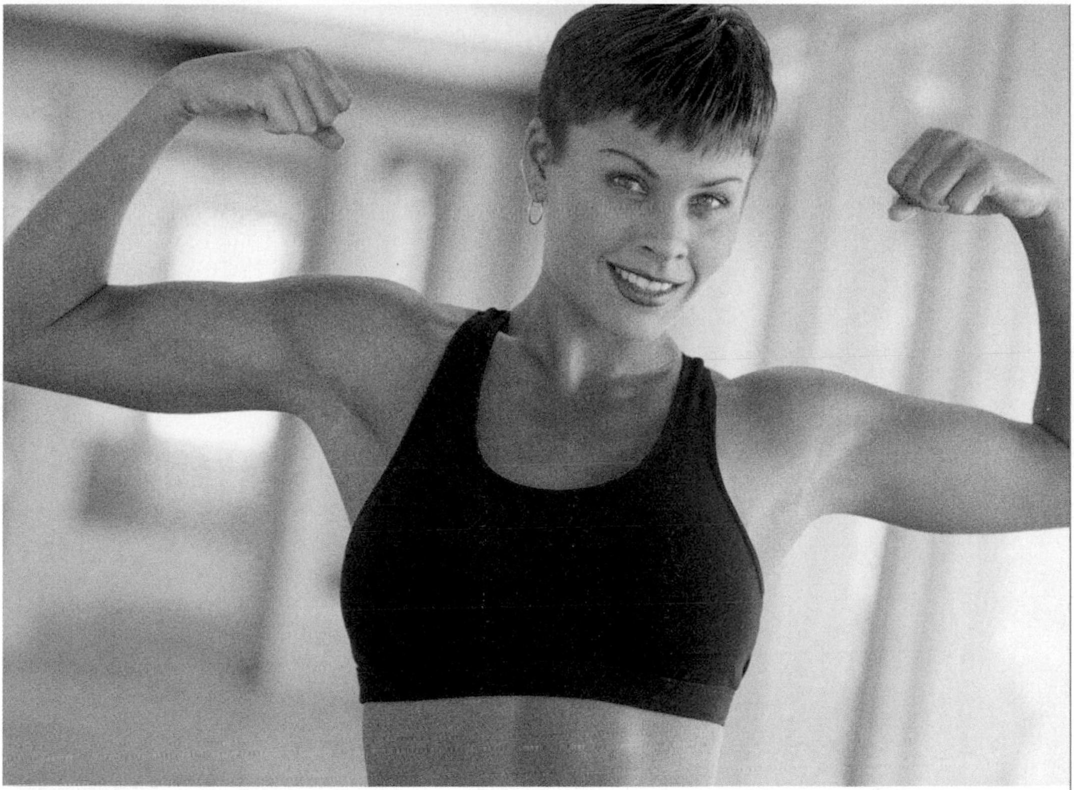

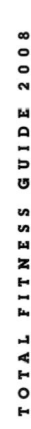

FITNESS FLAW:

Going at three speeds—hard, harder, and I'm gonna pant like an overheated Irish wolfhound.

High-intensity, high-impact aerobic activities can be great for calorie burning, but not for joint saving. "Constantly pounding the body with high-intensity exercise often won't give your body an adequate amount of recovery time. That can result in you reaching a plateau or worse, an overuse injury," Dr. Bryant says.

The Fix: Limit anything that has a lot of jumping, bounding, or repetitive stress (running, boot camp classes). And don't push your heart rate up to 90 percent of your maximum (estimated as 220 minus your age) more than 2 or 3 days a week, particularly if you're doing high-impact activities. Instead sub in swimming, walking, elliptical trainers, resistance training, or rest. "Signs you're overdoing it include muscle soreness lasting more than a day or two, fatigue lasting more than a few hours after a workout, frequent injury, loss of motivation, and increased or decreased appetite," Huehls says.

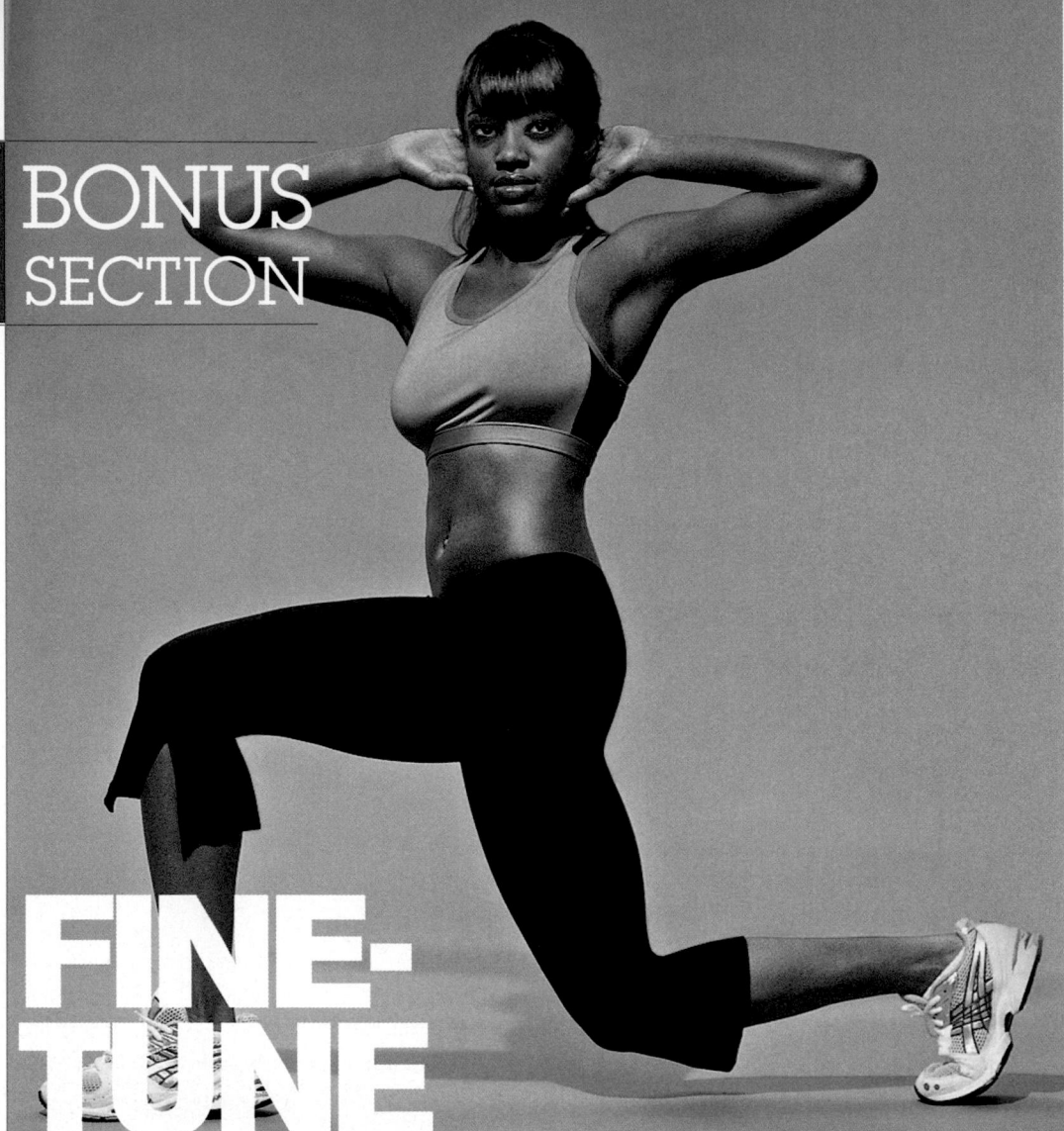

FINE-TUNE YOUR BODY

LITTLE TWEAKS IN YOUR WORKOUT CAN LEAD TO BIG RESULTS.

WHETHER IT'S SWITCHING LIPSTICK from matte to gloss or changing lanes from right to left, tiny shifts make a big difference. With exercise, altering moves even slightly means training muscles at different angles, working them harder, and breaking through plateaus, says Mike Mejia, a strength and conditioning specialist in New York. Try two or three sets of each of these tweaks of popular moves.

SQUAT TWEAK
1¼ SQUAT

Stand with your feet hip-width apart and push back into a regular squat until your thighs are parallel to the floor. Rise up a quarter of the way, pause for a second, go back down into the parallel position, pause again, then straighten all the way up. That's one rep. Do 10 to 12.

New results When you do a regular squat, your thighs work hardest in the parallel position. The 1¼ squat is a greater challenge because you spend more time closer to that sweet spot.

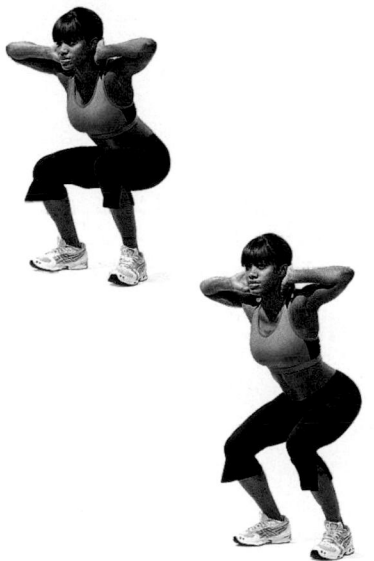

LUNGE TWEAK
TWISTING LUNGE

Stand with your hands behind your ears and step your left leg forward. Lunge down until your legs form two right angles. At the bottom of the movement, twist your torso as far left as you can. Hold for 1 second, return to neutral, and then to start. Alternate legs for five or six reps each leg.

New results The lunge works your thighs and glutes, but the twist forces you to stabilize yourself, working your legs harder. Plus, you fire up your obliques to improve your balance.

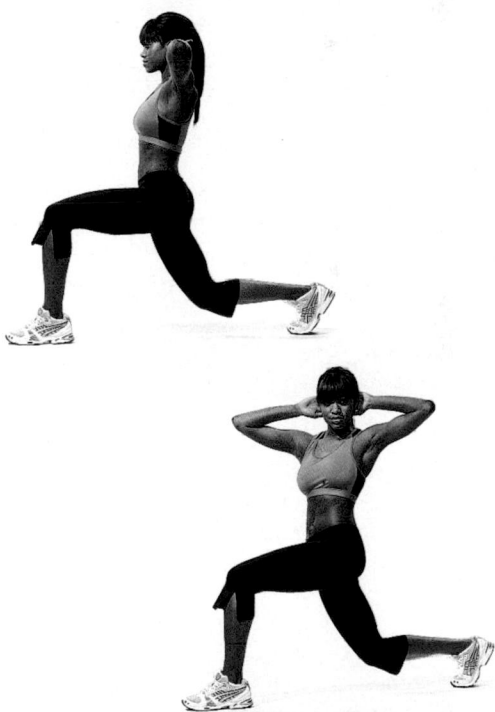

CRUNCH TWEAK
60-DEGREE CRUNCH

Place a rolled bath towel under your lower back as you lie on the floor. Bend knees to 90 degrees, keeping feet flat and fingers behind ears. Crunch up as high as you can while pressing your lower back into the towel. Pause at the top for 2 seconds and repeat, doing 12 to 15 reps.

New results The towel extends your range of motion, allowing you to work your deepest ab muscles without taxing your back.

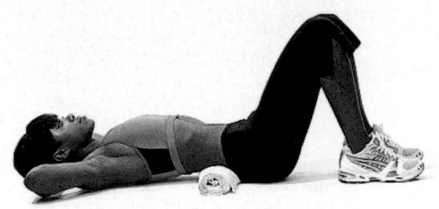

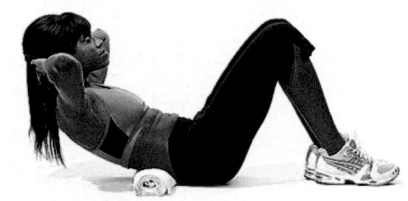

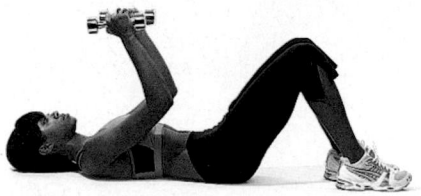

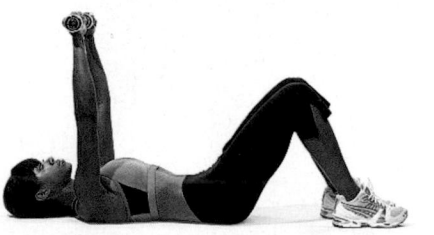

CHEST-PRESS TWEAK
INTERNALLY ROTATING
CHEST PRESS

Lie on a bench with knees bent, holding a dumbbell in each hand. Bend your elbows with palms facing each other. Press straight up, rotating arms at the top so thumbs come together and palms face forward. Rotate palms back in and lower.

New results Rotating your chest press engages more of your pectoral muscles and provides a more intense contraction.

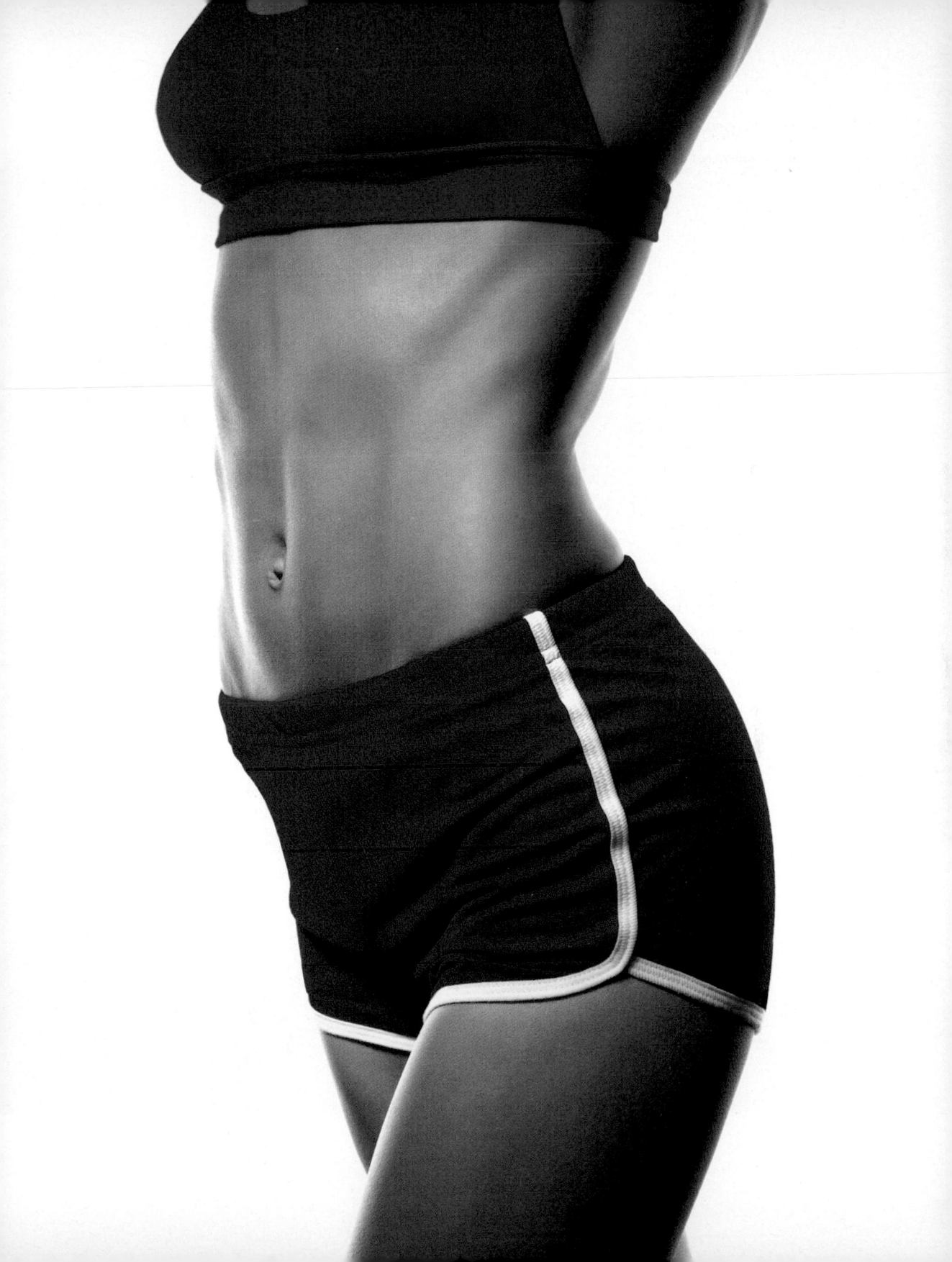

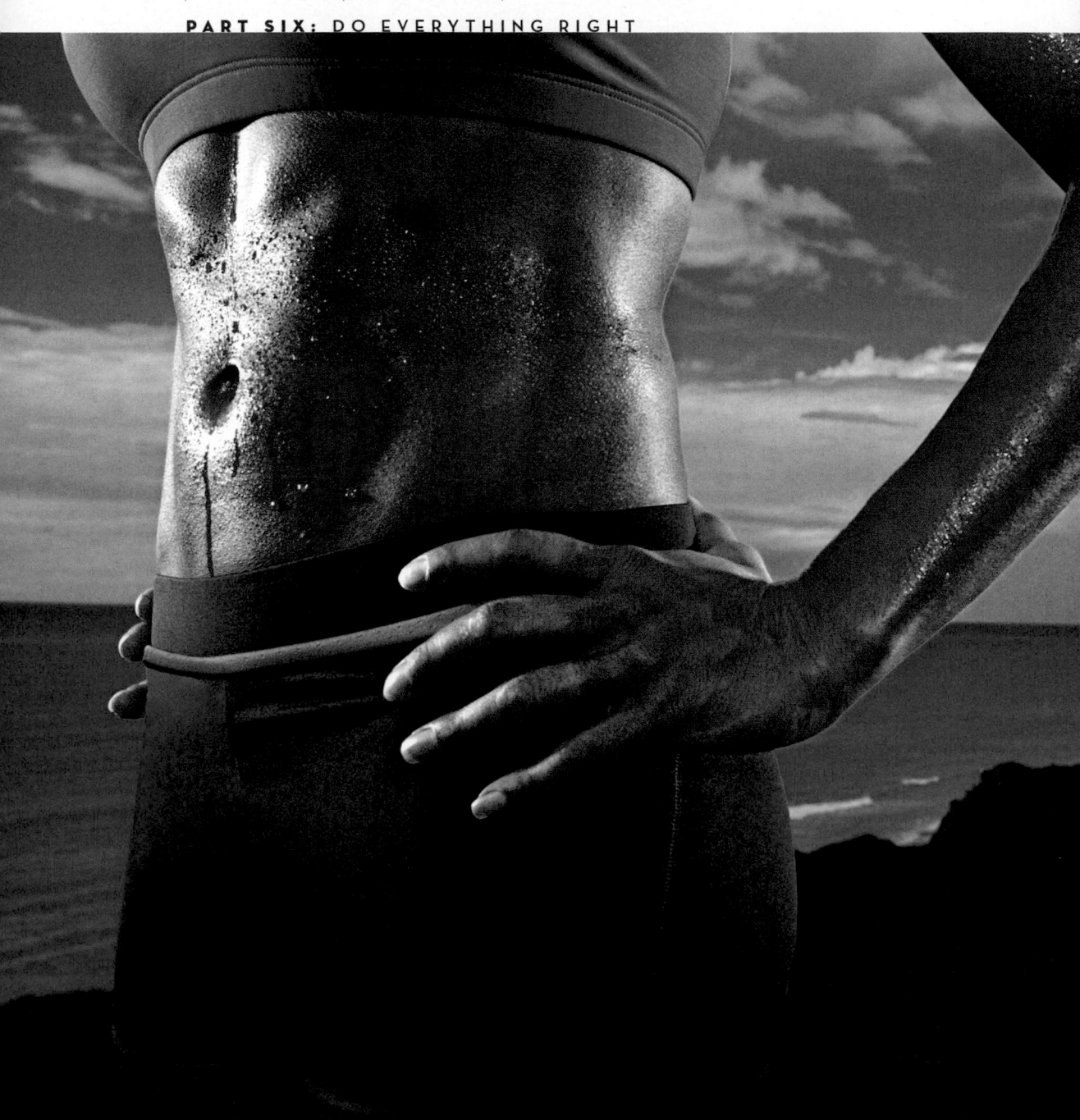

CHAPTER THIRTY-FIVE

NO MUSCLE LEFT BEHIND

FIND AND ELIMINATE YOUR WEAK LINK IN 5 EASY STEPS.

BY SELENE YEAGER

TOTAL FITNESS GUIDE 2008

W|H

PAIR A HOT GOING-OUT GETUP with questionable shoes or a hideous belt (braided, perhaps?) and you'll get not-so-smoking results. Your muscles work on the same only-as-good-as-their-weakest-link principle: If one group isn't up to snuff, your entire body suffers, from poor performance to overuse injuries to a droopy butt (even after your 300th donkey kick). "Your muscles work in unison, like a chain," explains Bill Hartman, C.S.C.S., a physical therapist in Indianapolis who specializes in building balanced bodies. "One can't function properly without the other. For example, if your hips are weak—and many women's are—all those kickbacks you do will just hurt your back."

Take these five 30-second tests to reveal which muscles you've been missing. Once you ID your neglected parts, add the suggested moves to your routine to balance things out—and create a top-shelf body.

Test 1

SPLIT SQUAT

Stand with your feet hip-width apart and your hands on your hips. Take a giant step forward with your left leg and let your right heel come off the floor. Drop your hips, keeping your left knee directly above your ankle, until your left thigh is parallel to the floor. Press back to start. If your right knee drifts inward or wobbles:

Your weak link Outer hips and hamstrings. These muscles become too mushy to support your legs properly when you spend the better part of the day parked in an office chair.

Get your fix Add these moves to your strength routine 3 nonconsecutive days a week.

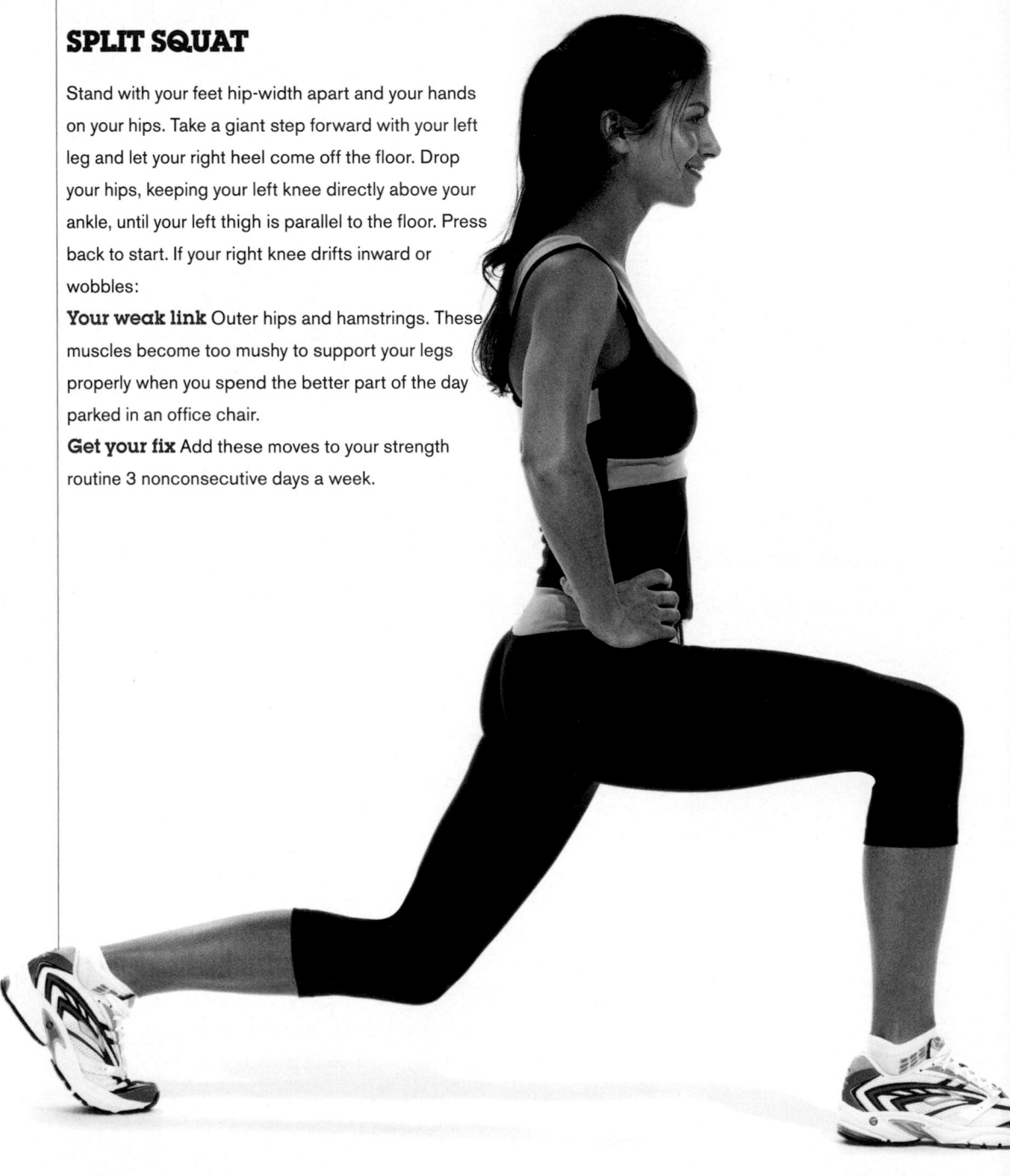

HAMSTRING CURL

WORKS GLUTES AND HAMSTRINGS

Lie on your back, legs extended, with heels resting on top of a stability ball. Press your heels into the ball and lift your hips off the floor until your body forms a straight line. Bend your knees and roll the ball in toward your butt. Roll back out to start. Do 1 set of 15 reps.

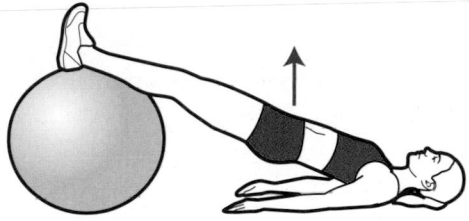

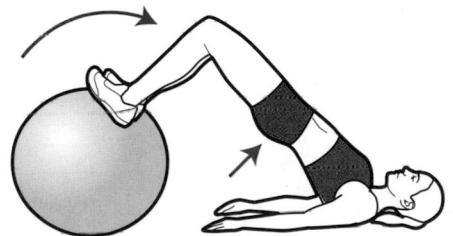

SIDE STEP

WORKS OUTER HIPS

Grab an exercise band and stand with your legs about hip-width apart. Loop the band around both legs, just above your ankles, and tie to secure. With knees slightly bent, take a giant step to the right with your right foot. Next, take a small step to the right with your left foot, keeping tension in the band. That's 1 rep. Do 10. Then repeat, stepping to the left. Do 6 sets on each side.

Body Bonus Stronger hip muscles protect your knees from injury and let you execute squats and lunges more effectively. Which adds up to one perky, firm excuse to lie bum side up at the beach.

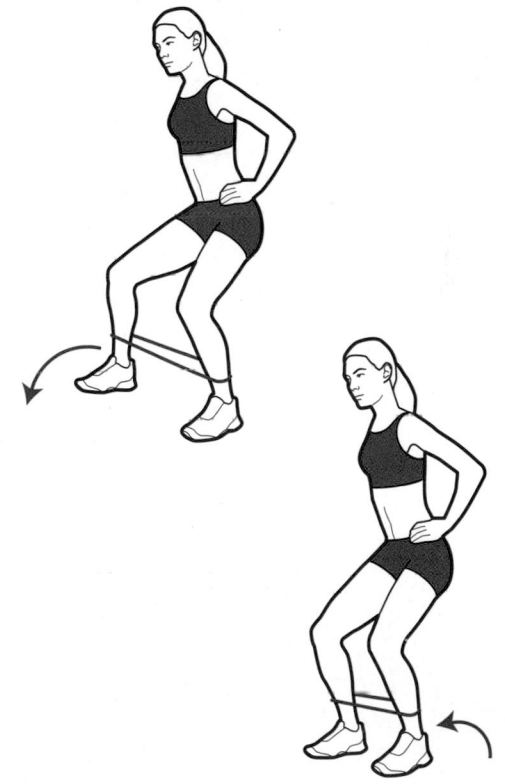

TOTAL FITNESS GUIDE 2008

W|H

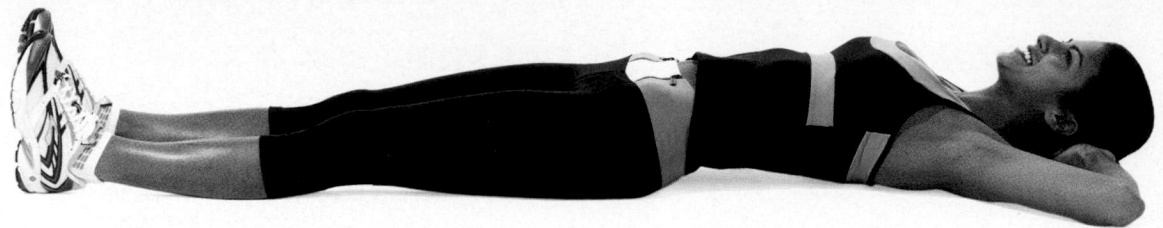

Test 2

LYING PEC STRETCH

Lie flat on your back with your legs extended. Place your palms under your head. Let your arms relax. Your elbows should be able to rest flat on the floor. If they don't reach or the stretch is uncomfortable:

Your weak link Stiff chest and shoulder muscles (especially your rotator cuffs) and weak upper-back muscles. About your posture? Just don't let Tyra see.

Get your fix Perform the Y stretch twice a day (in the morning and postworkout). Add the Y lift to your strength routine 3 nonconsecutive days a week.

Y STRETCH

STRETCHES ROTATOR CUFFS

Grab a pair of 3-pound dumbbells and lie with your shoulders and back on a stability ball. Position your feet hip-width apart. Extend your arms up until they are in line with your ears and form a Y. Hold for 30 seconds.

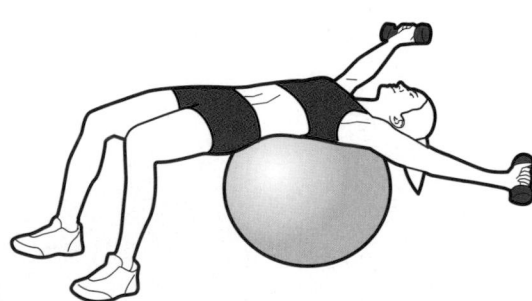

Y LIFT

WORKS MID- AND UPPER BACK

Grab a pair of 3-pound dumbbells and lie facedown on a stability ball with your navel on top of the ball. Let your arms hang down, palms facing each other. Lift your arms up and out on a diagonal until they're in line with your ears and form a Y. Hold for 6 seconds. Lower arms and repeat. Do 1 set of 6 reps.

Body Bonus In just a couple of weeks, you'll appear taller—no heels required.

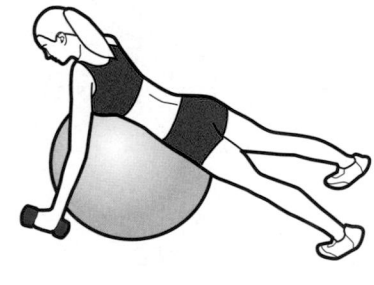

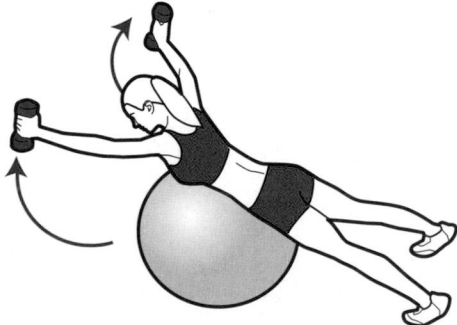

Test 3

BACK SCRATCH

Stand tall with your arms at your sides. Bend your left elbow and try to place the back of your left hand on your right shoulder blade. If you can't reach without pain or contorting yourself:

Your weak link Stiff rotator cuffs (the shoulder stabilizers). They're common in women who lift weights.

Get your fix Do this move twice a day (in the morning and postworkout).

LYING SHOULDER STRETCH
WORKS ROTATOR CUFFS

Lie on your left side. Extend your left arm straight out from your body so you're balancing on your left shoulder. Bend your left arm 90 degrees so it forms an L, with your palm facing your feet. Grab the outside of your left wrist with your right hand and press your left arm toward the floor in the direction of your feet. When you feel a stretch, hold for 30 seconds. Switch sides.

Body Bonus Your shoulders will naturally roll back, making you look longer and leaner. Flexible rotator cuffs will also improve your range of motion for, say, acing a serve.

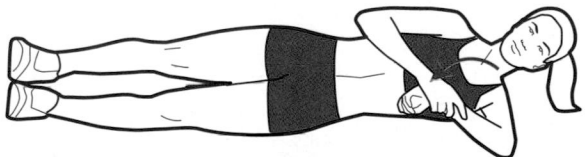

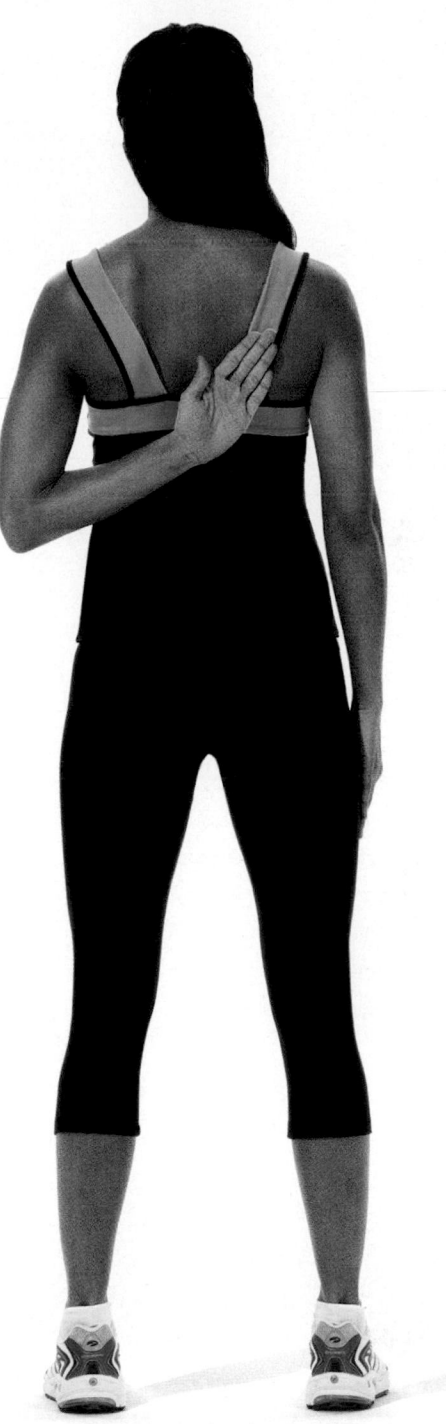

TOTAL FITNESS GUIDE 2008

W|H

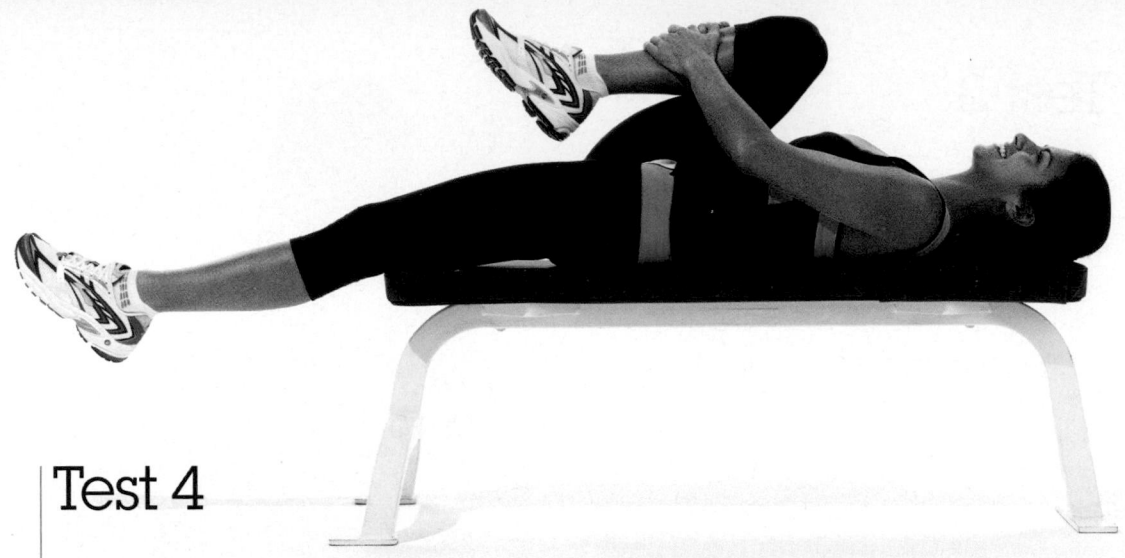

Test 4

RECLINING JACKKNIFE

Lie on your back on a bench. Bring both knees in toward your chest. Grab your right knee and hold it there while extending and lowering your left leg by relaxing your hips. Repeat, grabbing your left knee. If either leg can't lower to the bench:

Your weak link Glutes (underused) and hips (too tight). This causes your pelvis to tilt forward, your lower back to arch, and your butt to jut out.

Get your fix Perform the stability ball lunge twice a day to open up your scrunched hips. Tone your glutes by adding the drawbridge to your strength routine 3 nonconsecutive days a week.

STABILITY BALL LUNGE

STRETCHES GROIN AND HIPS

Place the right side of your butt on the edge of a stability ball. Extend your left leg behind you so you're in a lunge position. Squeeze your glutes and gently press your hips forward as you sink into the ball. Hold for 30 seconds. Switch sides.

DRAWBRIDGE

WORKS GLUTES

Lie on your back with your knees bent and feet flat on the floor, arms at your sides. Grasp your right knee with both hands and pull it to your chest. Simultaneously press your left heel into the floor and lift your hips. Hold for 6 seconds. Lower and repeat for 6 reps. Repeat, holding your left knee.

Body Bonus Never again ask, "Does my butt look fat?"

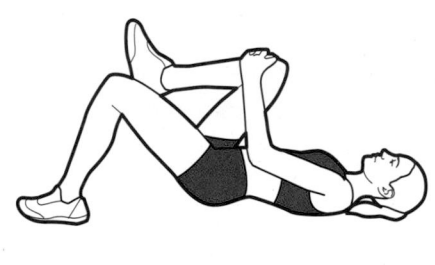

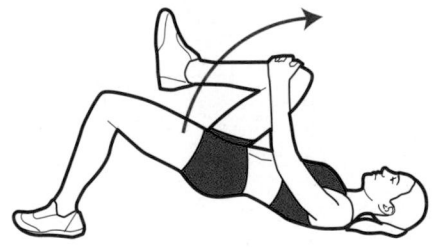

Test 5

OVERHEAD REACH

Fold a towel so it's about an inch thick. Lie on your back with the towel under your lower back. Extend both arms behind your head, palms facing each other. Without bending your elbows or lifting your back off the towel, try to touch the floor with the thumb sides of your hands. If you can't reach:

Your weak link Short, stiff lats–the back muscles that wrap around your torso–from all those hours spent hunched over a keyboard or a bike.

Get your fix Perform the roll-out twice a day to lengthen your midback and shoulder muscles. Add the reach, roll, and lift to your strength routine 3 nonconsecutive days a week.

ROLL-OUT

STRETCHES LATS

Grab a stability ball and kneel so you're facing it, about an arm's length away. Place your hands on top of the ball, shoulder-width apart. Roll your forearms along the ball and lower your head through your upper arms as far as comfortably possible. When you feel a stretch, hold for 30 seconds.

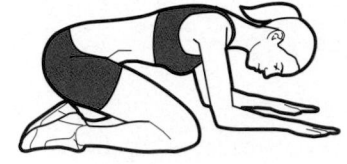

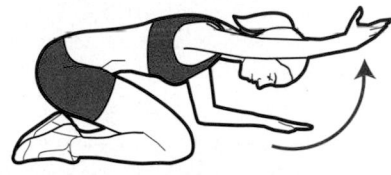

REACH, ROLL, AND LIFT

WORKS MIDBACK

Sit back on your heels. Rest your forearms on the floor, palms down. Slide your right palm forward until your arm is straight. Turn your palm toward the ceiling and raise that arm as far as possible without lifting your torso. Hold for 6 seconds. Lower your palm back to the floor. Raise and hold for 6 reps. Repeat with your left arm.

Body Bonus That hint of belly bulge will disappear as your midback straightens–goodbye, tankini. Hello, something stringier.

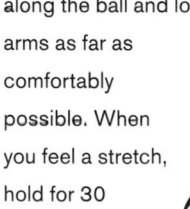
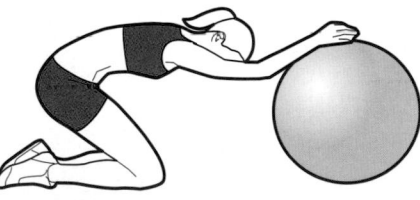
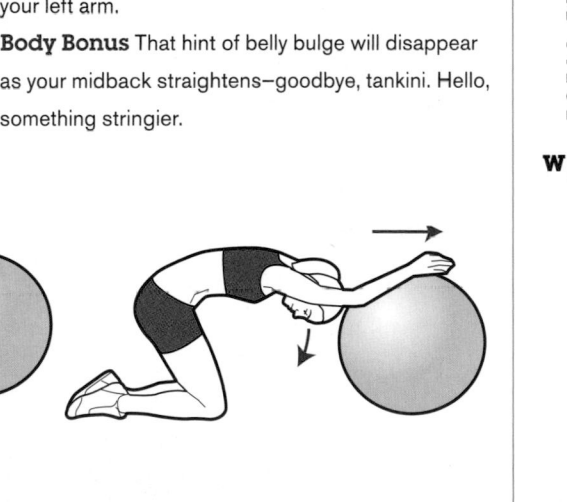

CREDITS

ADAPTED FROM

The Abs Diet for Women by David Zinczenko © 2005 Rodale Inc. Permission granted by Rodale, Emmaus, PA 18098. Available wherever books are sold or directly from the publisher by calling (800) 848-4735 or visit Rodale's Web site at rodalestore.com.

The Wedding Workout DVD © 2006 Rodale Inc. Permission granted by Rodale, Emmaus, PA 18098. Available directly from the publisher by calling (800) 848-4735 or at womenshealthdvds.com.

Train for Your Body Type DVD © 2006 Rodale Inc. Permission granted by Rodale, Emmaus, PA 18098. Available directly from the publisher by calling (800) 848-4735 or at womenshealthdvds.com.

Portions of this publication appeared originally in *Women's Health* magazine.

PHOTOS

Almay pages 80, 160

Bananastock pages iii, 110, 159, 169

Ondrea Barbe cover

Randi Berez pages 82, 92

Beth Bischoff pages 250–253, 286–289

Brand X Pictures page 219

Corbis pages 316, 354

Sasha Eisenman pages x, 22, 25, 28, 324

Michael Edwards pages 11–21, 115–121, 126–131, 133–137, 162–163, 175–176, 178, 180, 182–184, 185, 187 (top), 191–197, 201–209, 212–215, 241–245, 254, 256–261, 275–283, 326–335, 338–341, 350–352

Darryl Estrine pages 36, 170, 198, 200, 210, 248, 272, 284

Folio pages 342, 344

General Mills page 62

Digital Vision/Getty Images pages 216, 246

Eyewire/Getty Images pages 108, 314, 345–346, 349

Getty Images page 76

Photodisc/Getty Images pages 158, 161

Brian Hagiwara pages 60, 75, 89

John Hamel pages 48, 112

Jeff Harris page 102

Hilmar page 132

Lisa Hubbard pages 69, 85 (salmon)

Pearl Izumi pages 42

Jonathon Kantor pages 79, 353

Ture Lillegraven page 336

Steven Lippman page 138

Nicola Majocchio pages 124, 150, 153–154

Mitch Mandel/Rodale Images pages 47, 140-149, 308–313

Rita Maas pages 70, 73, 87 (stir-fry)

Sonja Pacho pages 262, 264–271

Plamen Petkov page 94

David Prince pages 65, 67, 74, 85 (turkey), 90 (salad), 91 (chicken)

Howard Puckett page 71

Rubberball Productions 347

Tina Rupp pages 72, 90 (bean salad)

ILLUSTRATIONS

INDEX

lying lat pullover, 180, **180**
modified eagle stretch, 329, **329**
1¼ bent-over row, 177, **177**
one-leg crossover, 335, **335**
partner row, 222, **222**
plank row, 184, **184**
prone gluteals, 271, **271**
push and row, 14, **14**
pushup position bird dog, 321, **321**
reach, roll, and lift, 361, **361**
reverse dumbbell fly, 183, **183**
reverse overhead throw, 195, **195**
reverse pushup, 186, **186**
Romanian deadlift, 176, **176**
seated ball stabilizer, 131, **131**
seated stability ball row, 339, **339**
spider, 326, **326**
stability ball back extension, 126, **126**
standing bar row, 181, **181**
stomach massage, 340, **340**
supine row, 323, **323**
swimming, 214, **214**
T pushup, 187, **187**
unilateral squat and cable row, 196, **196**
warrior I, 18, **18**, 328, **328**
wobble board balance and sit, 128, **128**
Y lift, 358, **358**
test for weakness in, 358
Back extension, 143, **143**
Back lunge, 308, **308**
with knee lift, 310, **310**
Back scratch test, 359, **359**
Bagels, whole-grain, 96
Balance
exercises
bridge, 237
plank, 237
side lunge, 237
single-leg squat, 237
stability ball twist, 19, **19**
tree, 19, **19**
fitness test (flamingo reach), 7, **7**
Balance squat and pull, 13, **13**
Ballet, 227, 340
Ballet squat, 243, **243**
Bally's Built to Fit program, 45
Barbell, lifting form for, 123
Bariatric physician, 46
Basal metabolic rate (BMR), 167
Beans, 78–79
Beef
Grilled Beef and Arugula Salad, 65, **65**
Grilled Flank Steak with Chile-Tomato Salsa, 73, **73**
Belly fat, 32
Bench press, 238
incline dumbbell, 116, **116**
Bent over row, 158
Berries, 96

Beta-carotene, 108–9
Biceps, exercises for
angled biceps curls, 159
bow, 327, **327**
butterfly, 327, **327**
chinup, 202, **202**
dumbbell military press, 203, **203**
hammer curls, 159
1¼ bent-over row, 177, **177**
Biceps curl, 149, **149**
angled, 159
Blood sugar, stabilizing, 51–59
BMR, 167
Body fat, 32–33, <u>35</u>
BodyGem, <u>348</u>
Body type
bone structure determination, 32, <u>32</u>
ecto apple, 181–83
ecto pear, 174–76
endo apple, 186–87
endo pear, 179–80
genetic basis, 173
identifying, 174
meso apple, 184–85
meso pear, 177–78
Body-weight exercises, 317–23
Bone structure, 32, <u>32</u>
Bottoms Up workout, 241–43
Bounce-back plan
2-month break, 26–27, 29
2-week break, 24, 26
2-year break, 29
after delivery, <u>27</u>
after injury, <u>26</u>
after surgery, <u>26–27</u>
Bow, 327, **327**
Brain, training, 190
Bread, whole-wheat, 78
Breastfeeding, nutritional supplements during, <u>104</u>
Bridge, 237
Bridge abduction, 242, **242**
Bridge press, 16, **16**
Bridge with roll, 266, **266**
Brooks Podium boy shorts, 293
Burpees, 245, **245**
Butt. *See* Gluteal muscles
Butterfly, 327, **327**
B vitamins, 109

C

Cable pull-through, 303, **303**
Cable with high-rope attachment, 253
Calcium, 107, 109
Calf muscles
exercises for
calf raise, 161
leg lift, 161
modified glute-ham raise, 301, **301**

Saxon side bend, 282, **282**
side bridge with abduction, 277, **277**, 318, **318**
side stepup with triceps kickback, 133, **133**
stability ball chest press, 129, **129**
stability ball chest press with hip extension, 197, **197**
stability ball dumbbell press, 185, **185**
stability ball pass-off, 281, **281**
stability ball rotation, 280, **280**
step-out lunge, 197, **197**
step up, 122, **122**
step walkover, 176, **176**
unilateral Romanian deadlift, 275, **275**
unilateral squat and cable row, 196, **196**
windshield wiper, 322, **322**
wobble board balance and sit, 128, **128**
wraparound ankle touch, 319, **319**
Core strength, benefits of
athletic performance improvement, 273
better digestion, 264
better posture, 263–64
clear head, 264
energy increase, 264
leaner look, 264
reduced back injury, 273
Cottage cheese, 99
Country Life Vitamin B$_{12}$, <u>104</u>
Cranberries, 99
Crunch
circle, 261, **261**
dynamic V, 259, **259**
hanging side, 253, **253**
knee cross, 283, **283**
knee-drop, 163, **163**
pace, 346
pullover, 123, **123**
raised-hips, 260, **260**
reverse, 205, **205**
reverse to modified dragon flag, 276, **276**
seated ab, 141, **141**
side double, 260, **260**
60-degree, 352, **352**
Swiss ball, 120, **120**
weighted bicycle, 130, **130**
Curl (fusion), 265, **265**
Curtsy lunge, 186, **186**, 243, **243**
Cycling, yoga exercises for
forward bend hang, 334, **334**
one-leg crossover, 335, **335**
spinal twist, 335, **335**

D

Dairy products, 93
Dance
African, 228
ballet, 227
capoeira, 231
hip-hop, 232
Deadlift, 182, **182**

Romanian, 176, **176**, 209, **209**
single-leg Romanian, 242, **242**
unilateral Romanian, 275, **275**
Deltoids, exercises for, 215, **215**
Diabetes, 55
Diastasis, <u>27</u>
Diet
deadline, 83–93
swap list, 92–93
Dietary Reference Intakes (DRIs), 105, 107
Diet doctor, 46
Dietitian, 46
Digestion, improvement from core strengthening, 264
Dip, 201, **201**
Dog pose flow, 137, **137**
Dogs, as exercise motivator, 44
Double arm reach, 283, **283**
Double-side jackknife, 258, **258**
Double-stop pushup, 320, **320**
Downward dog, 6, **6**, 137, **137**
Drawbridge, 360, **360**
DRIs, 105, 107
Dumbbell chest press, 206, **206**
Dumbbell military press, 203, **203**
Dumbbell pullover, 117, **117**
Dumbbell row, 204, **204**
with single leg, 115, **115**
Dumbbell squat, 208, **208**
Dynamic lunges, <u>121</u>
Dynamic stretching, 237, 240
Dynamic V-crunch, 259, **259**

E

Ecto morph body type
ecto apple, 181–83
ecto pear, 174–76
Eggs, 67, 99
Elevated reverse lunge, 175, **175**
Elliptical trainer, 152
Endo morph body type
endo apple, 186–87
endo pear, 179–80
Energy bar, <u>345</u>
Energy increase, from core strengthening, 264
Erector spinae muscles, exercises for
modified glute-ham raise, 301, **301**
1¼ barbell squat, 299, **299**
reverse hyper-extension, 295, **295**
Romanian deadlift, 302, **302**
Esquiva, 231
Exfoliation, 292
Extended side angle, 331, **331**
Extended triangle, 17, **17**, 331, **331**

F

Fat, dietary
percentage in diet, 54
swap list, 93

TOTAL FITNESS GUIDE 2008

W|H